Epicardial Interventions in Electrophysiology

Editors

JASON S. BRADFIELD
KALYANAM SHIVKUMAR

CARDIAC ELECTROPHYSIOLOGY CLINICS

www.cardiacEP.theclinics.com

Consulting Editors
RANJAN K. THAKUR
ANDREA NATALE

September 2020 • Volume 12 • Number 3

ELSEVIER

1600 John F. Kennedy Boulevard • Suite 1800 • Philadelphia, Pennsylvania, 19103-2899

http://www.theclinics.com

CARDIAC ELECTROPHYSIOLOGY CLINICS Volume 12, Number 3
September 2020 ISSN 1877-9182, ISBN-13: 978-0-323-72278-0

Editor: Stacy Eastman
Developmental Editor: Donald Mumford

Cardiac Electrophysiology Clinics (ISSN 1877-9182) is published quarterly by Elsevier Inc., 360 Park Avenue South, New York, NY 10010-1710. Months of issue are March, June, September, and December. Subscription prices are $231.00 per year for US individuals, $388.00 per year for US institutions, $249.00 per year for Canadian individuals, $438.00 per year for Canadian institutions, $303.00 per year for international individuals, $469.00 per year for international institutions and $100.00 per year for US, Canadian and international students/residents. To receive student/resident rate, orders must be accompanied by name of affiliated institution, date of term, and the signature of program/residency coordinator on institution letterhead. Orders will be billed at individual rate until proof of status is received. Foreign air speed delivery is included in all Clinics subscription prices. All prices are subject to change without notice. **POSTMASTER:** Send address changes to Cardiac Electrophysiology Clinics, Elsevier Health Sciences Division, Subscription Customer Service, 3251 Riverport Lane, Maryland Heights, MO 63043. **Customer Service: 1-800-654-2452 (US and Canada). From outside of the US and Canada, call 314-477-8871. Fax: 314-447-8029. E-mail: JournalsCustomerService-usa@elsevier.com (for print support); JournalsOnlineSupport-usa@elsevier.com (for online support).**

Reprints. For copies of 100 or more of articles in this publication, please contact the Commercial Reprints Department, Elsevier Inc., 360 Park Avenue South, New York, NY 10010-1710. Tel.: 212-633-3874; Fax: 212-633-3820; E-mail: reprints@elsevier.com.

Cardiac Electrophysiology Clinics is covered in *MEDLINE/PubMed (Index Medicus)*.

Contributors

CONSULTING EDITORS

RANJAN K. THAKUR, MD, MPH, MBA, FHRS
Professor of Medicine and Director, Arrhythmia
Service, Thoracic and Cardiovascular Institute,
Sparrow Health System, Michigan State
University, Lansing, Michigan, USA

ANDREA NATALE, MD, FACC, FHRS
Executive Medical Director of the Texas
Cardiac Arrhythmia Institute, St. David's
Medical Center, Austin, Texas, Professor, Dell

Medical School, University of Texas at Austin,
Austin, Texas, USA; National Medical Director,
Cardiac Electrophysiology, California,
Consulting Professor, Division of Cardiology,
Stanford University, California, USA; Clinical
Professor of Medicine, Case Western Reserve
University, Cleveland, Ohio, USA; Director,
Interventional Electrophysiology, Scripps
Clinic, San Diego, California, USA

EDITORS

JASON S. BRADFIELD, MD
Associate Professor of Medicine,
Director, Specialized Program for
Ventricular Tachycardia,
UCLA Cardiac Arrhythmia Center,
David Geffen School of Medicine at UCLA,
UCLA Health System, Los Angeles,
California, USA

KALYANAM SHIVKUMAR, MD, PhD
Professor of Medicine (Cardiology), Radiology
and Bioengineering, Director, UCLA Cardiac
Arrhythmia Center and EP Programs, Director
and Chief, UCLA Interventional CV Programs
and Cardiac Catheterization Laboratories,
David Geffen School of Medicine at UCLA,
UCLA Health System, Los Angeles, California,
USA

AUTHORS

MARTIN AGUILAR, MD
Fellow, Cardiovascular Division, Brigham and
Women's Hospital, Boston, Massachusetts, USA

AMIN AL-AHMAD, MD
Texas Cardiac Arrhythmia Institute, St. David's
Medical Center, Austin, Texas, USA

ALISARA ANANNAB, MD
Texas Cardiac Arrhythmia Institute, St. David's
Medical Center, Austin, Texas, USA;
Department of Cardiovascular Intervention,
Central Chest Institute of Thailand, Nonthaburi,
Thailand

FABRIZIO R. ASSIS, MD
ARVC Program, Division of Cardiology, Johns
Hopkins School of Medicine, Baltimore,
Maryland, USA

HUSEYIN AYHAN, MD
Texas Cardiac Arrhythmia Institute, St. David's
Medical Center, Austin, Texas, USA;
Department of Cardiology, Faculty of Medicine,
Yıldırım Beyazıt University, Ankara, Turkey

KUDRET AYTEMIR, MD
Department of Cardiology, Hacettepe
University Faculty of Medicine, Ankara, Turkey

MOHAMED BASSIOUNY, MD
Texas Cardiac Arrhythmia Institute, St. David's
Medical Center, Austin, Texas, USA

NOEL G. BOYLE, MD, PhD
UCLA Cardiac Arrhythmia Center, UCLA
Health System, David Geffen School of
Medicine at UCLA, Los Angeles, California,
USA

JASON S. BRADFIELD, MD
Associate Professor of Medicine,
Director, Specialized Program for
Ventricular Tachycardia,
UCLA Cardiac Arrhythmia Center,
David Geffen School of Medicine at UCLA,
UCLA Health System, Los Angeles,
California, USA

DAVID J. BURKHARDT, MD
Texas Cardiac Arrhythmia Institute, St. David's
Medical Center, Austin, Texas, USA

UGUR CANPOLAT, MD
Texas Cardiac Arrhythmia Institute, St. David's
Medical Center, Austin, Texas, USA;
Department of Cardiology, Hacettepe
University Faculty of Medicine, Ankara,
Turkey

RACHEL DEBENHAM, MD
Resident, Internal Medicine, University of
Colorado School of Medicine, Aurora,
Colorado, USA

DOMENICO G. DELLA ROCCA, MD
Texas Cardiac Arrhythmia Institute, St. David's
Medical Center, Austin, Texas, USA

LUIGI DI BIASE, MD, PhD
Arrhythmia Services, Department of Medicine,
Montefiore Medical Center, Albert Einstein
College of Medicine, Bronx, New York, USA;
Texas Cardiac Arrhythmia Institute, St. David's
Medical Center, Austin, Texas, USA;
Department of Clinical and Experimental
Medicine, University of Foggia, Foggia, Italy

TIMM MICHAEL DICKFELD, MD, PhD
Section of Cardiac Electrophysiology and
the Maryland Arrhythmia and Cardiac
Imaging Group (MACIG), University of
Maryland School of Medicine, Baltimore,
Maryland, USA

MICHELA FAGGIONI, MD
Icahn School of Medicine at Mount Sinai,
New York, New York, USA; James J Peters
Veterans Affairs Medical Center, Bronx, New
York, USA

GIOVANNI B. FORLEO, MD, PhD
Department of Cardiology, Azienda
Ospedaliera-Universitaria "Luigi Sacco,"
Milano, Italy

PAUL A. FRIEDMAN, MD
Chair and Professor, Division of Cardiovascular
Diseases and Internal Medicine, Mayo Clinic,
Rochester, Minnesota, USA

JOSEPH G. GALLINGHOUSE, MD
Texas Cardiac Arrhythmia Institute, St. David's
Medical Center, Austin, Texas, USA

ZACHARY HALE, MD
Division of Cardiac Electrophysiology, Texas
Heart Institute, Houston, Texas, USA

JUSTIN HAYASE, MD
UCLA Cardiac Arrhythmia Center, UCLA
Health System, David Geffen School of
Medicine at UCLA, Los Angeles, California,
USA

RODNEY P. HORTON, MD
Texas Cardiac Arrhythmia Institute, St. David's
Medical Center, Austin, Texas, USA

AUSTIN HOWARD, MD
Division of Cardiac Electrophysiology, Texas
Heart Institute, Houston, Texas, USA

ARVINDH N. KANAGASUNDRAM, MD
Vanderbilt Heart and Vascular Institute,
Nashville, Tennessee, USA

ROSHAN KARKI, MBBS
Fellow, Division of Cardiovascular Diseases
and Internal Medicine, Mayo Clinic, Rochester,
Minnesota, USA

AMMAR M. KILLU, MBBS
Assistant Professor, Division of Cardiovascular
Diseases and Internal Medicine, Mayo Clinic,
Rochester, Minnesota, USA

PIER D. LAMBIASE, PhD, FRCP, FHRS
Professor of Cardiology, St Bartholomew's
Hospital, Barts Heart Centre, Barts Health NHS
Trust, Institute of Cardiovascular Science,
University College of London, London, United
Kingdom

CARLO LAVALLE, MD
Department of Cardiology, Policlinico
Universitario Umberto I, Roma,
Italy

ANTHONY LI, MBBS, MD
Cardiology Academic Group, St. George's
University of London, London, United Kingdom

FRANCIS E. MARCHLINSKI, MD
Cardiac Electrophysiology, Cardiovascular Division, Hospital of the University of Pennsylvania, Philadelphia, Pennsylvania, USA

NILESH MATHURIA, MD, FHRS
Division of Cardiac Electrophysiology, Texas Heart Institute, Houston, Texas, USA

SANGHAMITRA MOHANTY, MD
Texas Cardiac Arrhythmia Institute, St. David's Medical Center, Austin, Texas, USA

SHUMPEI MORI, MD, PhD
UCLA Cardiac Arrhythmia Center, David Geffen School of Medicine at UCLA, Los Angeles, California, USA

DANIELE MUSER, MD
Cardiac Electrophysiology, Cardiovascular Division, Hospital of the University of Pennsylvania, Philadelphia, Pennsylvania, USA

ANDREA NATALE, MD, FACC, FHRS
Executive Medical Director of the Texas Cardiac Arrhythmia Institute, St. David's Medical Center, Austin, Texas, Professor, Dell Medical School, University of Texas at Austin, Austin, Texas, USA; National Medical Director, Cardiac Electrophysiology, California, Consulting Professor, Division of Cardiology, Stanford University, California, USA; Clinical Professor of Medicine, Case Western Reserve University, Cleveland, Ohio, USA; Director, Interventional Electrophysiology, Scripps Clinic, San Diego, California, USA

RUI PROVIDÊNCIA, MD, PhD
Senior Lecturer and Honorary Consultant, St Bartholomew's Hospital, Barts Heart Centre, Barts Health NHS Trust, Institute of Health Informatics, University College of London, London, United Kingdom

ALEJANDRO JIMENEZ RESTREPO, MD
Section of Cardiology, Marshfield Clinic Health System, Marshfield, Wisconsin, USA

TRAVIS D. RICHARDSON, MD
Vanderbilt Heart and Vascular Institute, Nashville, Tennessee, USA

JORGE ROMERO, MD
Arrhythmia Services, Department of Medicine, Montefiore Medical Center, Albert Einstein College of Medicine, Bronx, New York, USA

MOUHANNAD M. SADEK, MD
Arrhythmia Service, Division of Cardiology, The Ottawa Hospital, Ottawa, Ontario, Canada

ANU SAHORE, MD
Texas Cardiac Arrhythmia Institute, St. David's Medical Center, Austin, Texas, USA

PASQUALE SANTANGELI, MD, PhD
Cardiac Electrophysiology, Cardiovascular Division, Hospital of the University of Pennsylvania, Philadelphia, Pennsylvania, USA

ANNAHITA SARCON, MD
Division of Electrophysiology, University of California, San Francisco, San Francisco, California, USA

KALYANAM SHIVKUMAR, MD, PhD
Professor of Medicine (Cardiology), Radiology and Bioengineering, Director, UCLA Cardiac Arrhythmia Center and EP Programs, Director and Chief, UCLA Interventional CV Programs and Cardiac Catheterization Laboratories, David Geffen School of Medicine at UCLA, UCLA Health System, Los Angeles, California, USA

WILLIAM G. STEVENSON, MD
Professor of Medicine, Vanderbilt Heart and Vascular Institute, Nashville, Tennessee, USA

HARIKRISHNA TANDRI, MD
ARVC Program, Division of Cardiology, Johns Hopkins School of Medicine, Baltimore, Maryland, USA

NICOLA TARANTINO, MD
Arrhythmia Services, Department of Medicine, Montefiore Medical Center, Albert Einstein College of Medicine, Bronx, New York, USA

USHA B. TEDROW, MD, MSc
Cardiovascular Division, Brigham and Women's Hospital, Associate Professor of Medicine, Harvard Medical School, Director, Clinical Cardiac Electrophysiology Fellowship, Clinical Director, Ventricular Arrhythmia Program, Boston, Massachusetts, USA

VENKATAKRISHNA N. THOLAKANAHALLI, MD, FHRS
Director, Advanced Interventional Cardiac Electrophysiology, Left Atrial Appendage Closure Program, EP Laboratory, Minneapolis VA Health Care System, Professor of Medicine, University of Minnesota, Minneapolis, Minnesota, USA

CHINTAN TRIVEDI, MD, MPH
Texas Cardiac Arrhythmia Institute, St. David's Medical Center, Austin, Texas, USA

RODERICK TUNG, MD
Department of Medicine, Section of Cardiology, The University of Chicago Medicine, Center for Arrhythmia Care, Pritzker School of Medicine, Chicago, Illinois, USA

WENDY S. TZOU, MD, FHRS, FACC
Associate Professor of Medicine, Director, Cardiac Electrophysiology, University of Colorado School of Medicine, Aurora, Colorado, USA

YANG YANG, MD
Division of Cardiology, Baylor College of Medicine, Houston, Texas, USA

XIAO-DONG ZHANG, MD, PhD
Arrhythmia Services, Department of Medicine, Montefiore Medical Center, Albert Einstein College of Medicine, Bronx, New York, USA

Contents

 Video content accompanies this article at http://www.cardiacep.theclinics.com.

Justin Hayase, Shumpei Mori, Kalyanam Shivkumar, and Jason S. Bradfield

The pericardial cavity and its boundaries are formed by the reflections of the visceral and parietal pericardial layers. This space is an integral access point for epicardial interventions. As the pericardial layers reflect over the great vessels and the heart, they form sinuses and recesses, which restrict catheter movement. The epicardial vasculature is also important when performing nearby catheter ablation. The phrenic nerve and esophagus are other important structures to appreciate so as to avoid collateral injury. In addition, the Larrey space, or left sternocostal triangle, is a key avascular window through which pericardial access can be safely achieved.

Percutaneous epicardial access continues to have a growing role within cardiac electrophysiology. The classic approach has typically been with a Tuohy needle via a subxiphoid approach guided by fluoroscopic landmarks and tactile feedback. Recent developments have highlighted the role of the micropuncture needle, electroanatomic mapping, and real-time pressure sensors to reduce complications. Further, different access sites, such as the right atrial appendage, have been described and may offer a novel approach to percutaneous epicardial access. In addition, future directions of percutaneous access may involve direct visualization, near-field impedance monitoring, and real-time virtual imaging.

Accessing the epicardial space without a sternotomy or a surgical pericardial window to treat ventricular arrhythmias in Chagas disease became a medical necessity in South America. Since the introduction of the dry percutaneous epicardial access approach, epicardial access has been standard procedure for management of ventricular arrhythmias in ischemic and nonischemic cardiomyopathies and atrioventricular accessory pathways after failed conventional endocardial ablation. Understanding the epicardial space and neighboring structures has become an important subject of teachings in electrophysiology. The evolution of complex

Contents

ablation procedures to treat atrial and ventricular arrhythmias and device interventions requires thorough understanding of pericardial anatomy.

Ventricular arrhythmias (VAs) occurring in the absence of structural heart disease or ion channelopathies are referred to as idiopathic. They can clinically present with frequent monomorphic premature ventricular contractions, nonsustained ventricular tachycardia (VT), or sustained VT, and generally share a benign prognosis. Approximately 4% to 10% of idiopathic VAs have an epicardial site of origin, represented in most cases by the left ventricular summit and, less frequently, by the cardiac crux. Epicardial foci can be addressed by catheter ablation via the coronary venous system tributaries. In rarer instances, a direct epicardial access from a subxiphoid approach is needed.

Catheter ablation can effectively reduce the frequency of ventricular tachycardia in ischemic cardiomyopathy by ablating sites of reentry within complex regions of myocardial scar. In cases of near transmural infarction, this arrhythmia substrate may be nearer the epicardium than the endocardium, and epicardial ablation may be necessary. An epicardial substrate location can potentially be predicted by imaging that suggests transmural infarction. Percutaneous epicardial ablation improves outcomes in selected patients, but is higher risk and avoided in patients with prior coronary artery bypass grafting.

In patients with nonischemic cardiomyopathy, epicardial ablation is critical in targeting epicardial paravalvular substrate. Epicardial access and ablation can be performed safely with attention to epicardial structures, such as the coronary arteries, phrenic nerve, and epicardial fat. This review explores the indications, techniques, complications, and outcomes of epicardial ablation in patients with nonischemic cardiomyopathy. Although epicardial ablation adds to the complexity and risk of the ablation procedure, it is a vital tool that, combined with endocardial mapping and ablation, improves outcomes in patients with nonischemic cardiomyopathy suffering from ventricular arrhythmias.

 Video content accompanies this article at http://www.cardiacep.theclinics.com.

Arrhythmogenic right ventricular cardiomyopathy (ARVC) is an inherited heart muscle disease characterized by progressive fibrofatty replacement of the myocardium, right ventricular enlargement, and malignant ventricular arrhythmias. Ventricular tachycardia (VT) may be seen in all stages of the disease and is associated with sudden cardiac death. In patients who failed antiarrhythmic medical therapy, catheter ablation has become an attractive therapeutic option to reduce VT burden and implantable cardioverter-defibrillator interventions. In this article, the authors aim to address the overall concepts of epicardial catheter ablation in ARVC, focusing on substrate characterization and ablation strategies.

 Video content accompanies this article at http://www.cardiacep.theclinics.com.

Brugada syndrome is an inherited cardiac condition characterized by a typical electrocardiogram signature of coved-type ST-segment elevation in the right precordial leads and ventricular arrhythmias leading to sudden cardiac death, in the absence of unequivocal structural heart disease. Brugada syndrome specifically affects the right ventricle, which predisposes to cardiac arrest. Besides medical management with quinidine, emerging data indicate that catheter ablation can help reduce the ventricular arrhythmia burden in these patients. This review explores the mechanisms of ventricular arrhythmia, current approaches and evidence for ablating the epicardial arrhythmogenic substrate in this condition.

Supraventricular arrhythmias are the most common cardiac arrhythmias encountered; however, it is uncommon that supraventricular tachycardias require percutaneous epicardial access for successful mapping and ablation. There are particular scenarios where epicardial access and ablation should be considered. Certain accessory pathways particularly in the posteroseptal region may require epicardial access for successful ablation. These pathways may also be approached from within the coronary sinus system. In addition, tachycardias near the phrenic nerve in the right atrium or left atrium may require epicardial access for successful ablation or to allow displacement of the phrenic nerve facilitating safe catheter ablation.

The observations afforded by epicardial mapping have not only increased the appreciation of distinct epicardial structures in the left atrium but also underscore the need to address the substrate transmurally. Although epicardial access and ablation have attendant risks, comparative studies with hybrid surgical approaches are lacking. In the search to find unifying mechanisms of atrial fibrillation, a conceptual shift that emphasizes the substrate in 3 dimensions, with the epicardium distinct from the endocardium, holds promise for future investigation and evolving therapeutic tools.

Hybrid surgical ventricular tachycardia (VT) ablation combines surgical epicardial access/exposure with contemporary mapping and ablation techniques adapted from percutaneous catheter ablation procedures. Patients considered for a hybrid surgical approach for VT are those who have had prior cardiac surgery or failed percutaneous epicardial access due to pericardial adhesions. They often represent the most challenging end of the spectrum of patients and usually have undergone multiple unsuccessful ablations. In this review, the indications, preprocedure work-up, ablation techniques, and outcomes from hybrid surgical access VT ablations are discussed as well as key technical details that present unique challenges to its success.

Epicardial Ablation via Arterial and Venous Systems

Venkatakrishna N. Tholakanahalli

The intracoronary artery and venous routes provide unique roadmaps for mapping and interventions for ventricular arrhythmias and certain atrial arrhythmias. The unique anatomic location of these vessels on the epicardial surface enables mapping/interventions without the need to access the pericardial space. These anatomic routes also track deep into certain intramural regions, with interventions that are not accessible from either epicardial or endocardial routes. To map smaller vessels, multipolar catheters and wires are used to record local electrograms. Endocardial/epicardial ablation at adjacent sites is sometimes required to enhance successful outcomes. This article describes tools, techniques, and site-specific mapping and interventions.

Epicardial Ablation Biophysics and Novel Radiofrequency Energy Delivery Techniques

Rachel Debenham and Wendy S. Tzou

Important physiologic and anatomic differences exist between the epicardium and endocardium, particularly of the ventricles, and these differences affect ablation biophysics. Absence of passive convective effects conferred by circulating blood as well as the presence of epicardial fat and vessels and absence of intracavitary ridges and structures affect ablation lesion size when performing epicardial catheter-based ablation, whether using radiofrequency or cryothermal energy. Understanding differential effects in each environment is important in informing strategies to increase ablation lesion depth. When using actively cooled radiofrequency ablation, local impedance can be altered to selectively augment energy delivery.

Epicardial Ablation Complications

Nicola Tarantino, Domenico G. Della Rocca, Michela Faggioni, Xiao-Dong Zhang, Sanghamitra Mohanty, Alisara Anannab, Ugur Canpolat, Huseyin Ayhan, Mohamed Bassiouny, Anu Sahore, Kudret Aytemir, Annahita Sarcon, Giovanni B. Forleo, Carlo Lavalle, Rodney P. Horton, Chintan Trivedi, Amin Al-Ahmad, Jorge Romero, David J. Burckhardt, Joseph G. Gallinghouse, Luigi Di Biase, and Andrea Natale

The percutaneous epicardial approach has become an adjunctive tool for electrophysiologists to treat disparate cardiac arrhythmias, including accessory pathways, atrial tachycardia, and particularly ventricular tachycardia. This novel technique prompted a strong impulse to perform epicardial access as an alternative strategy for pacing and defibrillation, left atrial appendage exclusion, heart failure with preserved ejection fraction, and genetically engineered tissue delivery. However, because of the incremental risk of major complications compared with stand-alone endocardial ablation, it is still practiced in a limited number of highly experienced centers across the world.

Roshan Karki, Paul A. Friedman, and Ammar M. Killu

The pericardial space provides a unique vantage point to access different cardiac structures for diagnosis and treatment of arrhythmias and other nonelectrophysiologic conditions, such as heart failure. There have been notable innovations to improve safety of percutaneous pericardial access and its use for various procedures. Percutaneous pericardial device therapies for pacing and defibrillation have been in development, success of which will be a significant advance in treatment of bradyarrhythmias, cardiac resynchronization therapy, and prevention of arrhythmic deaths. There is need for continued efforts in development and expansion of this technique and a systematic approach to monitor efficacy and safety outcomes.

CARDIAC ELECTROPHYSIOLOGY CLINICS

SERIES OF RELATED INTEREST

Cardiology Clinics
Available at: https://www.cardiology.theclinics.com/
Heart Failure Clinics
Available at: https://www.heartfailure.theclinics.com/
Interventional Cardiology Clinics
Available at: https://www.interventional.theclinics.com/

THE CLINICS ARE AVAILABLE ONLINE!
Access your subscription at:
www.theclinics.com

Foreword
Epicardial Interventions in Electrophysiology

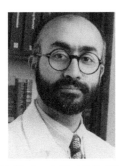

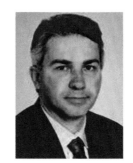

Ranjan K. Thakur, MD, MPH, MBA, FHRS   Andrea Natale, MD, FACC, FHRS

Consulting Editors

Since the emergence of clinical cardiac electrophysiology as a subspecialty of cardiology in the 1970s, the field has evolved in the direction of catheter-based invasive therapeutic interventions. These interventions have allowed us to approach arrhythmia substrates that were previously unknown or incompletely understood and incurable.

Epicardial ablation was initially used for ventricular tachycardia in the setting of Chagas disease, and this ablation access was first used by our colleagues in South America, where Chagas disease is common. In March 2010, Drs Shivkumar and Boyle edited an issue of the *Cardiac Electrophysiology Clinics* focused on Epicardial Interventions. A decade has elapsed, and much has been learned about ablation of various arrhythmias using the epicardial approach.

In this issue of the *Cardiac Electrophysiology Clinics*, Drs Bradfield and Shivkumar have assembled a panel of international experts to update the readership on arrhythmias that can be approached in the epicardial space. Contents include a discussion of the epicardial space, access and safe maneuvering of catheters in this space, and ablation of various forms of ventricular tachycardia, rare supraventricular tachycardias that fail endocardial ablation, and atrial fibrillation. In addition, they discuss the complications of ablation from the epicardial approach and the future evolution of this technique.

Despite the developments in this field, this technique remains in limited use because most practicing electrophysiologists don't encounter these complex arrhythmias in sufficient frequency to maintain adequate expertise in resorting to it when required. So, the technique remains limited to tertiary-care, high-volume ablation centers. However, that may change in the future. We hope the readership will enjoy reading this update of a still evolving field.

Ranjan K. Thakur, MD, MPH, MBA, FHRS
Sparrow Thoracic and Cardiovascular Institute
Michigan State University
1440 East Michigan Avenue, Suite 400
Lansing, MI 48912, USA

Andrea Natale, MD, FACC, FHRS
Texas Cardiac Arrhythmia Institute
Center for Atrial Fibrillation at
St. David's Medical Center
1015 East 32nd Street, Suite 516
Austin, TX 78705, USA

E-mail addresses:
thakur@msu.edu (R.K. Thakur)
andrea.natale@stdavids.com (A. Natale)

Card Electrophysiol Clin 12 (2020) xiii
https://doi.org/10.1016/j.ccep.2020.06.002
1877-9182/20/© 2020 Published by Elsevier Inc.

Preface

Epicardial Interventions in Electrophysiology: Transformation to an Established Approach

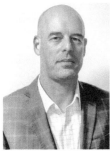

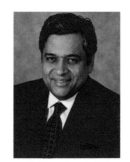

Jason S. Bradfield, MD   Kalyanam Shivkumar, MD, PhD

Editors

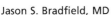

Percutaneous epicardial interventions in electrophysiology were initially utilized as a bail-out strategy to manage ventricular tachycardia in difficult-to-ablate nonischemic cardiomyopathy patients, in particular, patients with Chagas disease who had a predilection for epicardial and midmyocardial substrates. Subsequent clinical studies demonstrated the benefit of this approach in additional subsets of patients and led to more widespread use. This topic was reviewed by *Cardiac Electrophysiology Clinics* a decade ago.

The current literature in this area has grown, and it now supports the use of epicardial mapping/ablation in nonischemic cardiomyopathy, subsets of ischemic cardiomyopathy (failed endocardial ablation and/or transmural scar), and even in some patients with idiopathic ventricular tachycardia, supraventricular tachycardia, and atrial fibrillation. For this reason, Clinical Cardiac Electrophysiology fellowship trainees interested in joining or developing complex ablation programs have been drawn to learning epicardial interventions. In addition, in recent years with the development of percutaneous left atrial appendage interventions, practitioners have been further drawn to this skill set. Interest will undoubtedly continue to grow with future novel interventions for ablation, pacing, defibrillation, structural interventions, drug delivery, and gene therapy, among others.

In this series, we provide a much needed, state-of-the art review of the spectrum of epicardial interventions in electrophysiology and beyond. We are honored to have international leaders in the field contribute to the effort. Epicardial anatomy and access techniques are essential foundational reading. Subsequent comprehensive articles assess mapping and ablation of the spectrum of supraventricular and ventricular arrhythmias, novel mapping and ablation techniques, as well as the utility of perioperative imaging, optimization of ablation lesion technology, and the associated risks of these interventions. Finally, the future of epicardial interventions is discussed to complete the series. We thank the authors for crystalizing the state-of-the-art for the reader.

Jason S. Bradfield, MD
UCLA Cardiac Arrhythmia Center
100 medical Plaza, Suite 660
Los Angeles, CA 90095, USA

Kalyanam Shivkumar, MD, PhD
UCLA Cardiac Arrhythmia Center
100 UCLA Medical Plaza, Suite 660
Los Angeles, CA 90095, USA

E-mail addresses:
JBradfield@mednet.ucla.edu (J.S. Bradfield)
kshivkumar@mednet.ucla.edu (K. Shivkumar)

Card Electrophysiol Clin 12 (2020) xv
https://doi.org/10.1016/j.ccep.2020.06.003
1877-9182/20/© 2020 Published by Elsevier Inc.

Anatomy of the Pericardial Space

Justin Hayase, MD, Shumpei Mori, MD, PhD, Kalyanam Shivkumar, MD, PhD,
Jason S. Bradfield, MD*

KEYWORDS

- Pericardial space • Epicardium • Pericardial sinuses • Pericardial recesses

KEY POINTS

- Via the pericardial space, electrophysiologists can gain access to epicardial structures that cannot otherwise be reached with endovascular catheter methods.
- Anatomic boundaries and nearby structures must be respected when manipulating catheters within the pericardial space.
- The oblique and transverse sinuses as well as pericardial recesses are located posteriorly and superiorly, which restrict catheter manipulation in these areas.
- Adipose tissue surrounds the epicardial vessels, providing insulation against vascular injury but also impeding effective ablation lesion formation.
- Adjacent structures, such as the esophagus, phrenic nerve, and vasculature, must always be identified so as not to cause inadvertent collateral injury during epicardial interventions.

 Video content accompanies this article at http://www.cardiacep.theclinics.com.

INTRODUCTION

As technology and techniques have improved in electrophysiology, epicardial interventions have become increasingly used. As such, it is imperative for practicing electrophysiologists to have an expert understanding of the anatomic intricacy whenever entering the pericardial space.

The pericardial cavity is a potential space between the visceral and parietal pericardial layers, which meet at lines of attachment on the surfaces of the heart and the great vessels. Normally, up to 50 mL of fluid can be present within the pericardial sac.[1] The parietal pericardium (composed of an outer fibrous layer and inner serous layer) is an acellular layer up to 2 mm in thickness, which is contiguous with the adventitia of the aorta and pulmonary artery. The parietal pericardium is anchored to the posterior sternum by superior and inferior sternopericardial ligaments and to the diaphragm by its attachment to the central tendon. These anchoring sites help to maintain the heart's position within the thoracic cage. The visceral pericardium (also called the epicardium) is a single mesothelial cell layer that directly overlies the epicardial surface. The small amount of fluid within the potential space serves to lubricate the surface between the parietal and visceral layers, allowing smooth mechanical function of the beating heart.[2]

When entering the pericardial space, it is critical to grasp (1) the boundaries created by the pericardial reflections that form the sinuses and the recesses, (2) epicardial vasculature and how it is contained within the visceral pericardium, and (3) neighboring extrapericardial structures at risk of collateral damage. This

UCLA Cardiac Arrhythmia Center, David Geffen School of Medicine at UCLA, 100 Medical Plaza, suite 660, Los Angeles, CA 90095, USA
* Corresponding author.
E-mail address: JBradfield@mednet.ucla.edu

Card Electrophysiol Clin 12 (2020) 265–270
https://doi.org/10.1016/j.ccep.2020.04.003

article discusses each of these in detail and thus provides a working anatomic knowledge base for the safe performance of epicardial interventions.

THE PERICARDIAL SINUSES AND RECESSES

The pericardial reflections are all located superior and posterior to the heart, which means that entering the pericardial space provides access to the anterior, apical, and lateral surfaces of the ventricles.[3] This anatomy can be appreciated in Video 1, which processes through the heart in a left anterior oblique plane. In the video, there are no divisions within the pericardial space until the posterior surface of the heart and great vessels are reached. The major pericardial sinuses and recesses are shown in **Fig. 1**A, which provides

an overview of the important boundaries demarcating these spaces.

The oblique sinus lies posterior to the left atrium and ventricle (**Fig. 1**B, D). The oblique sinus is bounded on the right by the reflection against the inferior vena cava, superiorly by the reflection connecting the right and left pulmonary veins, and to the left by the reflection of the left-sided pulmonary veins (see **Fig. 1**A).[4] Inferiorly, the oblique sinus communicates with the remainder of the pericardial cavity. In cadaveric work by Chaffanjon and colleagues,[5] the average width of the oblique sinus was 41 ± 7 mm. Immediately posterior to the oblique sinus courses the esophagus, which is discussed in more detail later.

Just above the oblique sinus, the transverse sinus is bounded anteriorly by the great arteries,

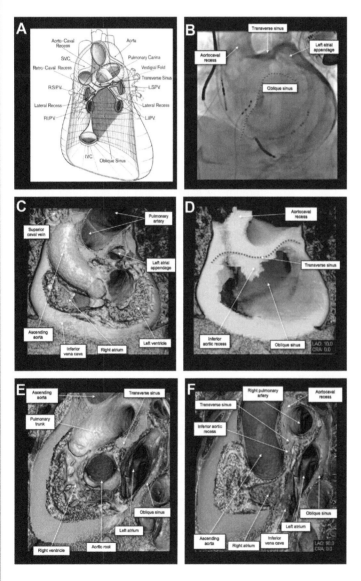

Fig. 1. Pericardial sinuses and recesses overview. (*A*) The pericardial space. (*B*) Fluoroscopic pericardiogram in left anterior oblique view showing contrast within the pericardial sinuses and recesses. (*C–F*) Three-dimensional reconstruction from computed tomography images with the pericardial space highlighted in blue. Left anterior oblique view with cardiac structures shown (*C*) and cardiac structures removed (*D*) with the transverse sinus indicated by the red hatched line. Left lateral sagittal plane view through the aortic root and pulmonary trunk (*E*) and more rightward plane (*F*) through the ascending aorta. IVC, inferior vena cava; LIPV, left inferior pulmonary vein; LSPV, left superior pulmonary vein; RIPV, right inferior pulmonary vein; RSPV, right superior pulmonary vein; SVC, superior vena cava. ([A] *Illustration courtesy* UCLA Cardiac Arrhythmia Center, Wallace A. McAlpine MD collection.)

the pulmonary trunk, and the associated ascending aorta (**Fig. 1**E, F). The posterior transverse sinus is formed by the anteromedial wall of the right atrium and the anterior-superior wall of the left atrium (**Fig. 2**A, B). The right pulmonary artery branches off the pulmonary trunk and then courses to the right superior-posteriorly to the transverse sinus.[6] On the left, the vestigial fold involving the ligament of Marshall and the left atrial appendage guard the opening to the transverse sinus (**Fig. 2**C, D).

To the right and superiorly, the transverse sinus communicates with the aortocaval recess (**Fig. 2**E, F). The reflection from the superior vena cava (SVC) to the upper third of the ascending aorta forms the roof of the aortocaval recess. The aortocaval recess is in contact with the right paratracheal and anterior tracheal lymph nodes, which are important culprits in malignant pericardial diseases.[4] The aortocaval recess may also be referred to as the superior sinus, superior aortic recess, or recessus aorticus. To the right and inferiorly, the pericardial reflection courses from the aorta to the anteromedial wall of the right atrium, forming what has been identified as the inferior aortic recess (**Fig. 2**D, F).

The retrocaval recess is formed as the reflection of the SVC courses around to meet the reflection of the right superior pulmonary vein (**Fig. 1**A–D). The retrocaval recess is bounded anteriorly by the SVC, posteriorly by the right superior pulmonary vein, and superiorly by the right pulmonary artery.

The right and left lateral recesses (also known as the pulmonary venous recesses) are invaginations formed by the reflections of the right-sided and left-sided pulmonary veins, respectively. There is considerable anatomic variability in the lateral recesses, as described by Chaffanjon and colleagues.[5] It should be noted that the right lateral

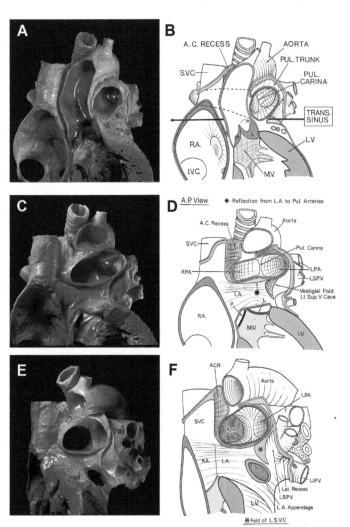

Fig. 2. Transverse sinus and aortocaval recess. (*A*, *B*) Anteroposterior view with coronal transection through the aortic root and left ventricle (LV). The transverse sinus crosses the midline posterior to the great vessels. The aortocaval recess is formed superiorly by the reflection between the aorta and SVC. (*C*, *D*) Anteroposterior view with removal of the aortic root and transection through the pulmonary artery at the pulmonary carina. (*E*, *F*) Left anterior oblique view with an oblique transection through the aortic arch and pulmonary carina. The vestigial fold (or ligament of Marshall) and left atrial appendage can be seen guarding the leftward entrance to the transverse sinus. AC, aortocaval; LA, left atrium; LPA, left pulmonary artery; MV, mitral valve; RA, right atrium; RPA, right pulmonary artery. (*Illustration courtesy UCLA Cardiac Arrhythmia Center, Wallace A. McAlpine MD collection.*)

recess may communicate with the oblique sinus approximately 4.6% of the time.[5]

Several cardiac ganglia are in close proximity to the pericardial sinuses and recesses and deserve mention. The retroatrial ganglia are very near the oblique sinus, the perigreat vessel ganglia reside close to the transverse sinus, and the aortocaval ganglion is situated near the aortocaval recess.[7] These anatomic relationships are important for the potential targeting of these ganglia for purposes of cardiac autonomic modulation in the management of arrhythmias.

EPICARDIAL VASCULATURE

In general, the great cardiac vein courses to the atrial side and lies superficial to the coronary arteries; however, there can be variability (**Fig. 3**).[4,8] The anterior interventricular vein lies anterolateral to the left anterior descending coronary artery. It then becomes the great cardiac vein as it courses lateral to the interventricular septum and crosses the left circumflex artery at the left ventricular summit. In this region, the great cardiac vein is most commonly superficial to the coronary artery, up to 61% of the time, although it can also run deep to the artery in approximately 37% of patients.[9] This relationship is important to remember when performing ablation of ventricular arrhythmias in the left ventricular summit because a catheter placed in the great cardiac vein may have to contend with an intervening coronary artery between it and the ventricular myocardium. The great cardiac vein then travels parallel to the left circumflex artery and becomes the coronary sinus at the valve of Vieussens, which is also the location of the vestigial ligament of Marshall or persistent left-sided SVC, if present.

Epicardial fat typically envelops the coronary vessels. This fat provides both advantages and disadvantages when performing nearby ablation. On one hand, the vasculature is insulated from damage by the adipose tissue; however, the epicardial fat also provides a physical barrier that can impede the formation of effective ablation lesions.[6] In addition, epicardial fat can affect voltage mapping, confounding its differentiation from scar tissue.[10] On average, epicardial fat comprises about 20% of the total heart's weight, and the amount of epicardial fat is directly correlated with obesity.[11]

NEIGHBORING STRUCTURES

The 2 phrenic nerves provide innervation to the pericardium and run between the parietal pericardium and the mediastinal pleura. The right phrenic nerve courses along the right anterolateral portion of the SVC and in very close proximity to the right superior pulmonary vein, which has significant implications for pulmonary vein and SVC isolation for catheter ablation of atrial fibrillation. The right phrenic nerve then continues downward, against the lateral wall of the right atrium before reaching

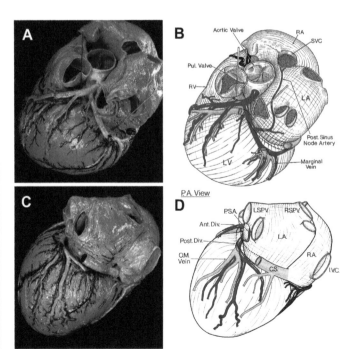

Fig. 3. Relationship between the cardiac veins and coronary arteries. (*A, B*) High posterior oblique view with dissection showing coronary vessels. Arteries are colored red and cardiac veins colored green. In this specimen, the great cardiac vein runs deep to the coronary arteries. (*C, D*) Posteroanterior view. In this specimen, the great cardiac vein courses superficial to the coronary arteries. Ant Div, anterior division/left anterior descending artery; CS, coronary sinus; LV, left ventricle; Post Div, posterior division/left circumflex artery; Pul, pulmonary; RV, right ventricle. (*Illustration courtesy* UCLA Cardiac Arrhythmia Center, Wallace A. McAlpine MD collection.)

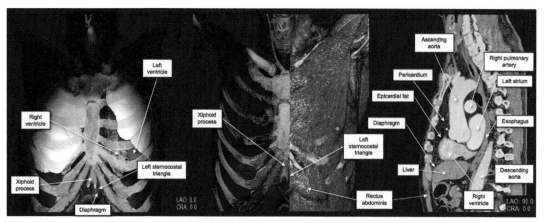

Fig. 4. Larrey space. (*Left*) Anteroposterior view of a three-dimensional computed tomography model showing the relationship between the xiphoid process, diaphragm, and left sternocostal triangle (also known as Larrey space). (*Middle*) Same as left panel with muscle plane included showing the rectus abdominis. (*Right*) Left lateral sagittal plane, which is sectioned along the vertical line indicated in the middle panel, of a computed tomography image showing the relationship between liver, rectus abdominis, and pericardial space, as well as other important extrapericardial structures.

the diaphragm adjacent to the lateral wall of the inferior vena cava. The left phrenic nerve travels down over the aortic arch, pulmonary trunk, and over the left atrial appendage before descending inferiorly over the lateral left ventricular free wall. This structure is important to keep in mind when placing epicardial left ventricular leads for cardiac resynchronization therapy or for catheter ablation. It may also course near the left coronary system as well as the great cardiac vein, which can have implications for ventricular arrhythmia ablation.[7]

The esophagus lies behind the oblique sinus and posterior to the left atrium. There can be variability in the course of the esophagus, which must be considered when performing ablation along the posterior wall of the left atrium. In an observational study of patients undergoing atrial fibrillation ablation who had computed tomography before ablation, the esophagus ran parallel to the left-sided pulmonary veins in 56% of patients, and, in 36% of the patients, the esophagus had an oblique course going from the left superior pulmonary vein to the right inferior pulmonary vein.[12] The mean width of contact between the esophagus and the left atrial posterior wall was 11 to 15 mm. An interposed fat pad was present in 98% of patients, but was discontinuous in 96%. Aside from these inherent anatomic considerations, left atrial enlargement can result in the sandwiching of the esophagus between the left atrium and the thoracic spine, which can also increase the risk of esophageal injury during posterior wall ablation.[13]

In addition, extrapericardial structures that can be damaged during percutaneous pericardial access must always remain at the forefront of electrophysiologists' awareness. Access approaches for pericardial access are discussed elsewhere in this issue; however, a few key anatomic considerations are important to address. The subxiphoid approach is the most common technique used for percutaneous access. When introducing a needle into the pericardial space via this method, 1 collateral structures such as the liver, abdominal viscera, diaphragm, and the epicardial coronary vessels must be kept in mind, particularly the inferior interventricular artery and vein (so-called posterior descending artery and middle cardiac vein, respectively). Notably, bleeding risk can be minimized by directing a needle through the left sternocostal triangle (also known as the Larrey space; **Fig. 4**), which is an avascular space except for the left superior epigastric artery running along the costal margin.[14–16] With this technique, the needle can pass through a window just inferior and to the left of the xiphoid process, through the rectus abdominis muscle, and avoid the liver and diaphragm as well as important vascular structures, such as the superior epigastric artery.[16]

SUMMARY

Entering the pericardial space allows electrophysiologists access to epicardial structures that cannot otherwise be reached via endovascular catheter methods. Although technological advancements have allowed the performance of safe access to the pericardium, certain anatomic boundaries and nearby structures must always be kept in mind. The oblique and transverse sinuses as well as pericardial recesses are located posteriorly and superiorly, and they restrict catheter manipulation in these areas. The epicardial vessels are often surrounded by adipose tissue, which can provide insulation against vascular injury but also impedes effective ablation lesion formation. In addition, adjacent structures, such as the esophagus, phrenic nerve, and vascular structures, must always be respected so as not to cause inadvertent collateral injury during epicardial interventions.

DISCLOSURE

None.

SUPPLEMENTARY DATA

Supplementary data to this article can be found online at https://doi.org/10.1016/j.ccep.2020.04.003.

REFERENCES

1. Zipes DP, Libby P, Bonow RO, et al. Braunwald's heart disease: a textbook of cardiovascular medicine. 11th edition. Amsterdam: Elsevier; 2019.

2. Spodick DH. Macrophysiology, microphysiology, and anatomy of the pericardium: a synopsis. Am Heart J 1992;124:1046–51.

3. Boyle NG, Shivkumar K. Epicardial interventions in electrophysiology. Circulation 2012;126:1752–69.

4. McAlpine WA. Heart and coronary arteries: an anatomical atlas for clinical diagnosis, radiological investigation, and surgical treatment. New York: Springer-Verlag; 1975.

5. Chaffanjon P, Brichon PY, Faure C, et al. Pericardial reflection around the venous aspect of the heart. Surg Radiol Anat 1997;19:17–21.

6. D'Avila A, Scanavacca M, Sosa E, et al. Pericardial anatomy for the interventional electrophysiologist. J Cardiovasc Electrophysiol 2003;14:422–30.

7. Lachman N, Syed FF, Habib A, et al. Correlative anatomy for the electrophysiologist, part II: cardiac ganglia, phrenic nerve, coronary venous system. J Cardiovasc Electrophysiol 2011;22:104–10.

8. Syed F, Lachman N, Christensen K, et al. The pericardial space: obtaining access and an approach to fluoroscopic anatomy. Card Electrophysiol Clin 2010;2:9–23.

9. Pejkovic B, Bogdanovic D. The great cardiac vein. Surg Radiol Anat 1992;14:23–8.

10. Tung R, Nakahara S, Ramirez R, et al. Distinguishing epicardial fat from scar: analysis of electrograms using high-density electroanatomic mapping in a novel porcine infarct model. Heart Rhythm 2010;7:389–95.

11. Rabkin SW. Epicardial fat: properties, function and relationship to obesity. Obes Rev 2007;8:253–61.

12. Lemola K, Sneider M, Desjardins B, et al. Computed tomographic analysis of the anatomy of the left atrium and the esophagus: implications for left atrial catheter ablation. Circulation 2004;110:3655–60.

13. Martinek M, Meyer C, Hassanein S, et al. Identification of a high-risk population for esophageal injury during radiofrequency catheter ablation of atrial fibrillation: procedural and anatomical considerations. Heart Rhythm 2010;7:1224–30.

14. Baudoin YP, Hoch M, Protin XM, et al. The superior epigastric artery does not pass through Larrey's space (trigonum sternocostale). Surg Radiol Anat 2003;25:259–62.

15. Tung R, Shivkumar K. Epicardial ablation of ventricular tachycardia. Methodist Debakey Cardiovasc J 2015;11:129–34.

16. Fukuzawa K, Nagamatsu Y, Mori S, et al. Percutaneous pericardiocentesis with the anterior approach: demonstration of the precise course with computed tomography. JACC Clin Electrophysiol 2019;5:730–41.

Techniques for Percutaneous Access

Zachary Hale, MD[a], Austin Howard, MD[a], Yang Yang, MD[b], Nilesh Mathuria, MD, FHRS[a],*

KEYWORDS

- Epicardial access • Catheter ablation • Percutaneous • Pericardial

KEY POINTS

- Percutaneous epicardial access is typically performed via a subxiphoid approach.
- Adjunctive techniques such as needle-in-needle technique, electroanatomic mapping assistance, and pressure sensor monitoring are emerging methods for improved success and reduced complication rates.
- Future methods for percutaneous epicardial access may include other sites of access, direct visualization, and novel parameters such as near-field impedance.

INTRODUCTION

The second century Greek physician Galen was the first to describe drainage of purulent pericarditis through direct visualization of the heart through a surgical incision and then stripping the overlying tissue. This technique was not improved on for more than a millennium until 1840 when Franz Schuh performed the first blind pericardiocentesis by inserting a surgical trocar into the third intercostal space just left of the sternum for a patient in tamponade.[1] Although revolutionary at the time, the risk of pneumothorax and ventricular puncture was extremely high and led to significant morbidity and mortality. The now-standard subxiphoid technique was first suggested by Marfan[2] in 1911 among a myriad of approaches, and its safety profile quickly led to its widespread adoption.

Sosa and colleagues[3] in 1996 first described percutaneous epicardial access in the context of electrophysiology studies, and this was largely inspired by subxiphoid pericardiocentesis methods practiced worldwide for treatment of cardiac tamponade. Given the notable difference in volume of fluid in the potential space, with only 15 to 50 mL of fluid in a normal pericardium, proper patient position, location selection, and puncture technique are crucial to avoiding right ventricle (RV) puncture and/or epicardial vessel damage.

CLASSIC TECHNIQUE

The procedure can be performed under general anesthesia or deep conscious sedation. After ensuring the patient is sterile, prepped, and draped in the supine position, the subxiphoid area may be anesthetized with 1% lidocaine in patients undergoing the procedure under conscious sedation. Fluoroscopic views are then adjusted to visualize access. Often, left anterior oblique (LAO)/right anterior oblique (RAO) views and/or anteroposterior (AP)/left lateral fluoroscopic views are used for access. Further, diagnostic electrophysiology catheters are placed toward the RV apex, which provides another fluoroscopic landmark during epicardial access. To minimize the likelihood of inadvertent trauma, a blunt-tipped 17-gauge (G) standard Tuohy needle originally designed for epidural access is used. The optimal entrance point is roughly 2 cm below and 1 cm

[a] Division of Cardiac Electrophysiology, Texas Heart Institute, Houston, TX, USA; [b] Division of Cardiology, Baylor College of Medicine, 6620 Main Street, 11th Floor, Houston, TX 77030, USA
* Corresponding author. PO Box 20345, MC 2-225, Houston, TX 77225-0345.
E-mail address: nimathuria@texasheart.org
Twitter: @NileshMathuria (N.M.)

Card Electrophysiol Clin 12 (2020) 271–280
https://doi.org/10.1016/j.ccep.2020.04.004

lateral to the xiphoid process. A small incision is frequently made before needle insertion to aid in positioning.

The needle should be positioned with the tip pointed toward the left shoulder of the patient, with the blunted end of the needle directed toward the heart. A decision must be made about whether an anterior or posterior approach is desired. The angle between the needle and the chest on the z-axis determines which part of the ventricle is initially accessed. Steeper angles initially reach the posterior portion of the ventricle, whereas shallower ones should allow more anterior portions of the ventricle to be immediately accessible. The initial approach should be more superficial (<30°). Once the desired trajectory is selected, the needle is carefully advanced under fluoroscopy. The initial course should make its way through superficial subcutaneous tissue and above the dome of the diaphragm. Once past this initial tissue, cardiac fluoroscopic landmarks can guide the operator to the level of the parietal pericardium. A small amount of contrast can be injected to confirm the location of the needle. Of note, excessive contrast administration can obscure cardiac landmarks. Subsequently, it comes to rest on the fibrous parietal pericardium. There should be some resistance to the needle advancing at this point; the gentle sensation of cardiac pulsations is also be felt by the operator at this point. A small contrast injection can then be done to show tenting of the parietal pericardium by the needle to ensure appropriate positioning of the needle at the desired location (**Fig. 1**A). The RAO view, which identifies the location of the needle along the basal-apical axis, is helpful to avoid damaging major epicardial vessels along the base of the heart. However, pericardial puncture is usually performed in the LAO view to ensure a more tangential approach to the RV. Having

catheters in the coronary sinus and RV apex can also help orient the operator to the location of the needle relative to the RV. Small adjustments in angle and trajectory may be needed, but, if large changes are needed, it is recommended to fully remove and reposition the needle to avoid laceration of chest wall and abdominal structures.

Before entering the potential space, the operator must be careful to take into account motion of the diaphragm during the respiratory cycle. Holding the needle still while the diaphragm contracts and moves inferiorly may cause the needle to inadvertently puncture the ventricle. For procedures performed under general anesthesia, careful control of respirations with apnea or decreased tidal volumes is helpful at this stage. Once ready, the operator can carefully advance the needle until a sudden decrease in resistance is felt. This sensation may be felt as a pop, which happens as the parietal pericardium is punctured. Withdrawing the needle slightly when the pop of pericardial puncture is felt can help minimize incidence of RV puncture or laceration by limiting the accidental advancement of the needle.

Once this potential space is entered, a small amount of contrast (5–10 mL) can be injected into the pericardium to allow visualization of the cardiac contour. A soft guidewire is then inserted through the needle. Carefully advancing the guidewire should allow it to move smoothly along the cardiac surface with little resistance. In contrast, the guidewire can be within the access needle at time of advancement in the pericardial space and advanced under fluoroscopy without contrast administration.[4] Using an LAO view, the guidewire should be visualized hugging the lateral border of the heart along the oblique sinus and then ideally advanced through the transverse sinus and around the RV (**Fig. 1**B). This approach ensures that the RV has not been punctured. Other signs

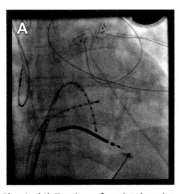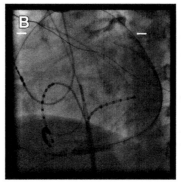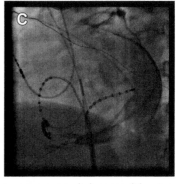

Fig. 1. (*A*) Tenting of parietal pericardium with Tuohy needle during percutaneous epicardial access, (*B*) epicardial access with guidewire (*white arrows*) in pericardial space encircling the cardiac border in LAO projection, (*C*) contrast injection via 5-Fr dilator confirming pericardial location.

of RV puncture at this stage include bloody aspirations through the needle, absence of contrast layering, or premature ventricular contractions during wire advancement. Aside from RV puncture, appropriate wire location also ensures that the pleural space and/or subdiaphragmatic space has not been accessed. The original Sosa technique also monitored for ST elevations by attaching a precordial lead to the Tuohy needle, but this is no longer in common practice.

Puncture or laceration can be managed conservatively if it is only with a Tuohy needle and generally does not lead to significant complications. If in the ventricle, the needle may be withdrawn slightly until blood can no longer be aspirated and the guidewire readvanced. This process may be repeated until there is confirmation of the guidewire in the pericardium. If unsuccessful, the needle should be fully withdrawn and a fresh attempt made. It is crucial to confirm positioning of the guidewire before proceeding because placement of a sheath into the RV generally requires operative repair for management of hemopericardium and abandonment of the intended procedure.

After confirmation of the guidewire in the pericardial space, a long 5-French (Fr) dilator can be advanced over the guidewire using standard Seldinger technique. Subsequent contrast administration to create a pericardiogram through this dilator can confirm a pericardial location and evaluate for adhesions before insertion of an ablation and/or mapping catheter (**Fig. 1**C).

ADJUNCTIVE STRATEGIES FOR PERICARDIAL ACCESS

Although the original Sosa and colleagues[3] method of epicardial access using the 17-G Tuohy needle with fluoroscopic guidance is still routinely used in current practice, there are several adjunctive strategies that have been developed to improve either procedural safety or feasibility of the access approach. When performing epicardial access, the following considerations can affect the decision for the optimal procedural approach:

- Reduce anatomic ambiguity during needle advancement
- Optimize positioning angle and site of entry for the procedure being performed
- Minimize the risk of puncture to critical epicardial structures (ie, epicardial coronary arteries and veins)
- Minimize the risk of myocardial injury and perforation, most commonly affecting the RV
- Early recognition of procedural complications

- Reduced ionizing radiation exposure to the patient and the operative staff

Needle-in-Needle Epicardial Access

The needle-in-needle method of epicardial access is similar in setup and approach to the Sosa method, but uses a smaller 21-G micropuncture needle for the pericardial puncture in an effort to limit the severity of inadvertent ventricular puncture.[5] A micropuncture needle, alone, yielded poor control and limited tactile feedback of the distal tip because of the depth traveled and flexibility of the needle. Instead, using an outer 18-G Cook needle (Percutaneous Entry Thinwall Needle, 18 G, 7 cm, Cook Medical, Bloomington, IN) provided strength and ease of the initial puncture, with an inner 21-G micropuncture needle (Cook Medical) or long spinal needle (Chiba Biopsy needle, 21 G, 20 cm, Cook Medical) and wire for the pericardial access to limit risk.

Method

1. The 18-G needle is inserted from the subxiphoid approach to a depth just proximal to the cardiac silhouette (**Fig. 2**).
2. The 21-G micropuncture needle is then inserted through the 18-G needle.
3. Using contrast and tactile feedback under fluoroscopy, the 21-G needle is advanced into the pericardial space.
4. An 0.46-mm (0.018-inch) guidewire (Hi Torque Steelcore 18 guidewire with mircoglide coating, 0.46-mm, 190 cm, Abbott Vascular, Santa Clara, CA) is then advanced into the micropuncture needle, into the pericardial space, ensuring the wire does not follow a particular cardiac chamber and remains lateral along the cardiac silhouette in the LAO projection.
5. The needles are then removed and a micropuncture dilator is advanced into the pericardium. This dilator is then exchanged for a 6-Fr or 8-Fr dilator and pericardial entry is again confirmed with contrast or fluid aspiration. The wire is then removed and a larger 0.89-mm (0.035-inch) floppy-tipped wire (0.89-mm Bentson wire, Cook Medical) is advanced into the pericardium, ensuring the same trajectory as the prior wire.
6. The sheath is then exchanged for an 8-Fr sheath. A second 0.89-mm wire may be introduced for expansion of the same puncture to 2 sheaths, if desired. The 8-Fr sheath is usually exchanged for a steerable sheath (Agilis, St. Jude Medical, Minneapolis, MN).

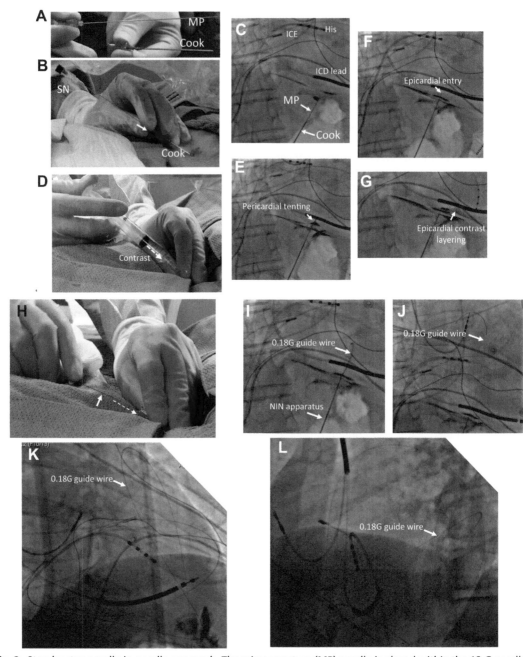

Fig. 2. Step-by-step needle-in-needle approach. The micropuncture (MP) needle is placed within the 18-G needle. Using the MP needle, contrast injection is used to aid epicardial access. Subsequent guidewire advancement through MP needle performed and confirmed to be in the pericardial space. NIN, needle-in-needle; ICD, implantable cardioverter defibrillator; ICE, intracardiac echo; SN, spinal needle. (*From* Kumar S, Bazaz R, Barbhaiya CR et al. "Needle-in-needle" epicardial access: Preliminary observations with a modified technique for facilitating epicardial interventional procedures. Heart Rhythm 2015;12:1691-7; with permission.)

In the original publication, Kumar and colleagues[5] compared the procedural success and complication rates with historical patients at the same institutions, using the Sosa method of large-bore access. Epicardial access was obtained in 100% (23 out of 23) with the needle-in-needle method, and 94% (297 out of 316) with the Sosa method. Major bleeding (defined as >80 mL) was similar at 8.7% (2 out of 23) versus 9.6% (28 out of 291) (*P* = 1), and with median blood loss of 170 mL and 160 mL, respectively.[5] This method has been shown to be safe and achievable for both posterior and anterior epicardial access.[6]

Potential advantages

Major complications during epicardial access seem to be reduced with micropuncture access compared with larger-bore access needles. Gunda and colleagues[7] reported differences in complication rates between large-bore needle (n = 185) and micropuncture needle (n = 219) access in patients undergoing epicardial access. Inadvertent right ventricular puncture without effusion or injury was seen in 7.6% versus 6.8%, respectively. However, major complications were less frequent with the micropuncture needle access (large pericardial effusion, 8.1% vs 0.9%; open heart surgical repair, 3.2% vs 0%).[7]

Potential disadvantages

This method requires the use of ionizing radiation, typically in the form of low-dose fluoroscopy. There is potential for limited tactile feedback and reduced visualization of the micropuncture needle and wire.[8]

Real-Time Pressure/Frequency Monitoring

The thorax and pericardial space have been shown to have similar mean pressure, but differ in pressure frequencies.[9] A novel epicardial access system called the EpiAccess system (EpiEP, Inc, New Haven, CT) was recently developed to monitor pressure frequency during access.[10] The system includes an 18-G Tuohy needle with an internal welded fiber-optic sensor to detect pressure frequency, and a computer monitor with a graphical user interface operating proprietary software to capture pressure frequency signals to display to the operator. The procedure is performed in the typical manner described by Sosa and colleagues[3] but captures real-time pressure frequency data during needle entry to reduce anatomic ambiguity. The signal is unique to the different tissues encountered during needle entry (**Fig. 3**):

1. There are low-amplitude waveforms detected from the subxiphoid epigastrium entry to the level of the fibrous pericardium.
2. A transition signal is observed when the needle is tenting the pericardium.
3. Once the needle enters the pericardial space, the pressure oscillates between +5 and −5 mm Hg.
4. When the needle is close to the right ventricular wall, or in the right ventricular cavity, the

pressures increase, oscillating between +20 and −20 mm Hg. Typically, premature ventricular contractions occur with ventricular injury.

The EpiAccess system was originally tested in 25 patients, and access was successfully obtained in all patients, with a mean access time of 4.4 ± 1.6 minutes. Inadvertent right ventricular puncture and pericardial effusion (>80 mL) occurred in 4% (1 patient) but did not result in tamponade. There were no other serious or minor complications noted.

Potential advantages

The needle is a modified Tuohy needle and provides a tactile feel similar to typical Tuohy needles. The unique system provides an early warning system when the RV has been penetrated. There seemed to be a shallow learning curve with inexperienced operators having no statistically different outcomes compared with experienced operators.

Potential disadvantages

The modified Tuohy needle differs slightly at the tip compared with typical Tuohy needles, resulting in decreased sharpness and diameter changes. This difference results in the operator having to use more force. A transition signal can be observed while tenting the diaphragm, which may confuse inexperienced operators. The 18-G access needle has a larger bore than other methods, which may result in more major complications.[7] Damage to adjacent structures, such as the liver, lung, or penetrating arteries, is not mitigated with this approach. This method also requires the use of ionizing radiation in the form of low-dose fluoroscopy. In addition, this method has only been tested in a small number of patients.

Electroanatomic Mapping Guidance

Electroanatomic mapping (EAM) has been shown to assist with epicardial access in a proof-of-concept publication by Bradfield and colleagues[11] in 8 patients undergoing epicardial access. The concept involved obtaining endocardial EAM definition using the Ensite NavX system (formally St. Jude Medical, now Abbott Laboratories, Abbott Park, IL) or Carto III (Biosense Webster, Diamond Bar, CA). Following this, an uninsulated 17-G Tuohy needle (Havel's, Inc, Cincinnati, OH) was connected to the system to allow visualization of the needle on the EAM system to assist in performance of the epicardial access in conjunction with standard techniques as described later. The needle tip serves as a unipolar electrode with the system reference patch as the indifferent

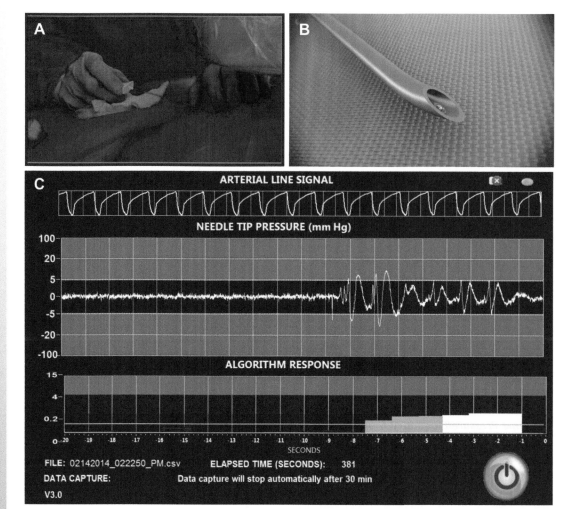

Fig. 3. Epicardial access with real-time pressure monitoring. Access is obtained in the (*A*) subxiphoid position with a (*B*) specialized Tuohy needle with an imbedded fiber-optic pressure sensor. (*C*) Real-time pressure monitoring reveals a sudden change from baseline to ±5 mm Hg consistent with pericardial pressures. Sudden increase to ±20 mm Hg would be concerning for RV puncture. (*From* Di Biase L, Burkhardt JD, Reddy V et al. Initial international multicenter human experience with a novel epicardial access needle embedded with a real-time pressure/frequency monitoring to facilitate epicardial access: Feasibility and safety. Heart Rhythm 2017;14:981-98; with permission.)

electrode in the Ensite NavX system, and as a bipolar electrode in the Carto III system.

1. EAM was performed endocardially with particular attention to capture the right ventricular apical endocardial borders, the inferior vena cava (IVC) and superior vena cava (SVC).
2. When available, computed tomography (CT) images of the IVC, SVC, and xiphoid process were synchronized with the endocardial borders of the IVC and SVC.
3. A 17-G Tuohy needle was connected to a sterile electrode clamp (alligator clip) and to the EAM system. Before attempting epicardial access, the needle was guided to the tip of the xiphoid process to ensure fidelity of the images and tracking to the needle.
4. Subxiphoid approach was then used to access the pericardial space using mapping points during advancement and verified under fluoroscopy.
5. A J-tipped wire was connected to the sterile electrode clamp and advanced into the pericardial space through the needle and visualized on the EAM system. The wire was tracked along the lateral aspect of the cardiac border and outside the endocardial EAM points and verified on fluoroscopy. The tip, but not the shaft, of the wire was accurately correlated with the fluoroscopic images.

Epicardial access was obtained in 100% (8 out of 8) of patients (**Fig. 4**). One patient had a prior history of a perforated right ventricular lead with subsequent cardiac tamponade and pericarditis and 2 epicardial access procedures. In this patient, the needle and wire were seen crossing the endocardial mapping points in the RV. The needle and wire were withdrawn and verified to be in the pericardial space on fluoroscopy without pericardial effusion; however, the procedure was aborted out of caution. No other clinically relevant complications occurred.

Potential advantages

The addition of EAM to fluoroscopy potentially adds anatomic reassurance and certainty. There is also the potential for limiting or even eliminating ionizing radiation during the procedure, although the patient does undergo a CT scan before the procedure. This scan can be performed with very low doses of radiation and has no medical staff exposure. The use of EAM incorporates a system that is already being used for many epicardial access procedures, likely incurs little to no additional cost, and presumably has a shallower learning curve than current practice.

Potential disadvantages

The use of EAM for epicardial access has only been studied in a limited number of patients to date. The limited data available suggest patients with prior epicardial access or potential adhesions may make access more challenging, as expected.

Carbon Dioxide Insufflation

Another potential avenue for reducing complications includes insufflating the pericardial space with CO_2 or injecting with iodinated contrast, which both increases visualization of the space and separates the pericardial layers further so that there is less chance for RV perforation. This method has been accomplished via transatrial entry into the epicardial space, in particular with intentional perforation of the right atrial appendage (RAA). This method was first done with the intent of drug delivery and sampling of pericardial fluid and then later for purposes of left atrial appendage (LAA) ligation with the Lariat device.[12–14] This method is accomplished by placing a catheter in the RAA, perforating the RAA with the back end

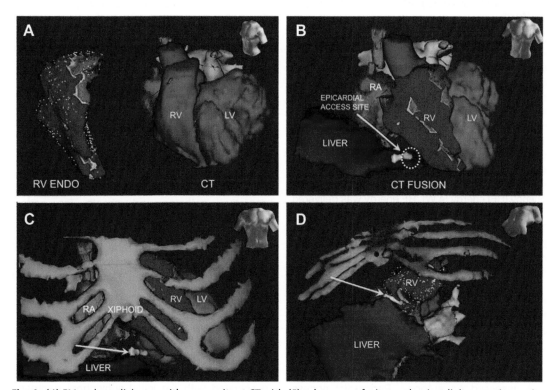

Fig. 4. (*A*) RV endocardial map with concomitant CT with (*B*) subsequent fusion and epicardial access site as visualized by EAM. (*C*) AP and (*D*) LAO caudal views of epicardial access site (*arrow*) with EAM/CT fusion. LV, left ventricle; RA, right atrium. (*From* Bradfield JS, Tung R, Boyle NG, Buch E, Shivkumar K. Our approach to minimize risk of epicardial access: standard techniques with the addition of electroanatomic mapping guidance. J Cardiovasc Electrophysiol 2013;24:723-7; with permission.)

of a guidewire, and then inserting a 2.4-Fr braided microcatheter (Renegade STC-18, 150 cm, Boston Scientific, Marlborough, MA) through the perforation. Through this microcatheter, iodinated contrast or CO_2 can be delivered, with the heavy iodinated contrast more suited to posterior approaches in supine patients, and the more buoyant CO_2 better suited for an anterior approach. The pericardial space is then accessed via the standard subxiphoid approach. Note that the iodinated contrast must also be removed from the space after the second access but that the CO_2 is resorbed by the body. The technique seems to be safe in humans, even in procedures requiring anticoagulation.[13] A similar idea has been used in ventricular tachycardia ablations but by perforating a small cardiac vein rather than the RAA.[15] Using the transatrial access for the procedure has also been attempted in animals but with the noted disadvantages of more bleeding and cardiac tamponade as well the requirement that the larger perforation be closed with a patent foramen ovale occluder.[16]

FUTURE DIRECTIONS
Radiofrequency Energy and Virtual Imaging Platform

In a study using a porcine model, 5 animals underwent epicardial access using a novel toolkit involving a specialized needle, preoperative multidetector CT imaging (VCT, General Electric Healthcare, Milwaukee, WI) of the thorax and upper abdomen, and a virtual imaging electromagnetic platform (Aurora, Northern Digital Instruments).[17] The needle is 19-G, 150 mm (6 inch), with an abbreviated bevel (25° angle, 1.7 mm [0.067 inch] length), an electrically insulted lumen and shaft, and an exposed 5-mm needle tip for delivery of radiofrequency (RF) energy (4 W). RF energy was delivered using a commercial generator (EPT-1000 XP, EP Technologies, San Jose, CA) to assist with parietal pericardial access. The imaging platform allows for real-time anatomic assessment of the needle with a spatial error of 0.6 mm.

The CT images were registered to the operative field. In this study to assess accuracy of the system, the epicardial coronary arteries were targeted with both an anterior (left anterior descending artery) and posterior (posterior depending artery) approach. RF energy was delivered on the epicardium and the location was assessed on autopsy. Pericardial access was achieved in 4 out of 5 animals on the first attempt, and in the final animal on repositioning. Postmortem analysis showed spatial inaccuracy of 4.2 ± 2.2 mm.

Potential advantages
The use of preoperative multidetector CT data and a virtual imaging platform may allow a more accurate assessment of the three-dimensional structures of the access tract, and limited ionizing radiation exposure to the medical staff during epicardial access. In addition, the use of RF energy to gain access to the parietal pericardium allows less use of force during needle entry. These elements could improve the safety of the procedure.

Potential disadvantages
This system has only been used in a limited number of animals without human use at the time of this writing. The needle used in this technique is 19 G, and large-bore access has been associated with more major complications.

Lateral Percutaneous Access

Isath and colleagues[18] describe in a canine model (n = 3) a novel lateral percutaneous epicardial access approach. Standard subxiphoid epicardial access was obtained and used to exchange for a novel balloon-tipped sheath, positioned laterally on the cardiac border under fluoroscopic guidance. The balloon is inflated with contrast medium for fluoroscopic visualization. Following this, a needle was introduced between a left lateral intercostal space and advanced to the balloon. The balloon can be seen tenting, then puncture of the balloon was performed.[18] A guidewire was then passed into the pericardial space and the needle was exchanged for the procedural sheath. There were no acute complications in this small case series.

Potential advantages
This novel system could allow safe lateral access, which may permit easier maneuverability of the operative catheter and sheath for certain arrhythmia conditions. The use of the balloon provides a physical barrier to limit inadvertent puncture of the myocardium and lateral epicardial coronary arteries. It also provides a more objective means of epicardial puncture feedback on balloon puncture.

Potential disadvantages
This trial is a small animal study with no use described in humans at the time of this writing. This method is unique because it allows for an alternative location of access but still has the risks associated with the initial subxiphoid approach and the additional lateral puncture. It is conceivable that the risk of pneumothorax may be increased in the later access. Fluoroscopy is required for the use of this method of access.

Direct Visualization

Direct visualization of the pericardium is another option for reducing inadvertent damage during epicardial access. This damage has been reported using surgical access for pericardioscopes[19] as well as with small fiber-optic devices.[20] Another promising approach for avoiding RV puncture includes pulling the pericardium away from the epicardium before puncture. This approach has been attempted by using a spiral tine at the distal tip of a needle[21] as well as with devices using a hollow tube and vacuum.[22] These approaches have seemingly been combined as well. Nakatsuma and colleagues[23] developed an experimental endoscopic device using both a fiber-optic camera and small forceps for grasping the pericardium. Similarly, the startup Perifect has developed the PeriCardioScope, a device combining video guidance, suction to safely lift the pericardium from the epicardium, and then safe needle entry into the space.

Near-Field Impedance

Bioimpedance is currently under investigation as a means of improving anatomic certainty during epicardial access. Investigators have performed a proof-of-concept study in an ovine model with the ability to accurately distinguish between tissues with differing average normalized impedance values for the anterior mediastinum (3.209 ± 0.227), pericardial space (1.760 ± 0.370), and the RV (1.024 ± 0.207; $P<.0001$).[24] These values were collected in a resting state using a POLARIS X decapolar catheter (Boston Scientific, Marlborough, MA) after access had been obtained using traditional access techniques. Current investigation is underway for use of near-field impedance during epicardial access in a porcine model using a modified 21-G micropuncture access needle; however, this work has not been published at the time of this writing.

SUMMARY

The classic subxiphoid approach remains the mainstay for percutaneous epicardial access. It is hoped that adjunctive techniques such as needle in needle, pressure monitoring, and electroanatomic mapping, as well as emerging technologies, will make the procedure safer and more effective, allowing further adoption by clinicians.

DISCLOSURE

The authors have nothing to disclose.

REFERENCES

1. Schuh F. Erfahrungen, über die Paracentese der Brust und des Herzbeutels. Medzinisches Jahrbuch Kaiserlichen Königlichen Staates Wein 1841;33:338.
2. Marfan AB. Ponction du péricarde par, l'epigastre. Ann de Méd et Chir Inf 1911;15:529.
3. Sosa E, Scanavacca M, d'Avila A, et al. A new technique to perform epicardial mapping in the electrophysiology laboratory. J Cardiovasc Electrophysiol 1996;7:531–6.
4. Long DY, Sun LP, Sang CH, et al. Pericardial access via wire-guided puncture without contrast: the feasibility and safety of a modified approach. J Cardiovasc Electrophysiol 2020;31(1):30–7.
5. Kumar S, Bazaz R, Barbhaiya CR, et al. "Needle-in-needle" epicardial access: preliminary observations with a modified technique for facilitating epicardial interventional procedures. Heart Rhythm 2015;12:1691–7.
6. Keramati AR, DeMazumder D, Misra S, et al. Anterior pericardial access to facilitate electrophysiology study and catheter ablation of ventricular arrhythmias: a single tertiary center experience. J Cardiovasc Electrophysiol 2017;28:1189–95.
7. Gunda S, Reddy M, Pillarisetti J, et al. Differences in complication rates between large bore needle and a long micropuncture needle during epicardial access: time to change clinical practice? Circ Arrhythm Electrophysiol 2015;8:890–5.
8. Romero J, Shivkumar K, Di Biase L, et al. Mastering the art of epicardial access in cardiac electrophysiology. Heart Rhythm 2019;16:1738–49.
9. Mahapatra S, Tucker-Schwartz J, Wiggins D, et al. Pressure frequency characteristics of the pericardial space and thorax during subxiphoid access for epicardial ventricular tachycardia ablation. Heart Rhythm 2010;7:604–9.
10. Di Biase L, Burkhardt JD, Reddy V, et al. Initial international multicenter human experience with a novel epicardial access needle embedded with a real-time pressure/frequency monitoring to facilitate epicardial access: feasibility and safety. Heart Rhythm 2017;14:981–8.
11. Bradfield JS, Tung R, Boyle NG, et al. Our approach to minimize risk of epicardial access: standard techniques with the addition of electroanatomic mapping guidance. J Cardiovasc Electrophysiol 2013;24:723–7.
12. Verrier RL, Waxman S, Lovett EG, et al. Transatrial access to the normal pericardial space: a novel approach for diagnostic sampling, pericardiocentesis, and therapeutic interventions. Circulation 1998;98:2331–3.
13. Greenbaum AB, Rogers T, Paone G, et al. Intentional right atrial exit and carbon dioxide insufflation to facilitate subxiphoid needle entry into the empty

pericardial space: first human experience. JACC Clin Electrophysiol 2015;1:434–41.

14. Rogers T, Ratnayaka K, Schenke WH, et al. Intentional right atrial exit for microcatheter infusion of pericardial carbon dioxide or iodinated contrast to facilitate sub-xiphoid access. Catheter Cardiovasc Interv 2015;86:E111–8.

15. Silberbauer J, Gomes J, O'Nunain S, et al. Coronary vein exit and carbon dioxide insufflation to facilitate subxiphoid epicardial access for ventricular mapping and ablation: first experience. JACC Clin Electrophysiol 2017;3:514–21.

16. Scanavacca MI, Venancio AC, Pisani CF, et al. Percutaneous transatrial access to the pericardial space for epicardial mapping and ablation. Circ Arrhythm Electrophysiol 2011;4:331–6.

17. Ludwig DR, Menon PG, Fill B, et al. A novel toolkit to improve percutaneous subxiphoid needle access to the healthy pericardial sac. J Cardiovasc Electrophysiol 2015;26:576–80.

18. Isath A, Abudan Al-Masry A, Sugrue A, et al. Lateral percutaneous epicardial access with a novel technique. JACC Clin Electrophysiol 2018;4:1115–6.

19. Zenati MA, Shalaby A, Eisenman G, et al. Epicardial left ventricular mapping using subxiphoid video pericardioscopy. Ann Thorac Surg 2007;84:2106–7.

20. Hack BJ, Ramon SG, Hagen ZA, et al. Direct vision in minimally invasive epicardial procedures: preliminary tests of prototype instrumentation. J Med Eng Technol 2015;39:272–80.

21. Pollak PM, Mahapatra S, Kanwal JK, et al. Novel pericardial access device: design features and in vitro evaluation. J Med Eng Technol 2011;35:179–84.

22. Seferovic PM, Ristic AD, Maksimovic R, et al. Initial clinical experience with PerDUCER device: promising new tool in the diagnosis and treatment of pericardial disease. Clin Cardiol 1999;22:l30–5.

23. Nakatsuma K, Yamamoto E, Watanabe S, et al. Ultra-thin endoscopy-guided pericardiocentesis: a pilot study in a swine model. J Invasive Cardiol 2016;28:78–80.

24. Burkland DA, Ganapathy AV, John M, et al. Near-field impedance accurately distinguishes among pericardial, intracavitary, and anterior mediastinal position. J Cardiovasc Electrophysiol 2017;28:1492–9.

Perioperative Imaging to Guide Epicardial Mapping and Ablation

Alejandro Jimenez Restrepo, MD[a],*, Timm Michael Dickfeld, MD, PhD[b]

KEYWORDS

• Imaging • Perioperative • Mapping • Epicardial

KEY POINTS

- To use perioperative imaging to enhance safety of epicardial access by understanding anatomic landmarks and key structures in the epicardial space, epigastrium, and mediastinum.
- To characterize arrhythmia substrates using perioperative imaging modalities in order to guide catheter ablation of atrial and ventricular arrhythmias in the epicardial space.
- To learn the value of computed tomography imaging in the evaluation of perivascular epicardial fat.
- To understand the value of perioperative imaging in structural interventions involving the epicardial space, such as left atrial appendage ligation and hybrid ablations.

INTRODUCTION

Accessing the epicardial space without a sternotomy or a surgical pericardial window to treat ventricular arrhythmias in Chagas disease (a predominantly epicardial infiltrative disease) became a medical necessity in the 1990s in South America. Since the introduction of the dry percutaneous epicardial access approach by Sosa and colleagues,[1] epicardial access is now regarded as a standard procedure in many centers for the management of ventricular arrhythmias in ischemic cardiomyopathies and nonischemic cardiomyopathies (NICMs) and atrioventricular accessory pathways after failed conventional endocardial ablation.

The understanding of the epicardial space and its neighboring structures has since become an important subject of comprehensive anatomic teachings in modern-day electrophysiology (EP). The evolution of complex ablation procedures to treat atrial and ventricular arrhythmias and device interventions to prevent cardioembolic stroke requires a thorough understanding of the pericardial anatomy to allow for safe access to the epicardial space.

This article presents the current state of perioperative imaging technologies, which assist in the evaluation of the epicardial space relevant to cardiac EP interventions.

PERIOPERATIVE IMAGING OF THE EPICARDIAL SPACE

Imaging modalities are important for 3 main reasons: (1) guiding safe access to the epicardial space, (2) evaluation of the underlying arrhythmia substrate, and (3) understanding of the anatomic landmarks and structures present in the epicardial space and the surrounding mediastinum. For the purposes of this article, the discussed technologies are divided into intraprocedural (fluoroscopy, 3-dimensional electroanatomic mapping [3DEAM], and intracardiac echocardiography [ICE]) and preprocedural (cardiac computed tomography [CCT] and cardiac magnetic resonance imaging [CMR]) modalities.

a Section of Cardiology, Marshfield Clinic Health System, 1000 North Oak Avenue, Marshfield, WI 54449, USA;
b Section of Cardiac Electrophysiology and the Maryland Arrhythmia and Cardiac Imaging Group (MACIG), University of Maryland School of Medicine, 22 South Greene Street, Room N3W77, Baltimore, MD 21201, USA
* Corresponding author.
E-mail address: ARestrepo@som.umaryland.edu

Card Electrophysiol Clin 12 (2020) 281–293
https://doi.org/10.1016/j.ccep.2020.06.001

Fluoroscopy

The first imaging technique employed to guide access to the epicardial space was fluoroscopic imaging, which is still the most common intra-procedural technique used to guide this procedure. Its availability, low cost, and widespread use in EP make it the obvious and preferred choice in most centers. The original subxiphoid percutaneous access technique[1] has had variations in the fluoroscopic views employed and materials used (types of needles, sheaths, guide wires, and so forth) but essentially follows the same principle of anatomically guiding a needle inserted percutaneously into the epicardial space, while avoiding injury of any internal organs or cardiac structures (mainly the liver, diaphragm, bowel, right ventricle [RV], and coronary arteries). Perpendicular views to the long axis of the access needle are preferred to ensure a safe trajectory, first to avoid the dome of the diaphragm as the needle enters the subcutaneous space below the xyphoid process (Larrey space) using a shallow angulation (no more than 20° in a left lateral projection) and later to guide an anterior (30°–35°) or posterior (45°) approach using a steep left anterior oblique or left lateral view and paying special attention to maintain the needle orientation just below the inferior heart border in order to avoid RV puncture. Contrast commonly is used to confirm the exact location of the needle along with tactile feedback to feel resistance (needle tenting on fluoroscopy) followed by advancement through the parietal layer of the pericardium. Once epicardial access is felt to be gained, it should be confirmed with contrast instillation to paint the outline of the epicardial space and advancement of a guide wire freely and across both right and left aspects of the cardiac silhouette in a left anterior oblique projection.[2] Under normal conditions, no significant amounts of blood should be retrieved from the pericardial space, because this may signify a coronary artery or RV laceration.[3] Once access is confirmed and bleeding issues are not suspected, a sheath can be introduced into the pericardial space to gain access for the desired procedure. Despite the limitations of fluoroscopy to visualize cardiac and abdominal structures, its value to guide percutaneous epicardial access cannot be underestimated. Abnormalities, such as cardiomegaly, extreme cardiac rotations, hepatomegaly, splenomegaly, colon or gastric dilatation, and diaphragmatic paralysis, can be taken into consideration, thus potentially avoiding complications from internal organ damage.

Three-Dimensional Electroanatomic Mapping

Although the 3DEAM modality has not been used as a stand-alone technique to gain percutaneous epicardial access, the combination of fluoroscopy and 3DEAM is implemented safely and easily using commercially available mapping systems and tools. The experience published by Bradfield and colleagues[4] demonstrated the feasibility of 3DEAM to guide percutaneous epicardial access using an electrode clamp attached to the access needle, allowing for its visualization in the 3-D mapping environment. Careful reconstruction of the cardiac chambers and nearby organs (using image integration with preprocedural CCT or CMR data sets) facilitates safe access and reduces the risk of complications.

3DEAM also can provide information regarding potential epicardial arrhythmia substrates even prior to gaining epicardial access, by means of unipolar endocardial voltage information to gain insight into potential mid-myocardial or epicardial scarring. This technique, however, offers only a generalized overview of scar burden and is unable to delineate intricate scar substrates, scar border zones, or conduction channels and is unable to delineate the extent of abnormal tissue involved in an arrhythmia circuit. In addition, this technique has been validated only in ventricular tachycardia (VT) substrates[5–7] and data on atrial tissue evaluation are lacking.

Intracardiac Echocardiography

ICE is favored in many centers due to its ease of use (single operator) and spatial resolution and currently is 1 of 3 imaging modalities (besides fluoroscopy and 3DEAM) allowing for real-time catheter visualization in the cardiac EP laboratory (at present, real-time CMR and computed tomography [CT]-guided procedures remain largely investigational and both require extensive modifications to the EP laboratory environment and equipment). Integration with 3DEAM systems also is possible to improve anatomic accuracy, by defining in great detail complex intracardiac structures, such as chordae tendineae, papillary muscles, and aortic cusps. In addition, ICE offers the ability to assess tissue characteristics, catheter-tissue interface (including catheter tip contact and response to ablation therapy), and monitor ventricular function and potential complications requiring urgent intervention (such as acute cardiogenic shock, steam pops, or pericardial effusion). Adjusting the ICE machine settings (gain, focus zone, depth, and dynamic range) can improve image quality and often allow for a more comprehensive evaluation of the tissue characteristics of endocardial, intramural, and epicardial aspects of the ventricular myocardium. This can guide a decision to proceed with epicardial access prior to gaining access into the left-side chambers and before systemic anticoagulation is initiated, thus reducing potential bleeding risks.

Endocardial, epicardial, and mid-myocardial scars (seen as tissue areas of increased echo brightness with to the normal surrounding myocardium) can be outlined and a specific geometry of the scar can be added to the anatomic maps for further characterization and correlation with voltage maps (**Figs. 1** and **2**). Bala and colleagues[8] described the value of ICE images to qualitatively evaluate the presence of epicardial and mid-myocardial scar in 18 patients with NICM undergoing VT ablation. They found a correlation between epicardial scar seen on ICE (based on visually increased echo brightness) and scar seen by epicardial bipolar mapping in all patients. No increased echo brightness was observed on ICE in a control group of patients (N = 30) with no left ventricular (LV) scarring. Not only is ICE able to allow visualization of

epicardial and mid-myocardial scar substrates, but also ICE images permit quantitative assessment of the tissue characteristics. Hussein and colleagues[9] reported the feasibility of using ICE imaging to quantify and differentiate normal myocardium from scar and border zone in 22 patients undergoing VT ablation for ischemic cardiomyopathy and NICM. Using commercially available software, signal intensity unit values were able to differentiate between normal myocardium and scar in all 15 patients with voltage defined ventricular scar zones (including 4 patients with mid-myocardial and 1 with transmural scar extending to the epicardium).

The main limitations of ICE include added procedural costs (the technology is not utilized broadly worldwide) and lack of operator experience for catheter manipulation required to obtain optimal fields of view to sample the regions of interest. Current and future advances in ICE probe and software technology, including 3-D automatic reconstruction, automatic border detection, and quantitative real-time tissue analytics, will facilitate the adoption of this technology beyond its current clinical use.

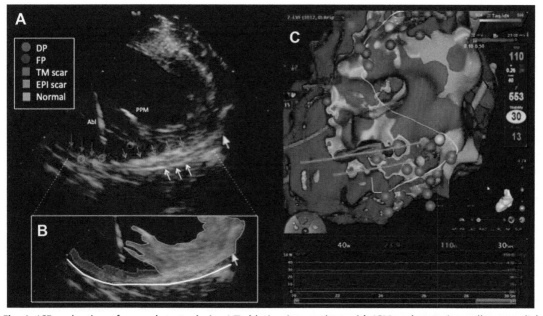

Fig. 1. ICE evaluation of scar substrate during VT ablation in a patient with ICM and posterior wall myocardial infarction. (*A*) Long axis view of the LV showing the PPM and a large area of transmural scar (*red arrows*) behind it, followed by an area of epicardial scar (*orange arrows*) underneath the PPM and healthy myocardium toward the apex. The parietal pericardium also is seen (*white arrows*). (*B*) Tissue analysis based on wall thickness and signal intensity demarcating the TM scar (*red*), epicardial scar (*orange*), healthy myocardium (*green*), and parietal pericardium (*white*). (*C*) 3DEAM with ICE integration of the PPM, epicardial scar (*orange lines*), annotated areas of diastolic potentials (*orange tags*), and fractionated potentials (*purple*). Note the ablation is conducted endocardially near the transition zone between TM scar (corresponding to bipolar endocardial voltage of 0.1–0.5 mV) and epicardial scar with underlying healthy myocardium. PPM< posterior papillary muscle. DP, diastolic potential; EPI, epicardial; FP, fractionated potential; TM, transmural.

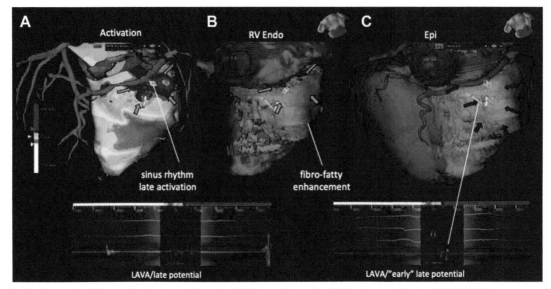

Fig. 2. Example of image fusion to guide epicardial mapping and ablation in a patient with ARVC. Maps are presented in an inferior view. (*A*) Fusion imaging between 3DEAM (activation map) and CCT with coronary artery reconstruction. The endocardial activation map shows areas of LAVA and late potentials in sinus rhythm (*bottom insert*). (*B*) CCT reconstructed RV endocardium (*blue*) and epicardial area of fibrofatty enhancement (ochre) in the RV free and inferior walls. (*C*) Fused CCT-3DEAM during epicardial mapping in sinus rhythm. Areas of LAVA and "early" late potentials are seen in the epicardial area corresponding to fibro-fatty replacement on CCT and located at a safe distance from the right coronary artery. Endo, endocardial; Epi, epicardial. (*Courtesy of* Pierre Jais. Université de Bordeaux, Bordeaux, France.)

Cardiac Computed Tomography

CCT is the most widely available and cost-effective imaging technology for preoperative anatomic evaluation in cardiac EP. Current CT scanners can produce within seconds high-quality images with remarkable spatial resolution. Postprocessing of CCT data sets to generate volume-rendered cardiac images, which can be used in the EP laboratory environment for preprocedural planning and intraprocedural navigation (using image integration techniques), demonstrates high reliability using current commercially available software.[10] Although not routinely employed by all centers performing epicardial ablations, preoperative evaluation of CCT images can help identify potential anatomic variants, which can pose an increased risk of complications or lead to failure to gain access, including gastric or bowel distension in the epigastric space, partial or complete congenital absence of the pericardium, chest wall deformities, hepatomegaly with left liver lobe prominence, pericardial calcifications or adhesions, heart rotations, RV dilatation, and unusual coronary artery trajectories or anomalies. The anatomic information obtained beforehand allows an operator to plan whether additional tools or techniques may be required to gain entry into the epicardial space freely (adhesiolysis, balloon dilatations, surgical window, and so forth).

Preoperative CCT can be used in innovative ways to guide epicardial access. Ebrille and colleagues[11] described a method of obtaining CT-guided epicardial access using a left parasternal approach in a patient with superimposed bowel in the epigastric space, by placing a CT grid in the patient's chest prior to scanning. The grid then was marked on the patient skin using a surgical marker and, using a 3-D CT rendition of the CT scan (which included the grid, chest wall, and internal organs), a safe path for needle entry into the epicardial space was achieved and epicardial ablation was conducted safely. Alternatively, with reconstruction of cardiac and visceral anatomy as a reference, Bradfield and colleagues[4] demonstrated the feasibility of using 3-D integration of preprocedural CCT anatomy (including the chest wall, sternum, heart, and solid organs) with intraprocedural 3DEAM and real-time needle visualization to guide safe epicardial subxiphoid access in 8 patients. For epicardial ablations, depiction of the coronary arteries anatomic trajectory and location of epicardial fat pads, cardiac veins, esophagus, and phrenic nerve (PN) course are essential to avoid collateral injury. In a study by Yamashita and colleagues,[12] 18% of patients undergoing epicardial mapping and ablation had local abnormal ventricular activities

(LAVAs), which could not be abolished due to their proximity to coronary arteries or PN. Displacement of the PN by means of epicardial balloon dilatation has become standard practice in some centers performing epicardial atrial and ventricular ablations, and image integration of the segmented PN from the preprocedural CCT with the putative ablation target sites on 3DEAM can help identify those patients who may require preemptive balloon instrumentation. Large-bore balloons (18 mm or greater) can be advanced into the oblique sinus in order to displace the esophagus or in the transverse sinus to displace the PNs. The effect is to increase the distance between the atrial or ventricular wall and those structures in order to decrease the risk of thermal injury during ablation procedures.[13,14] A study by Kumar and colleagues[13] showed that in 13 patients undergoing ablation for atrial arrhythmias originating from the superior vena cava (adjacent to the right PN) and epicardial left VTs (originating near the left PN trajectory), PN nerve displacement using large-bore balloons (n = 2), a combination of steerable sheath and EP catheter(n = 2), or both (n = 4) eventually were successful in displacing the PN and allowing for safe radiofrequency (RF) delivery on all cases. Although other means of esophageal displacement currently are available (usually by direct instrumentation of the esophageal lumen),[15,16] the epicardial access remains a viable alternative for esophageal displacement in selected cases.[14,17] CCT thus becomes essential to understand these important anatomic interactions.

CCT can provide useful information regarding the presence of subepicardial substrate for ventricular arrhythmias. Parameters, such as contrast enhancement and wall thickness, correlate well with the presence of scar on 3DEAM (see **Fig. 4**). Tian and colleagues[18] showed in 11 patients undergoing VT ablation that reduced wall thickness, wall motion abnormalities, and hypoperfusion correlated well with abnormal bipolar endocardial voltage less than 1.5 mV (r = 0.77) and integrated perfusion maps embedded in the 3DEAM correctly predicted transmurality, subepicardial involvement, and intramural substrates in 81.7% of the analyzed segments. Also, in a study by Esposito and colleagues,[19] delayed enhancement CCT identified LV scar and defined mural distribution in 39 of 43 patients referred for VT ablation. Epicardial scar substrates were seen in 7 patients (5 of whom underwent epicardial mapping) and correlated best with unipolar epicardial maps (average Kappa = 0.902). Finally, Yamashita and colleagues[20] evaluated the relationship between wall thinning on CCT and LAVAs in 42 patients

undergoing endo/epicardial VT ablation. Although severe wall thinning commonly was seen and highly predictive of the presence of epicardial LAVA in patients with ischemic scar and endocardial LAVA in patients postmyocarditis, severe wall thinning and LAVA rarely were seen in patients with NICM.

CCT also is useful to localize epicardial fat (**Fig. 3**), which can affect RF delivery to target areas in the ventricular myocardium and prevent a successful ablation. In 40 consecutive patients undergoing CCT evaluation, Sourwine and colleagues[21] demonstrated that thick epicardial fat (>5 mm) is more common near coronary vessels and along the RV and the ventricular base and that certain clinical characteristics (age >50, presence of coronary artery disease, and an elevated body mass index) are predictive of the presence of regional epicardial fat thickness greater than 5 mm. In arrhythmogenic RV cardiomyopathy (ARVC), myocardial fatty infiltration contributes to the arrhythmogenic substrate. Komatsu and colleagues[22] correlated the presence of fibrofatty myocardial replacement on CCT and 3DEAM epicardial voltage maps in 16 patients with ARVC undergoing VT ablation. Epicardial fat correlated well with regions of epicardial low voltage (K = 0.69) and registration of the CCT with the 3DEAM allowed for direct visualization of the coronary arteries and their relationship with epicardial fat distribution. These studies suggest a potential benefit for CCT-derived fat map reconstructions integrated with 3DEAM to guide epicardial substrate VT ablations.

Few limitations for preoperative CCT use exist, mainly related to intravenous contrast allergy and nephrotoxicity in some patients. The amount of x-ray radiation exposure with modern-day scanners is very low and, thus, usually acceptable from a safety perspective. Postprocessing of CT data sets is essential for image integration and 3-D visualization, and expertise with image segmentation and fusion techniques also is required (**Fig. 4**).

Cardiac Magnetic Resonance Imaging

Preoperative CMR in cardiac EP is used widely to evaluate both the anatomic and functional substrate before atrial and ventricular ablation procedures.[23–27] The preoperative information derived from such studies becomes relevant especially when mid-myocardial and epicardial arrhythmia substrates are identified and alternative approaches beyond conventional endocardial access are required. In certain cardiomyopathies with a high arrhythmia prevalence and mid-myocardial and epicardial tropism (Chagas

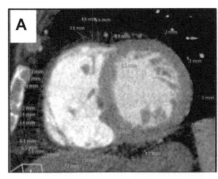
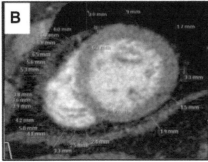
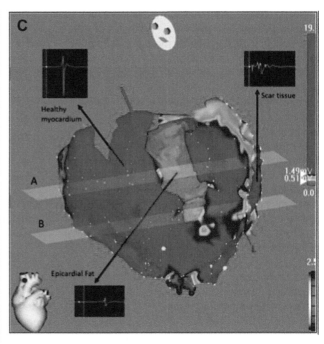

Fig. 3. CCT evaluation of epicardial fat. CCT ventricular short axis illustrating epicardial fat distribution and quantified fat thickness (in millimeters) in midventricular (*A*), and apical (*B*) short axis views. (*C*) CCT Perivascular epicardial fat reconstruction (*green*) registered to bipolar epicardial 3DEAM overlaying the territory of the left anterior descending artery. This illustrates the epicardial topography to guide epicardial mapping and ablation. Also depicted are the EGMs recorded from healthy tissue, fat, and scar tissue on the epicardial surface. Note that both epicardial fat and scar tissue display low voltage but late potentials are recorded only from scar tissue. The sliced sections on the map correspond to the cross-sectional depth of (*A*) and (*B*). (*From* Sourwine M, Jeudy J, Miller B, Vunnam R, Imanli H, Mesubi O, Etienne-Mesubi M, See V, Shorofsky S, Dickfeld T. Location, variations, and predictors of epicardial fat mapping using multidetector computed tomography to assist epicardial ventricular tachycardia ablation. Pacing Clin Electrophysiol. 2017; 40(10):1059-1066; with permission.)

disease, sarcoidosis, arrhythmogenic rhythm ventricular cardiomyopathy, hypertrophic cardiomyopathy (HCM), and postmyocarditis), epicardial access frequently is required to achieve a successful ablation. Identification of epicardial substrate before an ablation procedure can help plan timing of pericardial access and equipment selection (**Fig. 5**).

Important translational anatomy studies[28–30] evaluating the myoarchitecture of the atrial chambers elegantly described the anatomic basis for both normal atrial conduction and for the genesis of common atrial arrhythmias. The venoatrial junction of the left atrium, the site of focal electrical activity and triggers for atrial fibrillation,[31,32] is composed of myocardial strands with variable endocardial and epicardial distributions.[22] In addition to subendocardial myofibers, there are distinct subepicardial atrial myofiber strands (interatrial, septopulmonary, septoatrial, and intercaval bundles), which, together with the coronary sinus (CS) musculature and the vein and ligament of Marshall,[33] provide a network of bilayer fibers that propagate conduction across the atria. In a study by Pashakhanloo and colleagues,[34] diffusion tensor magnetic resonance imaging (MRI) was able to accurately delineate with submillimeter resolution the bilayered myoarchitecture of the atria described in the anatomic literature in 8 ex vivo heart specimens. Due to inherent limitations however, this technology is not available for clinical use. Recent publications highlight the importance of these epicardial muscle fibers and the atrial bilayer network in the perpetuation of atrial flutters despite documented endocardial conduction block.[33,35,36] Due to the thin nature of the atrial wall, atrial epicardial myofibers usually are ablated successfully endocardially or from inside a cardiac vein.

In contrast, epicardial arrhythmia substrates in the ventricles usually require an epicardial approach for successful mapping and elimination, particularly in the setting of NICMs and infiltrative cardiomyopathies. The presence of epicardial scarring on CMR should prompt consideration for epicardial as well as endocardial access.[37,38]

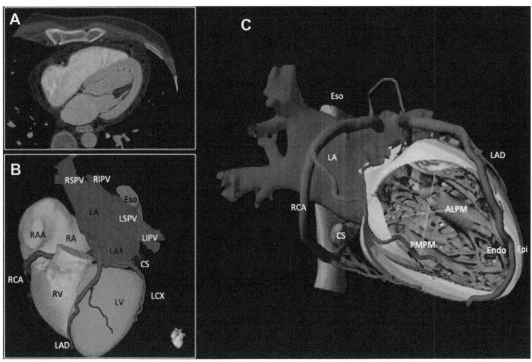

Fig. 4. Segmentation and 3-D volume rendering of CCT data sets. (*A*) Longitudinal axis segmentation of the cardiac chambers, esophagus, and CS. The left ventricle is segmented as a full thickness structure (*green*) with endocardium/papillary muscles (purple). (*B*) A 3-D volume model obtained from the segmentation in (*A*), including the coronary arteries. (*C*) A 3-D volume rendering of the cardiac endocardium/blood pool interfaces with full LV myocardium and coronary arteries. The anterolateral and posteromedial papillary muscles (ALPM and PMPM) are seen in great detail, along with the LV trabeculations.

Late gadolinium enhancement (LGE) CMR allows for detailed characterization of the topographic localization and extent of epicardial scar before a VT ablation procedure in order to plan the optimal approach (see **Fig. 3**). Piers and colleagues[24] demonstrated the value of LGE-CMR to predict successful ablation sites in 19 patients with NICM undergoing VT ablation. In 9 patients with VTs arising from basal anteroseptal scars, all but 1 had successful VT ablation targeting endocardial (N = 7) or the middle cardiac vein sites (N = 1). Conversely, in 8 patients with VTs originating from inferolateral scars, 5 of them required epicardial ablation for VT control. The CMR scar characteristics demonstrated anteroseptal scars to have a more transmural distribution and extension into the aortic root compared with inferolateral scars, which tended to be confined to the subepicardium. Maccabelli and colleagues[39] evaluated patients undergoing VT ablation secondary to myocarditis using preoperative CMR and endo-epicardial unipolar and bipolar voltage maps. LGE areas of scar correlating with arrhythmia substrates on 3DEAM were seen in the epicardium more often than the endocardium, and successful elimination of VT was seen in 20/26 patients (76.6%) during follow-up, supporting a first-time endo-epicardial approach.

Preprocedural CMR also has been used to characterize the epicardial VT substrate in patients with unique myocardial diseases. Xie and colleagues[26] described the value of CMR to characterize the epicardial substrate in patients with ARVC using LGE distribution compared with regional epicardial RV voltage signal amplitude and conduction channels defined by ripple mapping technology.[40] Muser and colleagues[41] showed, in a cohort of 31 patients undergoing VT ablation for CS, only modest correlation between scar defined by LGE CMR and low-voltage areas within endo-epicardial and epicardial scars defined by 3DEAM. The main utility of preprocedural CMR in this cohort of patients was the inverse correlation between LGE scar extent and arrhythmia-free survival, in agreement with other published studies.[42,43] There are no data on preprocedural MRI to guide VT ablation in hypertrophic cardiomyopathy, but from the reported case series, both endo-epicardial and endocardial-only approaches have been used with reasonable clinical success.[44–46]

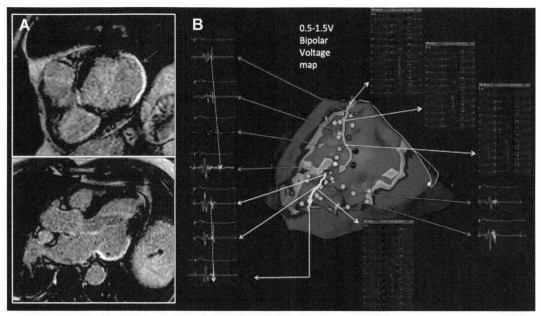

Fig. 5. Preprocedural CMR to identify arrhythmia substrate in CCM. (*A*) Sagittal (*top*) and axial (*bottom*) plane views of LV lateral aneurysm and epicardial scar (*orange arrows*) seen on LGE sequences. (*B*) Corresponding bipolar epicardial voltage map during substrate VT ablation. Note the identification of sequential LAVA (EGM panels) in sinus rhythm (*blue arrows*) along the long axis of the scar (*purple and yellow arrows*), which also correspond to perfect pace map (PM) matches of greater than 93% (*white arrows*) along the scar (overlay ECG PM panels). These 2 observations confirm this region represents a conduction channel within the scar. (*Courtesy of* Luis Sáenz, International Arrhythmia Center at Fundación CardioInfantíl, Bogotá, Colombia.)

Nevertheless, preprocedural MRI offers the opportunity to individualize the ablation approach in these patients, by evaluating the presence of mid-myocardial substrate, LV aneurysm, or epicardial scar, which may represent potential ablation targets. Preoperative multimodality imaging, including CT and CMR, has been used to successfully guide substrate ablation for recurrent VT in Chagas cardiomyopathy (CCM),[47] but clinical data on routine use of preprocedural CMR-guided VT ablation in CCM are lacking. CMR studies in CCM confirm the value of LGE to characterize scar extent and location of the scar. Identification of scar by LGE also appears predictive of VT events in CCM.[48] In addition to LGE sequences, native and postgadolinium T1 imaging techniques can identify diffuse interstitial fibrosis,[49,50] which may play a role in the mid-myocardial and epicardial arrhythmia substrates in patients with diffuse myocardial fibrosis but absence of LGE due to fibrosis burden and distribution pattern. Finally, for early repolarization syndromes, such as J wave syndrome and Brugada syndrome, CMR does not provide critical information about the epicardial RV outflow tract tissue characteristics to guide VF substrate ablation,[51] and these procedures are guided mostly based on epicardial electrogram (EGM) analysis.

OTHER IMAGING MODALITIES TO GUIDE EPICARDIAL ABLATIONS

Nuclear imaging technologies have the ability to characterize myocardial scar substrates based on perfusion (201Tl single-photon emission CT [SPECT]), metabolic activity (18-fluorodeoxyglucose position emission tomography [PET]), and innervation (123I-meta-iodobenzylguanidine [mIBG] SPECT) and provide valuable data regarding arrhythmia circuits in patients undergoing VT ablation.[52–54] Preprocedural PET-CT was able to identify isthmi of metabolically active channels within myocardial scar and identify epicardial scar in patients with normal endocardial voltage.[52] Klein and colleagues[54] reported the value of 123I-mIBG SPECT scans to identify regions of abnormal innervation, which harbored the VT exit sites despite preserved bipolar voltage by 3DEAM. The main limitation of nuclear imaging is its low spatial resolution (12 mm for SPECT and 6 mm for PET), which makes the determination of topographic transmural scar location difficult.

Electrocardiographic imaging (ECGi) is a noninvasive mapping technology using surface ECG lead signals to provide information regarding epicardial and transmural activation patterns in atrial and ventricular arrhythmias. This technology uses the combination of electrical data from chest electrodes combined with heart-chest anatomic data obtained from preoperative imaging (CCT or CMR) to generate propagation maps during sinus and paced rhythm or arrhythmias (**Fig. 6**). ECGi maps can be obtained before or in some cases during the procedure and with limited processing can generate complete activation and propagation maps of an entire chamber, even for nonsustained arrhythmias. This information has the potential to greatly facilitate preprocedural planning. Several ECGi systems have been developed (some commercially available), which vary in the ECG electrode density and the algorithms used for generating activation maps. Wissner and colleagues[55] studied the accuracy of a noncontact mapping system to target focal ablation of idiopathic ventricular premature beats (VPBs) and VT. In 20 patients (21 VPBs), the ECGi system predicted correctly the chamber of origin (RV vs LV) in all but 1, and the regional site of origin (SOO) in all but 3 patients (accuracy of 95% and 86%, respectively) compared with invasive mapping data.[55] Erkapic and colleagues[56] presented prospective randomized data on VPB or VT ablation guided by either ECG algorithm or ECGi plus 3DEAM in 42 patients. The ECGi

algorithm outperformed ECG algorithm in localization of the chamber of origin (95.2% vs 76.2%, respectively) and the SOO (95.2% vs 38.1%, respectively) for the VT/VPBs.[56] Both of these studies evaluated a distinct VT patient population presenting with focal outflow tract tachycardias, where the mapping strategy is mainly focal SOO identification, and transmural lesions usually are achieved with endocardial only ablation. In contrast, Wang and colleagues[57] evaluated the feasibility of ECGi for determining endocardial and epicardial activation patterns in 4 patients undergoing scar-related VT ablation via an endo-epicardial approach. Using a 120-lead ECG torso array, computed ventricular epicardial and endocardial unipolar ECGs during VT accurately identified distinct epicardial and endocardial VT exit sites compared with the 3DEAM activation maps.[57] Misra and colleagues[58] evaluated the accuracy of a novel ECGi mapping system using a standard 12-lead ECG configuration to detect the origin of ventricular arrhythmias in patients undergoing VPB or VT ablation. Despite assuming homogeneous conduction velocities regardless of whether healthy or abnormal myocardium was involved, ECGi still was able to predict the chamber of origin and SOO in 5/6 reentrant VT circuits in 5 patients

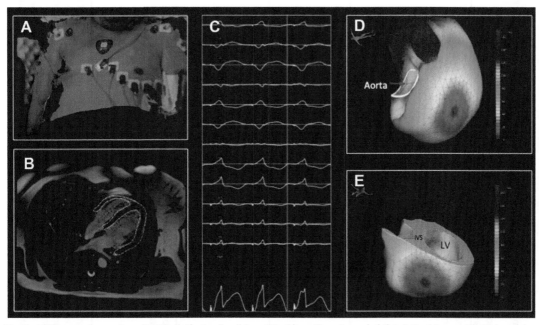

Fig. 6. ECGi mapping system (VIVO, Catheter Precision, Mt. Olive, New Jersey). (*A*) A 3-D picture with 12-lead electrodes in chest included and registered with preexisting CMR. (*B*) The CMR is segmented and a 3-D volume model is generated. (*C*) A 12-lead ECG signal analysis to determine the 3 vectorial components of ventricular activation (QRS onset [*red*], end of QRS [*blue*], end of T wave [*green*]). (*D*) Isochronal 3-D epicardial ventricular activation map obtained during pacing from the middle cardiac vein with (*E*) optional clipping plane to display intracavitary vectorial map.

Table 1
Suggested image guided procedural table for approaching ventricular arrhythmia ablations

Localization of Scar by Preprocedural Imaging	Access/Approach	Mapping Technique	Ablation Technique	Clinical Examples	Considerations
No scar/normal myocardium	Endocardial	3DEAM ± ECGi	Unipolar RF>>>bipolar RF > Cryo	Idiopathic VA from OT, PM, MB, LV summit	Epicardial or bipolar ablation may be required for LV summit VA. Consider cryo for papillary muscle VA if contact cannot be reliably achieved. ICE useful to assess catheter-tissue contact and monitor RF tissue effect
Endocardial	Endocardial	3DEAM>>>ECGi	Unipolar RF (NS > D5W or 1/2NS)	Ischemic heart disease	ICE useful to assess catheter-tissue contact and monitor RF tissue effect. ICE can visualize endo transition between scar and healthy tissue.
Epicardial	Endo/epicardial	3DEAM > ECGi	Unipolar RF (NS > D5W or 1/2NS)	ARVC, Chagas disease, nonischemic heart disease	Coronary arteries, PN, epicardial fat. Guide contact force vector toward the myocardium/instill saline/displace phrenic to reduce risk. ICE may show epicardial scar extent.
Intramural/abnormal myocardium	Endo/epicardial, CS, coronary arteries	Intracoronary arterial mapping (guide wire, cold saline), activation, and pace mapping with 3DEAM via GCV/AIV/MCV/LVB	Bipolar RF, unipolar RF (D5W or 1/2NS > NS), IC septal ETOH, needle RF	HCM, sarcoidosis, postmyocarditis	Uni/bipolar voltage on 3DEAM may be normal. ICE/fluoro to guide opposing catheter placement. ICE to monitor RF tissue effect

The identification scar topography allows for a decision of whether epicardial access likely is required, reducing the bleeding risks associated with such intervention while systemic anticoagulation is present during left sided mapping. Scar localization also can guide an anterior versus posterior pericardial approach. Segmentation of the PNs and coronary arteries from the preprocedural image data sets coregistered with 3DEAM can be used to reduce risk of collateral injury during epicardial mapping and ablation. 3DEAM techniques include activation, entrainment, and pace-mapping.

Abbreviations: 1/2NS, 0.45% sodium chloride solution; AIV, anterior interventricular vein; Cryo, cryoballoon ablation; ETOH, alcohol; Fluoro, fluoroscopy; D5W, 5% dextrose solution; GCV, greater cardiac vein; IC, intracoronary; LVB, lateral vein branches; MB, moderator band; MCV, middle cardiac vein; NS, 0.9% sodium chloride solution; OT, outflow tract; PM, papillary muscles; VA, ventricular arrhythmia.

requiring epicardial ablation (4 patients with ARVD and 1 with NICM).[58]

FUTURE IMAGING TECHNOLOGIES

The pericardial space is a 3-D structure, yet, currently only a biplanar approach is used to examine in detail. The 3-D understanding of the pericardium is based on gross anatomic post-mortem specimens, lacking accurate volumetric information. In a recent publication, Mori and Shivkumar[59] revealed a 3-D pericardial reconstruction model from a nongated CT scan of a patient with cardiac tamponade demonstrating the accurate volumetric representation of the oblique and transverse sinuses (along with the superior and inferior recesses). Future refinements in imaging techniques allowing for greater delineation between the visceral and parietal pericardium and its surrounding mediastinal structures may improve the clinical uses of preprocedural imaging evaluation for epicardial interventions. The integration of accurate 3-D volumetric data sets with 3-D printing technology[60] and virtual and augmented reality applications[61] can help develop patient-specific simulation models for preprocedural rehearsal of epicardial interventions in the future.[62] As seen with other applications using 3-D printing technology, these preprocedural simulated cases will be useful for equipment and material selection, defining choice of access and guiding intrapericardial navigation during mapping, ablation, and structural interventions.

SUMMARY

Preoperative imaging provides an opportunity to understand patients' unique anatomic features, which may impede successful percutaneous epicardial access. Additionally, the information obtained regarding region and location (endocardial, epicardial, or mid-myocardial) of myocardial scarring/fibrosis can guide the optimal procedural approach. A comprehensive stepwise procedural plan can be devised for access (endocardial and/or epicardial, subxyphoid vs parasternal vs pericardial window), equipment selection (Tuohy vs micropuncture needle for access or balloon or steerable sheath for PN displacement), mapping (3DEAM with or without ECGi or intravascular mapping), and ablation strategy (unipolar vs bipolar RF, normal vs low ionic RF irrigation, or alcohol septal ablation/coil embolization), minimizing complication risks and potentially improving procedural outcomes (**Table 1**).

DISCLOSURE

A.J. Restrepo—no disclosures; T.M. Dickfeld—Biosense Webster (Research Support), Catheter Precision (Research Support).

REFERENCES

1. Sosa E, Scanavacca M, d'Avila A, et al. A new technique to perform epicardial mapping in the electrophysiology laboratory. J Cardiovasc Electrophysiol 1996;7:531–6.
2. Romero J, Shivkumar K, Di Biase L, et al. Mastering the art of epicardial access in cardiac electrophysiology. Heart Rhythm 2019;16:1738–49.
3. Loukas M, Walters A, Boon JM, et al. Pericardiocentesis: a clinical anatomy review. Clin Anat 2012;25:872–81.
4. Bradfield JS, Tung R, Boyle NG, et al. Our approach to minimize risk of epicardial access: standard techniques with the addition of electroanatomic mapping guidance. J Cardiovasc Electrophysiol 2013;24:723–7.
5. Hutchinson MD, Gerstenfeld EP, Desjardins B, et al. Endocardial unipolar voltage mapping to detect epicardial ventricular tachycardia substrate in patients with nonischemic left ventricular cardiomyopathy. Circ Arrhythm Electrophysiol 2011;4:49–55.
6. Polin GM, Haqqani H, Tzou W, et al. Endocardial unipolar voltage mapping to identify epicardial substrate in arrhythmogenic right ventricular cardiomyopathy/dysplasia. Heart Rhythm 2011;8:76–83.
7. Soto-Becerra R, Bazan V, Bautista W, et al. Use of voltage mapping to characterize endoepicardial nonischemic scar distribution. Circ Arrhythm Electrophysiol 2017;10(11) [pii:e004950].
8. Bala R, Ren JF, Hutchinson MD, et al. Assessing epicardial substrate using intracardiac echocardiography during VT ablation. Circ Arrhythm Electrophysiol 2011;4(5):667–73.
9. Hussein A, Jimenez A, Ahmad G, et al. Assessment of ventricular tachycardia scar substrate by intracardiac echocardiography. Pacing Clin Electrophysiol 2014;37(4):412–21.
10. Jimenez A, Dickfeld T. Computed tomography in cardiac electrophysiology. In: Zipes D, editor. Cardiac electrophysiology: from cell to bedside. 7th Edition. Philadelphia: Elsevier; 2017. p. 1120.
11. Ebrille E, Killu AM, Anavekar NS, et al. Successful percutaneous epicardial access in challenging scenarios. Pacing Clin Electrophysiol 2015;38:84–90.
12. Yamashita S, Sacher F, Mahida S, et al. Role of high-resolution image integration to visualize left phrenic nerve and coronary arteries during epicardial ventricular tachycardia ablation. Circ Arrhythm Electrophysiol 2015;8(2):371–80.
13. Kumar S, Barbhaiya CR, Baldinger SH, et al. Epicardial phrenic nerve displacement during catheter

ablation of atrial and ventricular arrhythmias: procedural experience and outcomes. Circ Arrhythm Electrophysiol 2015;8:896–904.

14. Buch E, Nakahara S, Shivkumar K. Intra-pericardial balloon retraction of the left atrium: a novel method to prevent esophageal injury during catheter ablation. Heart Rhythm 2008;5:1473–5.

15. Bhardwaj R, Naniwadekar A, Whang W, et al. Esophageal deviation during atrial fibrillation ablation: clinical experience with a dedicated esophageal balloon retractor. JACC Clin Electrophysiol 2018; 4(8):1020–30.

16. Parikh V, Swarup V, Hantla J, et al. Feasibility, safety, and efficacy of a novel preshaped nitinol esophageal deviator to successfully deflect the esophagus and ablate left atrium without esophageal temperature rise during atrial fibrillation ablation: the DEFLECT GUT study. Heart Rhythm 2018;15(9): 1321–7.

17. Nakahara S, Ramirez RJ, Buch E, et al. Intrapericardial balloon placement for prevention of collateral injury during catheter ablation of the left atrium in a porcine model. Heart Rhythm 2010;7:81–7.

18. Tian J, Jeudy J, Smith MF, et al. Three-dimensional contrast-enhanced multidetector CT for anatomic, dynamic, and perfusion characterization of abnormal myocardium to guide ventricular tachycardia ablations. Circ Arrhythm Electrophysiol 2010;3(5):496–504.

19. Esposito A, Palmisano A, Antunes S, et al. Cardiac CT with delayed enhancement in the characterization of ventricular tachycardia structural substrate: relationship between CT-segmented scar and electro-anatomic mapping. JACC Cardiovasc Imaging 2016;9(7):822–32.

20. Yamashita S, Sacher F, Hooks DA, et al. Myocardial wall thinning predicts transmural substrate in patients with scar-related ventricular tachycardia. Heart Rhythm 2017;14(2):155–63.

21. Sourwine M, Jeudy J, Miller B, et al. Location, variations, and predictors of epicardial fat mapping using multidetector computed tomography to assist epicardial ventricular tachycardia ablation. Pacing Clin Electrophysiol 2017;40(10):1059–66.

22. Komatsu Y, Jadidi A, Sacher F, et al. Relationship between MDCT-imaged myocardial fat and ventricular tachycardia substrate in arrhythmogenic right ventricular cardiomyopathy. J Am Heart Assoc 2014;3(4) [pii:e000935].

23. Dickfeld T, Tian J, Ahmad G, et al. MRI-guided ventricular tachycardia ablation: integration of late gadolinium-enhanced 3D scar in patients with implantable cardioverter-defibrillators. Circ Arrhythm Electrophysiol 2011;4(2):172–84.

24. Piers SRD, Tao Q, van Huls van Taxis CFB, et al. Contrast-enhanced MRI-derived scar patterns and associated ventricular tachycardias in nonischaemic

cardiomyopathy: implications for the ablation strategy. Circ Arrhythm Electrophysiol 2013;6(5):875–83.

25. Berte B, Sacher F, Cochet H, et al. Postmyocarditis ventricular tachycardia in patients with only scar: a specific entity requiring a specific approach. J Cardiovasc Electrophysiol 2015;26:42–50.

26. Xie S, Desjardins B, Kubala M, et al. Association of regional epicardial right ventricular electrogram voltage amplitude and late gadolinium enhancement distribution on cardiac magnetic resonance in patients with arrhythmogenic right ventricular cardiomyopathy: implications for ventricular tachycardia ablation. Heart Rhythm 2018;15(7): 987–93.

27. Akoum N, Daccarett M, McGann C, et al. Atrial fibrosis helps select the appropriate patient and strategy in catheter ablation of atrial fibrillation: a DE-MRI guided approach. J Cardiovasc Electrophysiol 2011;22(1):16–22.

28. Cabrera JA, Ho SY, Climent V, et al. Morphological evidence of muscular connections between contiguous pulmonary venous orifices: relevance of the interpulmonary isthmus for catheter ablation in atrial fibrillation. Heart Rhythm 2009;6(8):1192–8.

29. Ho SY, Sánchez-Quintana D. The importance of atrial structure and fibers. Clin Anat 2009;22(1): 52–63.

30. Ho SY, Cabrera JA, Sánchez-Quintana D. Left atrial anatomy revisited. Circ Arrhythm Electrophysiol 2012;5(1):220–8.

31. Haissaguerre M, Jais P, Shah DC, et al. Spontaneous initiation of atrial fibrillation by ectopic beats originating in the pulmonary veins. N Engl J Med 1998;339(10):659–65.

32. Papez JW. Heart musculature of the atria. Am J Anat 1920;27:255–77.

33. Di Biase L, Romero J, Briceno D, et al. Evidence of relevant electrical connection between the left atrial appendage and the great cardiac vein during catheter ablation of atrial fibrillation. Heart Rhythm 2019; 16(7):1039–46.

34. Pashakhanloo F, Herzka DA, Ashikaga H, et al. Myofiber architecture of the human atria as revealed by submillimeter diffusion tensor imaging. Circ Arrhythm Electrophysiol 2016;9(4):e004133.

35. Garcia F, Enriquez A, Arroyo E, et al. Roof-dependent atrial flutter with an epicardial component: role of the septopulmonary bundle. J Cardiovasc Electrophysiol 2019;30:1159–63.

36. Briceño DF, Valderrábano M. Recurrent perimitral flutter due to vein of Marshall epicardial connections bypassing the mitral isthmus: response to ethanol infusion. Circ Arrhythm Electrophysiol 2014;7(5): 988–9.

37. Tung R, Shivkumar K. Epicardial ablation of ventricular tachycardia. Methodist Debakey Cardiovasc J 2015;11(2):129–34.

38. Kumareswaran R, Marchlinski FE. Practical guide to ablation for epicardial ventricular tachycardia: when to get access, how to deal with anticoagulation and how to prevent complications. Arrhythm Electrophysiol Rev 2018;7(3):159–64.

39. Maccabelli G, Tsiachris D, Silberbauer J, et al. Imaging and epicardial substrate ablation of ventricular tachycardia in patients late after myocarditis. Europace 2014;16(9):1363–72.

40. Xie S, Kubala M, Liang JJ, et al. Utility of ripple mapping for identification of slow conduction channels during ventricular tachycardia ablation in the setting of arrhythmogenic right ventricular cardiomyopathy. J Cardiovasc Electrophysiol 2019;30(3):366–73.

41. Muser D, Santangeli P, Pathak RK, et al. Long-term outcomes of catheter ablation of ventricular tachycardia in patients with cardiac sarcoidosis. Circ Arrhythm Electrophysiol 2016;9(8) [pii:e004333].

42. Kouranos V, Tzelepis GE, Rapti A, et al. Complementary role of CMR to conventional screening in the diagnosis and prognosis of cardiac sarcoidosis. JACC Cardiovasc Imaging 2017;10(12):1437–47.

43. Crawford T, Mueller G, Sarsam S, et al. Magnetic resonance imaging for identifying patients with cardiac sarcoidosis and preserved or mildly reduced left ventricular function at risk of ventricular arrhythmias. Circ Arrhythm Electrophysiol 2014;7(6):1109–15.

44. Dukkipati SR, d'Avila A, Soejima K, et al. Long-term outcomes of combined epicardial and endocardial ablation of monomorphic ventricular tachycardia related to hypertrophic cardiomyopathy. Circ Arrhythm Electrophysiol 2011;4(2):185–94.

45. Igarashi M, Nogami A, Kurosaki K, et al. Radiofrequency catheter ablation of ventricular tachycardia in patients with hypertrophic cardiomyopathy and apical aneurysm. JACC Clin Electrophysiol 2018;4(3):339–50.

46. Santangeli P, Di Biase L, Lakkireddy D, et al. Radiofrequency catheter ablation of ventricular arrhythmias in patients with hypertrophic cardiomyopathy: safety and feasibility. Heart Rhythm 2010;7(8):1036–42.

47. Valdigem BP, Pereira FB, da Silva NJ, et al. Ablation of ventricular tachycardia in chronic chagasic cardiomyopathy with giant basal aneurysm: carto sound, CT, and MRI merge. Circ Arrhythm Electrophysiol 2011;4(1):112–4.

48. Mello RP, Szarf G, Schvartzman PR, et al. Delayed enhancement cardiac magnetic resonance imaging can identify the risk for ventricular tachycardia in chronic chagas' heart disease. Arq Bras Cardiol 2012;98:421–30.

49. Everett RJ, Stirrat CG, Semple SI, et al. Assessment of myocardial fibrosis with T1 mapping MRI. Clin Radiol 2016;71(8):768–78.

50. Radenkovic D, Weingärtner S, Ricketts L, et al. T1 mapping in cardiac MRI. Heart Fail Rev 2017;22(4):415–30.

51. Nademanee K, Haissaguerre M, Hocini M, et al. Mapping and ablation of ventricular fibrillation associated with early repolarization syndrome. Circulation 2019;140(18):1477–90.

52. Dickfeld T, Lei P, Dilsizian V, et al. Integration of three-dimensional scar maps for ventricular tachycardia ablation with positron emission tomography-computed tomography. JACC Cardiovasc Imaging 2008;1(1):73–82.

53. Tian J, Smith MF, Ahmad G, et al. Integration of 3-dimensional scar models from SPECT to guide ventricular tachycardia ablation. J Nucl Med 2012;53:894–901.

54. Klein T, Abdulghani M, Smith M, et al. Three-dimensional 123I-meta-iodobenzylguanidine cardiac innervation maps to assess substrate and successful ablation sites for ventricular tachycardia: feasibility study for a novel paradigm of innervation imaging. Circ Arrhythm Electrophysiol 2015;8:583–91.

55. Wissner E, Revishvili A, Metzner A, et al. Non invasive epicardial and endocardial mapping of premature ventricular contractions. Europace 2017;19(5):843–9.

56. Erkapic D, Greiss H, Pajitnev D, et al. Clinical impact of a novel three-dimensional electrocardiographic imaging for non-invasive mapping of ventricular arrhythmias-a prospective randomized trial. Europace 2015;17(4):591–7.

57. Wang L, Gharbia OA, Nazarian S, et al. Non-invasive epicardial and endocardial electrocardiographic imaging for scar-related ventricular tachycardia. Europace 2018;20(Fl2):f263–72.

58. Misra S, van Dam P, Chrispin J, et al. Initial validation of a novel ECGI system for localization of premature ventricular contractions and ventricular tachycardia in structurally normal and abnormal hearts. J Electrocardiol 2018;51(5):801–8.

59. Mori S, Shivkumar K. Three-dimensional imaging of the pericardial space. HeartRhythm Case Rep 2020. https://doi.org/10.1016/j.hrcr.2019.12.009.

60. Bartel T, Rivard A, Jimenez A, et al. Medical three-dimensional printing opens up new opportunities in cardiology and cardiac surgery. Eur Heart J 2018;39(15):1246–54.

61. Jang J, Tschabrunn CM, Barkagan M, et al. Three-dimensional holographic visualization of high-resolution myocardial scar on HoloLens. PLoS One 2018;13(10):e0205188.

62. Seslar SP, Patton KK. Initial experience with a novel electrophysiology simulator. Pacing Clin Electrophysiol 2018;41(2):197–202.

Epicardial Ablation of Idiopathic Ventricular Tachycardia

Daniele Muser, MD, Pasquale Santangeli, MD, PhD*

KEYWORDS

- Idiopathic ventricular arrhythmias • Epicardial ablation • Catheter ablation
- Coronary venous system

KEY POINTS

- Up to 4% to 10% of idiopathic ventricular arrhythmias (VAs) originate from epicardial foci. These arrhythmias are typically linked to the perivalvular epicardium, including the left ventricular summit region and the cardiac crux.
- Mapping and ablation of epicardial VA can be performed through adjacent sites, such as the coronary venous system, the coronary cusps, the left or right ventricular endocardium, or through direct pericardial access.
- Given the proximity of major coronary vessels and the thick layer of epicardial fat at the region of the atrioventricular and interventricular grooves, catheter ablation of arrhythmic foci at these sites with a direct approach may be challenging.
- When direct ablation at the selected epicardial site is not feasible or unsuccessful, an approach from anatomically adjacent sites can be considered.
- In refractory cases, alternative ablation strategies have been proposed, including use of simultaneous unipolar radiofrequency ablation, bipolar radiofrequency ablation, alcohol arterial/venous ablation, or surgical epicardial ablation with direct visualization of the coronary vessels and dissection of the epicardial fat.

INTRODUCTION

Ventricular arrhythmias (VAs) in patients with structurally normal hearts are referred to as idiopathic VAs and typically have a favorable prognosis.[1] Frequent premature ventricular contractions (PVCs) account for approximately 90% of all idiopathic VAs, whereas sustained ventricular tachycardia (VT) and ventricular fibrillation (VF) are far less common.[2] Approximately 4% to 10% of patients have an epicardial site of origin,[3,4] with the most common site being the perivalvular epicardium at the left ventricular (LV) summit, followed by the cardiac crux region.[3] Radiofrequency

(RF) catheter ablation (CA) is increasingly being used for the treatment of idiopathic VA.[5] In patients with epicardial idiopathic VAs, direct epicardial ablation can be challenging owing to the presence of major coronary arterial vessels and epicardial fat. In most cases, LV summit arrhythmias can be targeted via the distal coronary venous system (CVS; great cardiac vein [GCV] and the junction of the GCV and the anterior interventricular vein [AIV]), whereas cardiac crux VAs can be targeted from the middle cardiac vein (MCV).[6,7] When ablation at the earliest epicardial site is not feasible, an anatomic approach targeting adjacent sites or alternative ablation strategies

Disclosures: None related to this topic.
Electrophysiology Section, Cardiovascular Medicine Division, Hospital of the University of Pennsylvania, Philadelphia, PA, USA
* Corresponding author. Hospital of the University of Pennsylvania, 9 Founders Pavilion – Cardiology, 3400 Spruce Street, Philadelphia, PA 19104.
E-mail address: pasquale.santangeli@pennmedicine.upenn.edu

including the use of bipolar/simultaneous unipolar ablation or surgical ablation can be considered. This article provides a summary of the electrophysiologic features and outcomes of CA of idiopathic VAs arising from epicardial foci.

CLINICAL PRESENTATION AND ELECTROCARDIOGRAM FEATURES

The clinical presentation of patients with idiopathic VA ranges from a completely asymptomatic state with the diagnosis made incidentally on routine electrocardiogram (ECG) to palpitations (about 50% of the cases) or other associated symptoms such as chest pain, fatigue, dyspnea, presyncope, and (rarely) syncope (<5%).[1] Similar to other idiopathic VAs, it is generally accepted that epicardial idiopathic VAs have a favorable clinical outcome, although in a minority of cases they lead to a reversible form of LV dysfunction (especially in cases of high burden of PVC) or are the trigger for polymorphic VT or VF.[8,9]

As mentioned, the LV summit region accounts for most epicardial VAs.[4] The LV summit represents the most superior aspect of the LV epicardium, delineated by the bifurcation of the left anterior descending (LAD) and the left circumflex (LCx) coronary arteries and transected laterally by the GCV at its junction with the AIV (**Fig. 1**).[10] The course of the GCV divides the LV summit region into a medial and more superior region (above the GCV), inaccessible to CA because of close proximity to the major coronary vessels and the presence of thick epicardial fat (inaccessible area), and a more lateral and inferior region (below the GCV), which may be approachable by CA being far from major coronary vessels (accessible area). Several ECG features have been described to predict an LV summit origin of VA but also to differentiate an origin from the accessible versus inaccessible region, which can influence the procedural approach.[7,10] Idiopathic VA originating from the LV summit typically has a right bundle branch block (RBBB) morphology with a positive concordance throughout the precordial leads or a left bundle branch block (LBBB) morphology with early ($\leq V_2$) precordial transition and a right inferior axis with deeper Q waves in aVL compared with aVR. The delayed initial activation of the LV epicardium is reflected by a slurring of the initial portion of the QRS complex, which can be quantitatively measured as (1) time to earliest rapid deflection in precordial leads (pseudodelta wave) greater than or equal to 34 milliseconds, (2) interval to peak of R wave in lead V_2 (intrinsicoid deflection time) greater than or equal to 85 milliseconds, (3) shortest interval to maximal positive or negative

deflection divided by QRS duration (maximum deflection index [MDI]) greater than or equal to 0.55 milliseconds, and (4) time to earliest QRS nadir in precordial leads (shortest RS complex) greater than or equal to 121 milliseconds.[7,10–12] An RBBB pattern and deep Q waves in aVL compared with aVR (especially in the presence of a QS pattern in lead I) predict an origin from the accessible area.[10] In particular, the presence of a dominant R wave in V_1 with an R/S ratio greater than or equal to 2.5 has been shown to be associated with an origin from the accessible area in up to 90% of cases.[10] In contrast, an LBBB pattern with less than or equal to V_2 transition, a Q-wave ratio in aVL/aVR less than 1.45, or a characteristic pattern break in V_2 (abrupt loss of R wave in lead V_2 compared with V_1 and V_3) suggest an origin from the septal aspect of the LV summit and are more commonly seen in cases of origin from the inaccessible area.[13,14]

The epicardial crux represents a posterior epicardial region of the heart located at the intersection between the posterior atrioventricular and interventricular grooves where the MCV takes off from the coronary sinus (CS). Idiopathic VA originating from the cardiac crux and MCV region typically show an LBBB morphology with early precordial transition less than or equal to V_2, a left superior axis with QS complexes and slurred downstroke deflections in inferior leads, and an MDI greater than or equal to 0.55.[4] From a procedural point of view, the cardiac crux region can be further subdivided into a basal region, which can be effectively targeted from the MCV or from the proximal CS, and an apical region, which may require subxiphoid epicardial access.[15] Arrhythmias coming from the basal crux typically show a superior axis with a QS pattern in lead III and an LBBB morphology with an early transition less than or equal to V_2, whereas apical crux VA can present either an RBBB or LBBB pattern. An R/S ratio less than 1 in lead V_6 with an R wave in aVR and aVL has invariably been associated with an origin from the apical crux.[15] Recently, our group described some ECG features that can differentiate a basal inferoseptal LV endocardial origin from an epicardial basal crux origin.[16] In particular, an initial R wave in leads II, III, and/or aVF; an R/S ratio less than 1 in lead V_1; a notching in lead II; a narrow QRS duration; and an MDI less than 0.55 were all associated with effective elimination of the arrhythmia from the inferoseptal LV endocardium (**Fig. 2**).[16]

ACTIVATION AND PACE MAPPING

When an epicardial origin is suspected because of specific ECG features or because of unsuccessful

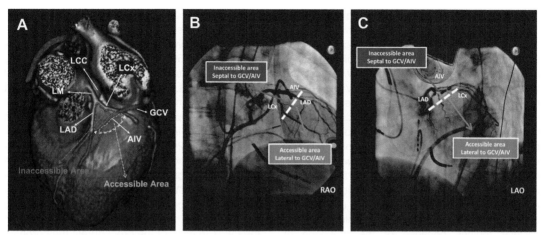

Fig. 1. Computed tomography reconstruction (*A*) and fluoroscopic views (*B, C*) of the heart showing the anatomy of LV summit and its relationship with adjacent structures. The LV summit is a triangular region of the LV epicardium with the apex at the bifurcation between the LAD and LCx coronary arteries, and the base formed by an arch connecting the first septal perforator branch of the LAD with the LCx (*A, white dotted line* and *arrows*). The LV summit is bisected by the AIV in 2 regions: (1) closer to the apex of the triangle (*red, inaccessible area*), and (2) more lateral toward the base of the triangle (*green, accessible area*). LAO, left anterior oblique; LCC, left coronary cusp; LM, left main; RAO, right anterior oblique.

endocardial mapping and ablation, detailed activation mapping of the coronary venous system (CVS) should be performed to confirm that the epicardium has the earliest activation. Coronary venous activation should be systematically compared with activation in the adjacent aortic sinus cusps and right ventricular outflow tract (RVOT)/LV outflow tract (LVOT) for inferior axis VA, and with the right ventricular (RV) and LV endocardium for superior axis VA.[16,17] Smaller-caliber linear multipolar catheters can be used to facilitate access to the distal CVS and compare

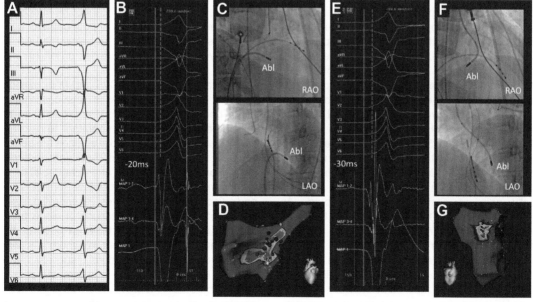

Fig. 2. A 46-year-old man symptomatic for frequent PVCs coming from the cardiac crux (*A*). Activation mapping showed an earliest activation on the epicardium (*B*) mapped through the MCV (*C*, fluoroscopic view; *D*, activation map) compared with the endocardium (*E*) in the basal inferoseptal region (*F*, fluoroscopic view; *G*, activation map). Radiofrequency ablation at the ostium of the MCV resulted in effective suppression of the PVCs. Abl, ablation.

the activation time within the CVS with other endo-cardial sites. A long sheath with or without additional inner catheters can enhance proximal support and facilitate catheter manipulation, especially when mapping the distal GCV/AIV region. When local activation within the CVS precedes the QRS onset by more than 20 milliseconds, CA may be attempted. Pace mapping can be used to further corroborate the site of origin, being particularly useful when no spontaneous or inducible clinical VAs are present.[18] However, when interpreting pace mapping data, operators should be aware of the limited spatial resolution (2–3 cm^2) particularly when higher outputs are used (which are often necessary to capture the epicardial perivalvular regions because of the presence of epicardial fat), presence of preferential conduction, and far-field capture of adjacent structures (**Fig. 3**).[19,20]

CATHETER ABLATION

RF CA should always be performed at the site where earliest activation is recorded and, ideally, a concordant pace map.[10] A coronary angiogram is always recommended before RF energy delivery at any epicardial site to ensure adequate distance (>5 mm in at least 2 orthogonal fluoroscopic projections and at any moment of the cardiac cycle) from major coronary vessels (see **Fig. 1**).[21] Ablation from the CVS may present other limitations, such as inability to achieve adequate power because of high impedance, which often cannot be overcome with open irrigation. At our center, we start with irrigated RF ablation typically at 20 W and titrating up to 40 W with the goal to achieve a decrease in the impedance of at least 10% from baseline value. Ablation power is reduced or ablation interrupted in case of impedance increase. Overall, observational studies have shown that ablation success rates from the CVS range between 50% and 70% (**Table 1**).[4,22,23] When CA at the best site within the CVS is unsuccessful or not feasible because of proximity to the coronary arteries, an approach targeting anatomically adjacent sites can be attempted. An anatomic approach has been shown to be effective when the distance between the 2 adjacent sites is less than or equal to 12.8 mm or when the difference between local activation times is less than or equal to 7 milliseconds (**Fig. 4**).[13,22,24] This approach typically requires long RF lesions (up to 3–5 minutes) with progressive titration of the RF power up to 40 W to maximize the likelihood of durable VA suppression. In LVOT VA, Yamada and colleagues[25] reported the necessity to attempt an anatomic approach in

17% of the procedures because of unsuccessful ablation or presence of anatomic obstacles precluding RF delivery. Overall, this approach was successful in 56% of the procedures, typically when the VA site of origin was the intramural LVOT or lateral LVOT.[25] In cases of VA with earliest activation within the distal GCV, Nagashima and colleagues[22] reported that an anatomic approach was attempted in 63% of the procedures and successful in only 26% of them. In all successful procedures, the local activation time was no more than 7 milliseconds later than the earliest activation site in the CVS. For LV summit VA, we recently reported a success rate of 49% with an anatomic approach. The targeted adjacent structure was the LVOT in 45% of the procedures; the coronary cusps in 32% of the procedures; and the RVOT, the most leftward septal aspect of which is frequently less than 1 cm from the AIV, in 23% of them. An anatomic distance less than or equal to 12.8 mm was the best predictor of success (sensitivity of 95% and specificity of 48%).[24] Notably, we did not find an interaction between the delta in activation time between the targeted adjacent structures and the efficacy of an anatomic ablation approach, with anatomic distance being the only predictor of success.

The left atrial appendage (LAA) anatomically overlies the LV summit and theoretically can be accessed to map and ablate summit arrhythmias. In our experience, LAA instrumentation for mapping and ablation of LV summit arrhythmias is futile because, in most cases, RF cannot be effectively be delivered safely because of poor catheter contact, presence of epicardial fat below the LAA, or proximity to the coronary arteries or left phrenic nerve.[26]

When ablation from the CVS and from multiple adjacent endocardial sites is unsuccessful, a direct percutaneous epicardial approach can be considered.[7] However, it is important to highlight that the outcomes of epicardial ablation are generally poor. In a recent series of 23 patients undergoing epicardial mapping and attempted ablation of LV summit VA after failed attempts from the CVS and adjacent endocardial sites, RF energy delivery could not be attempted because of close proximity to major coronary arteries in 39% of the cases, and, among patients in whom CA was attempted, acute procedural success was reached in only 35% , with long-term success in 29%.[7] An aVL/aVR Q-wave ratio was significantly greater in patients with successful epicardial ablation compared with that in the unsuccessful group. Moreover, an R wave to S-wave ratio in lead V1 greater than V2 and absence of initial Q-wave in V1 were documented in the successfully ablated

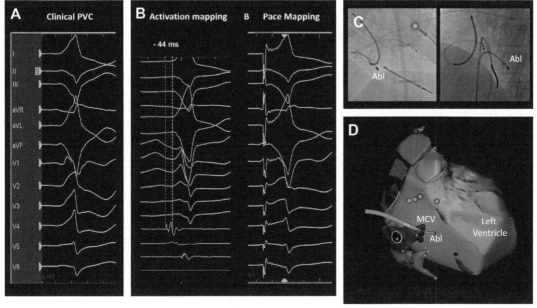

Fig. 3. A 50-year-old man presenting with frequent PVCs with a morphology consistent with an epicardial origin from the cardiac crux (*A*) confirmed by activation (*B*) and pace mapping (*C*) from the proximal portion of the MCV (*D*). Ablation at this site (*C*, fluoroscopic view; *D*, activation map) resulted in suppression of the PVC.

group. Once again, these features intuitively reflect a more lateral site of origin of VAs in the accessible area, distant from the main coronary arteries.[7]

INTRAMURAL ORIGIN

When activation time from multiple adjacent structures is suboptimal without a clearly earliest site and a more diffuse multisite breakthrough, an intramural origin of VA can be suspected.[27] In this setting, septal coronary venous perforator mapping may be used to identify ablation targets and guide ablation (**Fig. 5**).[28] At our institution, coronary venous mapping of septal perforators is performed by advancing a steerable 71-cm Agilis sheath (St. Jude Medical, Sylmar, CA) over a long guidewire into the CS in order to reach the GCV and perform coronary venography to delineate venous branches. Selective cannulation of septal perforator branches is performed by introducing a Glidecath hydrophilic-coated catheter (Terumo, Somerset, NJ) inside the Agilis sheath in order to guide the mapping guidewire. The guidewire (a 0.36-mm [0.014-inch] Vision Wire, Biotronik SE and Co KG, Berlin, Germany) is then advanced deep into the selected septal perforator branch with its proximal end connected to an alligator clip in a unipolar configuration and the skin serving as the reference electrode (filtered at 30–150 Hz) in order to allow activation and pace mapping through its noncoated tip. In the presence of

intramural foci, CA should be attempted at the sites of best activation first, followed by the sites of best pace map. Ablation from multiple adjacent sites is often required to eliminate the VA. Standard unipolar RF ablation may not be successful in eliminating the arrhythmias, even if sequentially delivered from multiple adjacent sites with high power and long-duration lesions (up to 3–5 minutes).[29] In these cases, bailout ablation strategies can be used (discussed later).[30]

BAILOUT CATHETER ABLATION STRATEGIES AND ALTERNATIVE APPROACHES

In refractory cases, alternative ablation strategies have been proposed, including use of simultaneous unipolar RF ablation, bipolar RF ablation, alcohol arterial/venous ablation or coil embolization, or surgical epicardial ablation with direct visualization of the coronary vessels and dissection of the epicardial fat.

The use of half-normal saline as cooling RF irrigant has been recently shown to be a safe and effective alternative, with up to 83% of acute procedural success in cases of VA refractory to standard normal saline CA. The use of half-normal saline has the capability to improve RF energy delivery to the myocardial tissue because of its higher electrical impedance compared with normal saline, which results in increased current density at the tissue-catheter interface.[31]

Table 1
Principal studies evaluating catheter ablation of idiopathic epicardial ventricular arrhythmias

Study	No. of Patients	Site of Earliest Activation Recorded (No. of Patients)	Earliest Activation Time, Pre-QRS (ms)	Site of Ablation (No. of Patients)	Reasons for Not Performing Ablation at the Earliest Activation Site Within CVS (No. of Patients)	Acute Procedural Success (%)	Complications (No. of Patients)	Follow-up (mo)	Long-term Success (% of Patients with Acute Procedural Success)
Daniels,[42] 2006	12	GCV (2) AIV-GCV junction (3) Proximal AIV (4) MCV (3)	47 ± 7	Inside CVS at earliest activation site (6) Percutaneous epicardial (6)	Inability to advance the ablation catheter to the site of earliest activation (6)	92	Pericarditis with mild effusion related to percutaneous epicardial ablation (1)	NA	NA
Obel et al,[43] 2006	5	Distal GCV (5)	NA	Inside CVS at earliest activation site (5)	—	100	None	Mean 25	100
Doppalapudi et al,[44] 2009	4	MCV (4)	Mean 28	Inside CVS at earliest activation site (1) Inside CVS proximal to the earliest activation site (1) Percutaneous epicardial (2)	Failed ablation at the earliest activation site (3)	75	NA	Mean 6	75

Study	n	Location	Age	Ablation site	Reasons for failure	%	Complications	Follow-up	Success %
Baman et al,[4] 2010	27	Distal GCV (26) MCV (1)	29 ± 8	Inside CVS at earliest activation site (20) Inside CVS proximal to the earliest activation site (5) Percutaneous epicardial (2)	Proximity to coronary arteries (1) Inability to advance the ablation catheter to the site of earliest activation (4) Inadequate power delivery (1) Proximity to phrenic nerve (1)	74	None	Median 13	90
Yamada et al,[45] 2010	14	Distal GCV/AIV (14)	37 ± 10	Inside CVS at earliest activation site (9) Not performed (5)	Inability to advance the ablation catheter to the site of earliest activation/ inadequate power delivery (5)	64	NA	12	64
Yamada et al,[10] 2010	25	Distal GCV/AIV (25)	Median 32	Inside CVS at earliest activation site (20) Percutaneous epicardial (5)	Inability to advance the ablation catheter to the site of earliest activation (1) Inadequate power delivery (4) Failed ablation at the earliest activation site (1)	65	None	Median 12	100
Yokokawa et al,[46] 2011	33	Distal GCV/AIV (32) MCV (1)	30 ± 6	Inside CVS at earliest activation site (10) Inside CVS proximal to the earliest activation site (4) Inside CVS proximal to the earliest activation site/LV endocardium/aortic cusps region (8) LV endocardium/aortic cusps region (4) Percutaneous epicardial (4) Not performed (3)	Inability to advance the ablation catheter to the site of earliest activation (5) Proximity to coronary arteries/phrenic nerve (3) Inadequate power delivery (3)	67	None	12–48	91

(continued on next page)

Table 1
(continued)

Study	No. of Pati-ents	Site of Earliest Activation Recorded (No. of Patients)	Earliest Activation Time, Pre-QRS (ms)	Site of Ablation (No. of Patients)	Reasons for Not Performing Ablation at the Earliest Activation Site Within CVS (No. of Patients)	Acute Proce-dural Success (%)	Compli-cations (No. of Patients)	Follow-up (mo)	Long-term Success (% of Patients with Acute Proce-dural Success)
Jaureguiet Abularach et al,[13] 2012	16	Distal GCV/AIV	12–75	Left sinus of Valsalva (5) Adjacent LV endocardium (2) Both of the above (2)	Inability to advance the ablation catheter to the site of earliest activation/proximity to coronary arteries/inadequate power delivery	56	Pericardial effusion (1) Narrowing of obtuse marginal coronary artery brunch (1)	NA	NA
Steven et al,[47] 2013	14	Distal GCV	39 ± 9	Inside CVS at earliest activation site (7)	Proximity to coronary arteries (6) Inadequate power delivery (1)	43	NA	NA	83

Study	N								
Li et al,[48] 2013	12	Distal GCV (4) Extended tributary of GCV distal to the origin of AIV (3) Proximal AIV (5)	37 ± 3	Inside CVS at earliest activation site (12)	—	100	None	Median 17	83
Kawamura et al,[15] 2014	18	MCV (14) Epicardial cardiac crux (4)	52 ± 18 ms	MCV (18) Epicardium (4)	Attempted in all	72	NA	26 ± 13	67
Frankel et al,[49] 2014	2	AIV	25	Septal RVOT (2)	Close proximity to coronary arteries (2)	100	None	Median 24	100

(continued on next page)

Table 1
(continued)

Study	No. of Patients	Site of Earliest Activation Recorded (No. of Patients)	Earliest Activation Time, Pre-QRS (ms)	Site of Ablation (No. of Patients)	Reasons for Not Performing Ablation at the Earliest Activation Site Within CVS (No. of Patients)	Acute Procedural Success (%)	Complications (No. of Patients)	Follow-up (mo)	Long-term Success (% of Patients with Acute Procedural Success)
Li et al,[50] 2014	30	Distal GCV (anterior-lateral mitral annulus) (8) Distal GCV (AIV opening proximal end) (6) Extended tributary of GCV distal to the origin of AIV (6) Proximal AIV (10)	36 ± 6	Inside CVS at earliest activation site (30)	—	100	NA	18 ± 13	93

Naga-shima et al,[22] 2014	30	GCV (30)	37 ± 8	Inside CVS at earliest activation site (15) Adjacent sites outside CVS (19) Percutaneous epicardial (2) Open-chest surgical ablation (3)	Proximity to coronary arteries (14) Inability to advance the ablation catheter to the site of earliest activation (3) Failed ablation at the earliest activation site (7)	53	Coronary artery occlusion requiring stenting of a marginal branch of the circumflex artery (2) GCV perforation (1)	Median 3	100
Mounta-ntonakis et al,[51] 2015	47	Distal GCV (25) AIV (19) MCV (3)	39 ± 18	Inside CVS at earliest activation site (18) Inside CVS proximal to the earliest activation site (14) Adjacent sites outside CVS (15)	Proximity to coronary arteries (21) inability to advance the ablation catheter to the site of earliest activation (4) Inadequate power delivery (2) Operator choice (2)	94 with ablation at the earliest CVS site 55 with ablation at adjacent CVS or non-CVS sites	Femoral artery Pseudoaneurysm (1) Pericardial effusion caused by CS perforation (1) Stenosis of the proximal circumflex coronary artery (1)	31 ± 21	76

(continued on next page)

Table 1
(continued)

Study	No. of Patients	Site of Earliest Activation Recorded (No. of Patients)	Earliest Activation Time, Pre-QRS (ms)	Site of Ablation (No. of Patients)	Reasons for Not Performing Ablation at the Earliest Activation Site Within CVS (No. of Patients)	Acute Procedural Success (%)	Complications (No. of Patients)	Follow-up (mo)	Long-term Success (% of Patients with Acute Procedural Success)
Santangeli et al,[7] 2015	23	Epicardial LV summit (21) AIV (2)	31 ± 10	Percutaneous epicardial (14)	Close proximity to coronary arteries (9)	22	Pericardial effusion caused by perforation of the GCV (1)	Median 36	60
Yamada et al,[29] 2015	24	Distal GCV	<−20 (22) >−20 (2)	Inside CVS at earliest activation site (24) AMC (9) Simultaneous unipolar RF ablation from AMC and GCV (3)	Failed ablation at the earliest activation site (9)	100	None	6	100
Lin et al,[52] 2016	16	GCV/AIV	30 ± 16 ms	Inside CVS at earliest activation site (16)	—	100	None	Median 16	88

Yamada et al,[53] 2016	23	GCV (16) Communicating branch of the GCV (7)	<−20	Inside CVS at earliest activation site (23) Inside CVS proximal to the earliest activation site (1) AMC (1) LCC (1)	Inadequate power delivery (1) Failed ablation at the earliest activation site (2)	100	None	Median 55 100
Yamada et al,[54] 2016	40	Distal GCV	<−20 (38) >−20 (2)	Inside CVS at earliest activation site (40) AMC (12) Simultaneous unipolar RF ablation from AMC and GCV (3)	Failed ablation at the earliest activation site (12)	100	None	Median 51 NA

Abbreviations: AMC, aorto-mitral continuity; LCC, left coronary cusp; NA, not available.

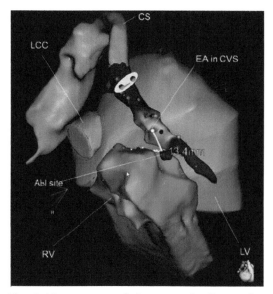

Fig. 4. Measurement of the anatomic distance between the earliest activation site in the CVS and the targeted adjacent site on the endocardium in a successful LV summit ablation case with an anatomic approach from the adjacent endocardial LV outflow tract. Although the earliest activation is mapped epicardially within the CVS ablation at the earliest site is not possible because of proximity to the left anterior descending coronary artery. The ablation catheter is maneuvered to the anatomically opposite LVOT endocardium with evidence of later activation. Ablation at that site effectively suppressed the arrhythmia. EA, earliest activation. (*Adapted from* Shirai Y., Santangeli P., Liang JJ., et al. Anatomical proximity dictates successful ablation from adjacent sites for outflow tract ventricular arrhythmias linked to the coronary venous system. Europace 2019;21(3):484–91; with permission.)

Bipolar RF ablation delivered from the coronary veins to the adjacent endocardium has also been proposed as alternative approach for treatment of refractory LV summit arrhythmias.[32] With bipolar CA, the current is delivered from 1 catheter to the other and may be less effective whenever there is an impedance mismatch between the 2 catheter tips (ie, CVS vs LV/RV endocardium) because the higher impedance of either electrode limits the current that can be applied to both electrodes because of uneven tissue heating at either catheter and the risk of steam pops. Simultaneous unipolar RF ablation can be a valid alternative to bipolar RF when there is impedance mismatch between the 2 catheter locations. In this case, RF energy is delivered from 2 separated open-irrigated catheters using 2 separate RF generators allowing for independent power titration at each ablation catheter and independent assessment of impedance trends during ablation at each location.[29,33] It has been reported that simultaneous unipolar CA is more likely to be required for the elimination of LVOT VA when the earliest activation at multiple endocardial and epicardial sites is more than −30 milliseconds pre-QRS and the distance between the endocardial and epicardial earliest activation site is more than 8 mm.[29]

Alternatives to RF energy include retrograde coronary venous and transarterial coronary ethanol infusion or coronary coil embolization.[34,35] Retrograde coronary venous ethanol infusion is typically performed by venogram-guided CVS mapping using a small-caliber multipolar catheter or an alligator clip connected to the angioplasty wire, then an angioplasty balloon (1.5–2 × 6 mm) is used to deliver 1 to 4 mL of 98% ethanol solution into a septal branch of the targeted vein.[34] In a similar manner, in transarterial coronary ethanol ablation, selective coronary angiography is performed after mapping in order to identify arterial branches supplying the target region that are sufficiently distal and without collateral flow to avoid unnecessary ventricular damage. The artery is then engaged with an angioplasty wire, a balloon is deployed at its ostium, and iced saline is injected through the central lumen in an attempt to terminate the VA. If the VA terminates with cold saline injection, ethanol injection is then performed and occlusion is verified with contrast injection after guidewire removal.[36]

Mapping of intramural VA arising from the basal septum with intracoronary guidewires and effective treatment with coil embolization has been reported in 2 cases. Coronary arteriography is performed to detect septal perforator branches, then a coronary guidewire is placed into septal perforators and subsequently exchanged over a microcatheter for a 0.36-mm (0.014-inch) Vision wires (Biotronik SE and Co KG, Berlin, Germany) that can be used for mapping purposes. Once the arrhythmic focus is detected in one of the territories supplied by a septal perforator, a Courier Microcatheter (Codman Neurovascular, Codman and Shurtleff, Inc, Raynham, MA) is positioned over the 0.36-mm (0.014-inch) coronary wire, the wire is removed, and coils are deployed in the septal perforator. In addition, complete occlusion of the septal perforator is shown by contrast injection.[35]

Intramyocardial ablation using RF ablation delivered through a system routinely used to treat coronary artery chronic total occlusions (ie, Stingray LP Coronary CTO Re-Entry System, Boston Scientific, Marlborough, MA) has also been reported by the University of California, Los Angeles, group. Similarly to coil embolization, after identifying the septal perforator with the earliest activation, a Stingray LP

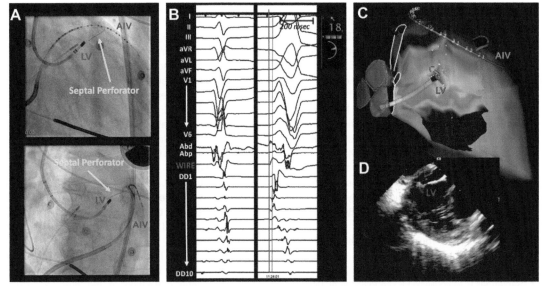

Fig. 5. Activation mapping from multiple adjacent sites including LVOT endocardium, AIV, and 1 of its septal perforator branches through guidewire mapping (*A*). The earliest activation is recorded from the guidewire consistent with an intramural site of origin of the PVC (*B*). Because RF energy cannot be delivered directly from the guidewire, CA is performed at the LV site anatomically opposite to the earliest activation site as shown by 3D electroanatomi mapping (*C*) and intracardiac echocardiography (*D*).

device is advanced into the proximal portion of the branch and the arterial wall is deliberately perforated using the hydrophilic-coated Stingray guidewire (0.36 mm), which is then advanced into the myocardium and RF energy is delivered by placing the proximal end of the guidewire in a saline bath along with an 8-mm tip catheter to deliver RF in power-controlled mode at 50 W.[37]

Surgical cryoablation has been described as an alternative for VA arising from the LV summit after unsuccessful attempt of either endocardial and epicardial CA.[38,39] The procedure requires accurate preoperative endocardial/epicardial mapping to identify the arrhythmogenic focus then a bipolar pacing lead can be placed in the overlying cardiac vein for guidance during surgery.[38] The procedure requires median sternotomy and is performed under cardiopulmonary bypass and even though coronary injury still remains a risk. For these reasons, it should be performed only in highly selected patients such as those who are highly symptomatic, have developed arrhythmia-induced cardiomyopathy, or those requiring cardiac surgery for other reasons. A less invasive surgical approach with a remotely navigated robotic system (da Vinci, Intuitive Surgical, Sunnyvale, CA) has been described by Mulpuru and colleagues[40] in order to overcome the inability to perform cryoablation close to coronary arteries. The technique involves dissection of the epicardial fat and manual displacement of the LAD to deliver cryoenergy below it under direct

visualization. A similar approach, called totally endoscopic robotic epicardial ablation, has recently been reported using RF energy instead of cryoenergy.[41]

SUMMARY

Idiopathic VAs originating from epicardial foci generally arise from the perivalvular epicardium superiorly at the LV summit region or inferiorly from the cardiac crux region and pose significant clinical challenges for mapping and ablation because of close proximity to important anatomic structures such as the major coronary vessels and the phrenic nerve, and the presence of insulating epicardial fat. Effective ablation can be achieved in up to 70% of patients from the CVS or from adjacent anatomic structures if within a critical anatomic distance. In refractory cases, alternative approaches, such as simultaneous unipolar RF ablation, bipolar RF ablation, alcohol arterial/venous ablation, arterial coil embolization, or surgical epicardial ablation with direct visualization of the coronary vessels and dissection of the epicardial fat, may be considered.

REFERENCES

1. Lerman BB. Mechanism, diagnosis, and treatment of outflow tract tachycardia. Nat Rev Cardiol 2015; 12(10):597–608.

2. Latif S, Dixit S, Callans DJ. Ventricular arrhythmias in normal hearts. Cardiol Clin 2008;26(3):367–80, vi.

3. Hayashi T, Liang JJ, Shirai Y, et al. Trends in successful ablation sites and outcomes of ablation for idiopathic outflow tract ventricular arrhythmias. J Am Coll Cardiol 2019. https://doi.org/10.1016/j.jacep.2019.10.004.

4. Baman TS, Ilg KJ, Gupta SK, et al. Mapping and ablation of epicardial idiopathic ventricular arrhythmias from within the coronary venous system. Circ Arrhythm Electrophysiol 2010;3(3):274–9.

5. Cronin EM, Bogun FM, Maury P, et al. 2019 HRS/EHRA/APHRS/LAHRS expert consensus statement on catheter ablation of ventricular arrhythmias. Heart Rhythm 2019. https://doi.org/10.1016/j.hrthm.2019.03.002.

6. Meininger GR, Berger RD. Idiopathic ventricular tachycardia originating in the great cardiac vein. Heart Rhythm 2006;3(4):464–6.

7. Santangeli P, Marchlinski FE, Zado ES, et al. Percutaneous epicardial ablation of ventricular arrhythmias arising from the left ventricular summit: outcomes and electrocardiogram correlates of success. Circ Arrhythm Electrophysiol 2015;8(2):337–43.

8. Hasdemir C. PVC-induced cardiomyopathy: the cutoff value for the premature ventricular contraction burden. Europace 2013;15(7):1063.

9. Viskin S, Rosso R, Rogowski O, et al. The "short-coupled" variant of right ventricular outflow ventricular tachycardia: a not-so-benign form of benign ventricular tachycardia? J Cardiovasc Electrophysiol 2005;16(8):912–6.

10. Yamada T, McElderry HT, Doppalapudi H, et al. Idiopathic ventricular arrhythmias originating from the left ventricular summit: anatomic concepts relevant to ablation. Circ Arrhythm Electrophysiol 2010;3(6):616–23.

11. Bazan V, Gerstenfeld EP, Garcia FC, et al. Site-specific twelve-lead ECG features to identify an epicardial origin for left ventricular tachycardia in the absence of myocardial infarction. Heart Rhythm 2007;4(11):1403–10.

12. Berruezo A. Electrocardiographic recognition of the epicardial origin of ventricular tachycardias. Circulation 2004;109(15):1842–7.

13. Jauregui Abularach ME, Campos B, Park K-M, et al. Ablation of ventricular arrhythmias arising near the anterior epicardial veins from the left sinus of Valsalva region: ECG features, anatomic distance, and outcome. Heart Rhythm 2012;9(6):865–73.

14. Hayashi T, Santangeli P, Pathak RK, et al. Outcomes of catheter ablation of idiopathic outflow tract ventricular arrhythmias with an r wave pattern break in lead V2: a distinct clinical entity. J Cardiovasc Electrophysiol 2017. https://doi.org/10.1111/jce.13183.

15. Kawamura M, Gerstenfeld EP, Vedantham V, et al. Idiopathic ventricular arrhythmia originating from the cardiac crux or inferior septum: epicardial idiopathic ventricular arrhythmia. Circ Arrhythm Electrophysiol 2014;7(6):1152–8.

16. Liang JJ, Shirai Y, Briceño DF, et al. Electrocardiographic and electrophysiologic characteristics of idiopathic ventricular arrhythmias originating from the basal inferoseptal left ventricle. JACC Clin Electrophysiol 2019;5(7):833–42.

17. Enriquez A, Malavassi F, Saenz LC, et al. How to map and ablate left ventricular summit arrhythmias. Heart Rhythm 2016. https://doi.org/10.1016/j.hrthm.2016.09.018.

18. Shirai Y, Liang JJ, Santangeli P, et al. Catheter ablation of premature ventricular complexes with low intraprocedural burden guided exclusively by pace-mapping. J Cardiovasc Electrophysiol 2019;30(11):2326–33.

19. Bogun F, Taj M, Ting M, et al. Spatial resolution of pace mapping of idiopathic ventricular tachycardia/ectopy originating in the right ventricular outflow tract. Heart Rhythm 2008;5(3):339–44.

20. Yamada T, Murakami Y, Yoshida N, et al. Preferential conduction across the ventricular outflow septum in ventricular arrhythmias originating from the aortic sinus cusp. J Am Coll Cardiol 2007;50(9):884–91.

21. Stavrakis S, Jackman WM, Nakagawa H, et al. Risk of coronary artery injury with radiofrequency ablation and cryoablation of epicardial posteroseptal accessory pathways within the coronary venous system. Circ Arrhythm Electrophysiol 2014;7(1):113–9.

22. Nagashima K, Choi E-K, Lin KY, et al. Ventricular arrhythmias near the distal great cardiac vein: a challenging arrhythmia for ablation. Circ Arrhythm Electrophysiol 2014;7(5):906–12.

23. Muser D, Santangeli P. Ventricular arrhythmias linked to the left ventricular summit communicating veins: a new mapping approach for an old ablation problem. Circ Arrhythm Electrophysiol 2018;11(1):e006105.

24. Shirai Y, Santangeli P, Liang JJ, et al. Anatomical proximity dictates successful ablation from adjacent sites for outflow tract ventricular arrhythmias linked to the coronary venous system. Europace 2019;21(3):484–91.

25. Yamada T, Yoshida N, Doppalapudi H, et al. Efficacy of an anatomical approach in radiofrequency catheter ablation of idiopathic ventricular arrhythmias originating from the left ventricular outflow tract. Circ Arrhythm Electrophysiol 2017;10(5):e004959.

26. Yakubov A, Salayev O, Hamrayev R, et al. A case of successful ablation of ventricular tachycardia focus in the left ventricular summit through the left atrial appendage: a case report. Eur Heart J Case Rep 2018;2(4):yty110.

27. Di Biase L, Romero J, Zado ES, et al. Variant of ventricular outflow tract ventricular arrhythmias

requiring ablation from multiple sites: intramural origin. Heart Rhythm 2019;16(5):724–32.

28. Briceño DF, Enriquez A, Liang JJ, et al. Septal coronary venous mapping to guide substrate characterization and ablation of intramural septal ventricular arrhythmia. JACC Clin Electrophysiol 2019;5(7): 789–800.

29. Yamada T, Maddox WR, McElderry HT, et al. Radiofrequency catheter ablation of idiopathic ventricular arrhythmias originating from intramural foci in the left ventricular outflow tract: efficacy of sequential versus simultaneous unipolar catheter ablation. Circ Arrhythm Electrophysiol 2015;8(2):344–52.

30. Koruth JS, Dukkipati S, Miller MA, et al. Bipolar irrigated radiofrequency ablation: a therapeutic option for refractory intramural atrial and ventricular tachycardia circuits. Heart Rhythm 2012;9(12): 1932–41.

31. Nguyen DT, Tzou WS, Sandhu A, et al. Prospective multicenter experience with cooled radiofrequency ablation using high impedance irrigant to target deep myocardial substrate refractory to standard ablation. JACC Clin Electrophysiol 2018;4(9): 1176–85.

32. Futyma P, Sander J, Ciąpała K, et al. Bipolar radiofrequency ablation delivered from coronary veins and adjacent endocardium for treatment of refractory left ventricular summit arrhythmias. J Interv Card Electrophysiol 2019. https://doi.org/10.1007/s10840-019-00609-9.

33. Yang J, Liang J, Shirai Y, et al. Outcomes of simultaneous unipolar radiofrequency catheter ablation for intramural septal ventricular tachycardia in nonischemic cardiomyopathy. Heart Rhythm 2018. https://doi.org/10.1016/j.hrthm.2018.12.018.

34. Kreidieh B, Rodríguez-Mañero M, Schurmann P, et al. Retrograde coronary venous ethanol infusion for ablation of refractory ventricular tachycardia. Circ Arrhythm Electrophysiol 2016;9(7). https://doi.org/10.1161/CIRCEP.116.004352.

35. Tholakanahalli VN, Bertog S, Roukoz H, et al. Catheter ablation of ventricular tachycardia using intracoronary wire mapping and coil embolization: description of a new technique. Heart Rhythm 2013;10(2):292–6.

36. Tokuda M, Sobieszczyk P, Eisenhauer AC, et al. Transcoronary ethanol ablation for recurrent ventricular tachycardia after failed catheter ablation an update. Circ Arrhythm Electrophysiol 2011;4(6): 889–96.

37. Romero J, Diaz JC, Hayase J, et al. Intramyocardial radiofrequency ablation of ventricular arrhythmias using intracoronary wire mapping and a coronary reentry system: description of a novel technique. Heartrhythm Case Rep 2018;4(7):285–92.

38. Choi E-K, Nagashima K, Lin KY, et al. Surgical cryoablation for ventricular tachyarrhythmia arising from the left ventricular outflow tract region. Heart Rhythm 2015;12(6):1128–36.

39. Liang JJ, Betensky BP, Muser D, et al. Long-term outcome of surgical cryoablation for refractory ventricular tachycardia in patients with non-ischemic cardiomyopathy. Europace 2018;20(3):e30–41. https://doi.org/10.1093/europace/eux029.

40. Mulpuru SK, Feld GK, Madani M, et al. A novel, minimally-invasive surgical approach for ablation of ventricular tachycardia originating near the proximal left anterior descending coronary artery. Circ Arrhythm Electrophysiol 2012;5(5):e95–7.

41. Aziz Z, Moss JD, Jabbarzadeh M, et al. Totally endoscopic robotic epicardial ablation of refractory left ventricular summit arrhythmia: first-in-man. Heart Rhythm 2016. https://doi.org/10.1016/j.hrthm.2016.09.005.

42. Daniels DV. Idiopathic epicardial left ventricular tachycardia originating remote from the sinus of valsalva: electrophysiological characteristics, catheter ablation, and identification from the 12-lead electrocardiogram. Circulation 2006;113(13):1659–66.

43. Obel OA, d'Avila A, Neuzil P, et al. Ablation of left ventricular epicardial outflow tract tachycardia from the distal great cardiac vein. J Am Coll Cardiol 2006;48(9):1813–7.

44. Doppalapudi H, Yamada T, Ramaswamy K, et al. Idiopathic focal epicardial ventricular tachycardia originating from the crux of the heart. Heart Rhythm 2009;6(1):44–50.

45. Yamada T, Mcelderry HT, Okada T, et al. Idiopathic left ventricular arrhythmias originating adjacent to the left aortic sinus of valsalva: electrophysiological rationale for the surface electrocardiogram. J Cardiovasc Electrophysiol 2010;21(2):170–6.

46. Yokokawa M, Latchamsetty R, Good E, et al. Ablation of epicardial ventricular arrhythmias from nonepicardial sites. Heart Rhythm 2011;8(10):1525–9.

47. Steven D, Pott C, Bittner A, et al. Idiopathic ventricular outflow tract arrhythmias from the great cardiac vein: challenges and risks of catheter ablation. Int J Cardiol 2013;169(5):366–70.

48. Li Y-C, Lin J-F, Li J, et al. Catheter ablation of idiopathic ventricular arrhythmias originating from left ventricular epicardium adjacent to the transitional area from the great cardiac vein to the anterior interventricular vein. Int J Cardiol 2013;167(6):2673–81.

49. Frankel DS, Mountantonakis SE, Dahu MI, et al. Elimination of ventricular arrhythmias originating from the anterior interventricular vein with ablation in the right ventricular outflow tract. Circ Arrhythm Electrophysiol 2014;7(5):984–5.

50. Li J-W, Chen X-L, Li Y-C, et al. Distinct ECG characteristics of idiopathic ventricular arrhythmias originating from four regions of left coronary veins. Int J Cardiol 2014;175(1):181–2.

51. Mountantonakis SE, Frankel DS, Tschabrunn CM, et al. Ventricular arrhythmias from the coronary

venous system: Prevalence, mapping, and ablation. Heart Rhythm 2015;12(6):1145–53.

52. Lin C-Y, Chung F-P, Lin Y-J, et al. Radiofrequency catheter ablation of ventricular arrhythmias originating from the continuum between the aortic sinus of Valsalva and the left ventricular summit: electrocardiographic characteristics and correlative anatomy. Heart Rhythm 2016;13(1):111–21.

53. Yamada T, Doppalapudi H, Litovsky SH, et al. Challenging radiofrequency catheter ablation of idiopathic ventricular arrhythmias originating from the left ventricular summit near the left main coronary artery. Circ Arrhythm Electrophysiol 2016; 9(10):e004202.

54. Yamada T, Doppalapudi H, Maddox WR, et al. Prevalence and electrocardiographic and electrophysiological characteristics of idiopathic ventricular arrhythmias originating from intramural foci in the left ventricular outflow tract. Circ Arrhythm Electrophysiol 2016;9(9):e004079.

Epicardial Ablation of Ventricular Tachycardia in Ischemic Cardiomyopathy

Travis D. Richardson, MD[a], Arvindh N. Kanagasundram, MD[a],
William G. Stevenson, MD[b],*

KEYWORDS

- Ventricular tachycardia • Myocardial infarction • Ischemic cardiomyopathy • Catheter ablation
- Epicardial access

KEY POINTS

- In most reported series of patients with ischemic cardiomyopathy (ICM) and ventricular tachycardia (VT) presenting for catheter ablation, epicardial ablation is performed in a minority of cases. However, in those with no prior cardiac surgery, who do undergo epicardial mapping, epicardial substrate is identified in up to one-third of patients and up to 8 of 10 patients with evidence of transmural infarction on imaging.
- Cardiac MRI, cardiac computed tomography, or nuclear scintigraphy suggesting transmural infarction may be predictive of the presence of epicardial substrate.
- When feasible, simultaneous epicardial and endocardial ablation of VT substrate may reduce VT recurrences compared with an endocardial alone approach.
- In patients with prior coronary artery bypass grafting, attempts at percutaneous epicardial access should likely be avoided, although surgical access can be considered.

INTRODUCTION

Catheter ablation is an increasingly common treatment for patients with ventricular tachycardia (VT) late after myocardial infarction, but recurrence is frequent.[1–4] VT is due to reentry within complex regions of myocardial scar.[5] Necrosis during myocardial infarction begins at the endocardium because of the gradient in tissue perfusion pressure; however, it has long been appreciated that the substrate for reentry within the resulting scar can extend all the way to the epicardium. During surgical ablations in the early 1990s, sites of both "exact" entrainment of VT, that is, sites of entrainment with concealed fusion, as well as VT termination were identified on the epicardium.[6,7] Furthermore, recent comprehensive in vivo and in vitro mapping studies have demonstrated that a significant portion of VT circuits may be located within intramural regions, limiting the utility of endocardial-only mapping and ablation.[8] In addition, animal models have demonstrated that lesion formation may be limited within areas of scarred myocardium; in an ischemic substrate, this may prevent ablation of deep substrate from an endocardial approach, even in thin-walled areas.[9] Thus, epicardial ablation is important in these patients and may reduce recurrence. Here, the authors review the evidence surrounding epicardial ablation in patients with ischemic cardiomyopathy (ICM).

FREQUENCY OF EPICARDIAL "SUBSTRATE" OBSERVED IN ISCHEMIC CARDIOMYOPATHY

In 1990, Svenson and colleagues[6] reported their experience performing surgical ablations for VT in 30 patients following myocardial infarction. In

[a] Vanderbilt Heart and Vascular Institute, Nashville, TN, USA; [b] Vanderbilt Heart and Vascular Institute, East South Tower, Suite 5209, 1215 21st Avenue South, Nashville, TN 37232-8802, USA
* Corresponding author.
E-mail address: william.g.stevenson@vumc.org

Card Electrophysiol Clin 12 (2020) 313–319
https://doi.org/10.1016/j.ccep.2020.05.003
1877-9182/20/© 2020 Elsevier Inc. All rights reserved.

that series, epicardial ablation was necessary to terminate at least 1 VT in 10 of 30 patients (33%). In contrast, a series by Sarkozy and colleagues[10] examined all percutaneous catheter ablations performed for VT in patients with ICM at a tertiary care center (444 patients). Epicardial mapping was performed in 14% of patients, and epicardial ablation was performed in 8.5%, with 0.5% not undergoing ablation of identified epicardial substrate because of proximity to an epicardial coronary vessel. The difference in frequency of epicardial substrate is at least in part explained by differences in patient selection (**Fig. 1**). In the catheter-based series, endocardial ablation was performed before epicardial mapping, and epicardial mapping was not performed if VT was no longer inducible; this was not always the case in the surgical series. Furthermore, 52% of patients in the catheter ablation series had undergone prior coronary artery bypass grafting (CABG), and percutaneous access was specifically avoided in these patients. Several series have examined epicardial substrate in selected patients without prior cardiac surgery. Di Biase and colleagues[11] examined a group of 44 patients with ICM, VT storm, and no prior history of CABG. They performed extensive endocardial substrate modification and then performed epicardial mapping in all of these patients. In 14 cases (33%), potential epicardial arrhythmia substrate was identified following endocardial ablation. In this series, substrate was defined as regions with electrograms having greater than 3 sharp deflections, amplitude less than 1.5 mV, or electrogram duration greater than 70 milliseconds. Tung and colleagues[12] examined a cohort of 34 patients with ICM and VT undergoing simultaneous epicardial and endocardial mapping. Of these, 22 (65%) underwent epicardial ablation. Of the 12 (35%) that did not undergo epicardial ablation, 9 had no identifiable targets, and in 3, mapping was interrupted because of pericardial access complications. Further supporting that epicardial substrate is frequent in this population, in a series of 24 patients with transmural scar based on cardiac MRI without a history of cardiac surgery, Acosta and colleagues[13] observed epicardial substrate (defined as electrograms with a delayed component) in 87.5% of cases (21 of 24). Although abnormal electrograms consistent with scar were recognized, in most cases, specific reentry circuit sites were not confirmed.

- In an unselected population of patients with ICM and VT presenting for catheter ablation, epicardial ablation is performed in a minority of cases.

- In patients with ICM and no prior cardiac surgery, epicardial substrate may be identified in up to one-third of unselected patients and up to 8 of 10 patients with evidence of transmural infarction.

It should also be noted that in most patients with ICM and epicardial substrate, endocardial substrate is also identified. In the surgical series by Svenson and colleagues,[6] all 10 patients with epicardial VT had at least 1 endocardial VT circuit. In the patients with epicardial circuits, a total of 36 VT morphologies were observed, only 13 of which were terminated with epicardial ablation. In the series by Sarkozy and colleagues,[10] 50% of patients with epicardial ablation also had endocardial circuits. Finally, in the series by Tung and colleagues,[12] 16 of 21 patients (76%) who underwent epicardial mapping also required endocardial ablation.

- Most patients who require epicardial ablation *also* have endocardial substrate

PREDICTORS OF EPICARDIAL SUBSTRATE

In contrast to non-ICM, the ECG morphology of VT in patients with prior myocardial infarction is not useful for identifying epicardial reentry substrates.[14] VTs with markedly slurred and broad QRS complexes can often be interrupted with endocardial ablation.

Region of Scar

Initial experience from surgical ablation of VT was suggestive that inferior and lateral myocardial infarctions were more likely to require epicardial ablation. In the series by Svenson and colleagues,[6] of the 10 patients with epicardial VT circuits identified, 9 of them had inferior infarctions involving either the right coronary or the left circumflex territory. However, more recent series have often found epicardial substrate with a similar frequency in anterior and inferior wall infarctions.[10,12,13] Epicardial substrate would not be expected in patients with infarction confined to the septum, an unusual entity.

- The region of myocardial infarction does not appear to be predictive of epicardial involvement.

Infarct Transmurality

Not surprisingly, it appears that infarct transmurality predicts the presence of epicardial substrate. In a series of 23 patients with ICM who underwent cardiac MRI before ablation, critical isthmus sites

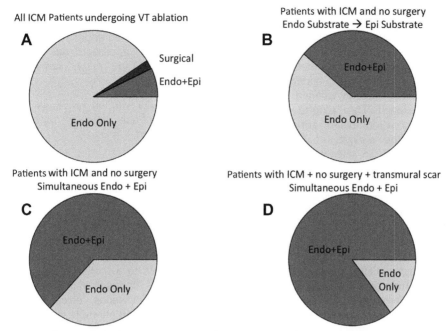

Fig. 1. Frequency of epicardial substrate in ICM. Pie charts represent the proportion of patients in each population found to have epicardial arrhythmogenic substrate based on the presence of abnormal electrograms. The population studied dramatically affects the frequency of observed epicardial substrate. (*A*) Series by Sarkozy and colleagues[10] examining all patients with ICM undergoing ablation for VT at 1 center that used epicardial mapping only after endocardial ablation failed. Surgical ablation refers to epicardial cryoablation performed in the operating room via anterior sternotomy or lateral thoracotomy. (*B*) Series by Di Biase and colleagues[11] examining the frequency of epicardial substrate identified after endocardial scar homogenization. (*C*) Series by Tung and colleagues[12] examining the frequency of epicardial substrate in patients undergoing simultaneous epicardial and endocardial mapping with no prior cardiac surgery. (*D*) Series by Acosta and colleagues[13] examining the frequency of epicardial substrate in patients undergoing simultaneous epicardial and endocardial mapping with no prior cardiac surgery and evidence of transmural infarct on pre-procedural imaging. Endo, endocardial; Epi, epicardial.

(as defined by several parameters) were identified at sites of near transmural scar (scar thickness, 66%–76%). Isthmus sites clustered around the core-border zone transition: 90% of pace map sites, 100% of concealed entrainment sites, and 80% of termination sites were located within 5 mm of greater than 75% transmural scar.[15] In the series by Acosta and colleagues,[13] patients also underwent cardiac MRI before enrollment; patients with less than 75% thickness scar underwent an endocardial-only ablation, and those with greater than 75% thickness underwent epicardial and endocardial ablation. There was no statistically significant difference between group outcomes suggestive that imaging was a potentially useful tool to assess the need for epicardial mapping. As described above, a high rate of epicardial substrate was observed in the patients with transmural scar.

- Imaging, such as cardiac MRI, cardiac computed tomography, or nuclear scintigraphy suggesting transmural infarction may identify patients more likely to have epicardial substrate.

OUTCOMES OF EPICARDIAL ABLATION IN ISCHEMIC CARDIOMYOPATHY

Although epicardial substrate may be present in a large portion of patients with transmural myocardial infarction, this does not necessarily mean that ablation of this substrate affects clinical outcomes. Acosta and colleagues[13] examined outcomes following simultaneous epicardial and endocardial ablation versus a historical cohort of endocardial-only ablation in patients with transmural myocardial infarction (based on imaging). They observed a reduction in VT recurrence with an initial endocardial-epicardial approach. In patients undergoing simultaneous endocardial-epicardial approach, 91.6% (22 of 24) were rendered noninducible for VT versus 75% of those undergoing endocardial-only approach (24 of 32) (*P* = .235). At 2 years of follow-up, recurrence was observed in 12.5% of patients undergoing endocardial-epicardial approach versus 40.6% of those with endocardial-only ablation (*P* = .011). Di Biase and colleagues[11] compared sequential groups of patients undergoing endocardial-only ablation with an activation/entrainment mapping approach to a group undergoing endocardial followed by epicardial ablation using a substrate modification approach. They reported that patients undergoing a combined approach had 81% arrhythmia-free survival at 2 years as compared with 53% in the endocardial-only group; however, the extent to which epicardial ablation contributed to the improved outcome was not clear. In multivariate analysis, a combined approach was associated with reduced likelihood of recurrence (hazard ratio 0.46, 0.21–0.87). However, the radiofrequency (RF) time in the group undergoing substrate modification was nearly double that of the standard ablation group (74 vs 39 minutes; *P*<.001). Tung and colleagues[12] reported increased rates of freedom from VT in patients undergoing simultaneous epicardial and endocardial ablation versus endocardial-only ablation at 12 months of follow-up (85% vs 56%), despite similar acute procedural success between the groups (94% vs 95%). Finally, when these data were examined in a metaanalysis, the overall relative risk (RR) of VT recurrence was 0.43 (0.28, 0.67) with a combined endocardial and epicardial versus an endocardial-alone approach, despite no difference observed in the likelihood of acute procedural success RR 1.01 (0.97, 1.05).[16] Despite association with lower VT recurrence rates, a combined epicardial and endocardial approach likely carries increased risk of procedural complications. In a metaanalysis by Romero and colleagues,[16] a trend toward increased complications was observed with an RR of 2.62 (confidence interval 0.91–7.52) for epicardial procedures. There are no prospective randomized trials of endocardial-only versus combined endocardial + epicardial ablation.

- When feasible, simultaneous epicardial and endocardial ablation of VT substrate may improve arrhythmic outcomes compared with an endocardial alone approach.

LEFT VENTRICULAR THROMBUS

In patients with remote myocardial infarctions, ventricular aneurysm formation can occur with the subsequent development of laminated ventricular thrombi. These patients have significant myocardial scar and thus occasionally present with VT that cannot be controlled by medical therapy alone. In this instance, catheter ablation has

been reported as a potential therapy; however, there is risk of thrombus disruption and potential embolization with an endocardial approach.[17] An epicardial-only approach has been effective without embolism in a small number of cases.[10,17,18]

- In patients with left ventricular thrombus, an epicardial-only ablation approach may be considered.

EPICARDIAL ACCESS IN THE SETTING OF PRIOR CARDIAC SURGERY

In patients with prior cardiac surgery or pericarditis, adhesions may develop between the visceral and parietal pericardium, which in some cases fuse together entirely. Not infrequently, percutaneous access to a portion of the pericardium is possible, but catheter maneuverability is often restricted. In 1 series, epicardial access was possible in 3 of 10 attempts in patients with prior CABG. In 2 of 3 cases whereby access was obtained, mapping the anterior LV was not possible because of adhesions.[10] Although data have been presented that epicardial access and manipulation of the sheath and catheter can be used to lyse adhesions in patients after prior cardiac surgery,[19,20] there are also anecdotal cases of coronary injury even in the absence of prior cardiac surgery. Jincun and colleagues[21] reported a case of subepicardial dissection with unroofing of the circumflex following catheter-based lysis of adhesions in a patient without prior cardiac surgery or pericarditis. The authors' practice is not to attempt percutaneous epicardial access in the face of prior coronary bypass surgery, aortic and mechanical prostheses, or pericardial adhesions. In these instances, the authors prefer a subxiphoid or lateral thoracotomy for a surgical window if feasible given the substrate location.[22,23] In some instances, a median sternotomy is used if more extensive exposure is required. Need for concomitant surgery (including coronary artery bypass, valve surgery, ventricular assist device placement, or septal myectomy) may also favor a hybrid surgical approach in certain cases. Cryothermy can be applied to targets identified by previous electrophysiology studies, presumptive exit sites based on 12-lead morphology, or visible scar. The authors favor concomitant electroanatomic mapping to define substrate (**Fig. 2**). Typical cryoapplications are performed for 3 minutes with a target minimum temperature of −60 C to −150 C depending on the system used. In selected patients with prior cardiac surgery without CABG (eg, valve repair or replacement), percutaneous

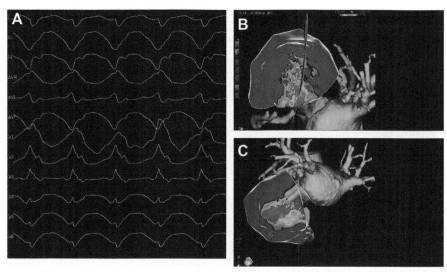

Fig. 2. Example of hybrid surgical approach. Example of the authors' approach in a patient with previous CABG, mechanical mitral valve replacement, and inferior infarct with recurrent VT after 2 prior endocardial ablations. Surgical access was obtained via a left thoracotomy. (*A*) Monomorphic VT with a right bundle branch block-like morphology and superior and rightward axis. (*B, C*) Electroanatomic voltage maps of the epicardium at the time of surgery revealing an area of scar and border zone in the basal inferolateral wall. Purple indicates bipolar voltage greater than 1.5 mV. (*C*) After surgical cryothermy applications, the voltage map shows a more homogenenous low-voltage appearance. Following cryoablation, epicardial pacing with a roving mapping catheter demonstrated no capture in the low-voltage area (pacing stim strength 10 mA at 2 milliseconds), and VT was no longer inducible.

access can sometimes be achieved and may be of less risk in the absence of bypass grafts. In any case, aggressive attempts to lyse adhesions by manipulating catheters and sheaths should likely be avoided.

- In patients with prior CABG, percutaneous attempts at epicardial access should likely be avoided.
- In selected patients with prior cardiac surgery without CABG, it may be reasonable to attempt percutaneous pericardial access, but aggressive lysis of adhesions should likely be avoided.

THE AUTHORS' APPROACH

Although evidence suggests that patients undergoing a combined endocardial-epicardial ablation may have better outcomes than those with an endocardial-only approach, these data have significant limitations. Most data are from patients without a history of prior cardiac surgery and thus may not be generalizable to all patients with ICM. Most data are from patients who have failed endocardial ablation and hence may be more likely to have epicardial arrhythmia substrate. Furthermore, obtaining epicardial access certainly

increases risk of complications, some of which can be catastrophic and require emergent surgical intervention.[16,21] Operators in reported series from experienced centers exercised discretion in choosing candidates suitable for attempted epicardial access; the risk of epicardial access in all-comers would possibly be greater than reported. Because of these considerations, it is the authors' practice that absent unusual circumstances (eg, left ventricular thrombus) they perform thorough endocardial mapping and ablation before considering an epicardial approach (**Fig. 3**). Generally, in patients in whom VT was inducible at procedure start, if VT is noninducible following endocardial ablation, they do not perform epicardial mapping. In patients in whom VT is not inducible or cannot be induced safely at procedure start, they will obtain epicardial access following endocardial ablation if epicardial substrate is suspected and there is no history of prior cardiac surgery. Catheters are removed from the left heart, and heparin is reversed before epicardial access. In the absence of pericardial bleeding, patients can be reanticoagulated if further endocardial mapping is desired.[24] In patients with a high risk of epicardial access complications (morbid obesity, large gastric bubble,

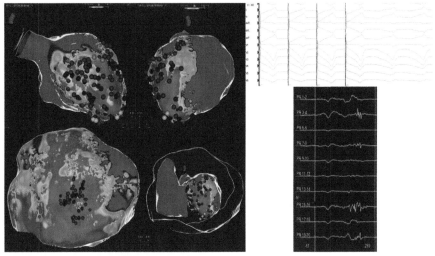

Fig. 3. Example of endocardial and epicardial lesion set. Example of approach in a patient with remote infarct due to dissection of the left anterior descending coronary artery with recurrent VT. Following extensive endocardial ablation (*top*, voltage maps; *bottom, right* voltage map), VT remained inducible. Epicardial mapping disclosed a site with late abnormal ventricular activation during sinus rhythm (*bottom right*, EGMs) and an entrainment response consistent with an exit site (*top right*, image). Ablation at this area terminated VT, which was then no longer inducible. Maps represent bipolar voltage collected with a multipolar catheter; voltage range displayed 0.1 to 1.5 mV. Red dots represent sites of RF ablation; gray dots are sites of no pace excitability before ablation; black dots are sites of no pace excitability after ablation; light pink dots are sites of ablation with poor impedance fall.

pectus excavatum), the authors reserve epicardial access for repeat procedures and also consider surgical access.

DISCLOSURE

T.D. Richardson: No relevant disclosures; A.N. Kanagasundram: Speaking honoraria: Biosense Webster, Janssen Pharmaceuticals; W.G. Stevenson: Speaking honoraria: Abbott, Boston Scientific, Johnson and Johnson, Biotronik; consulting: Novartis; Patent for irrigated needle ablation consigned to Brigham and Women's Hospital.

REFERENCES

1. Al-Khatib SM, Stevenson WG, Ackerman MJ, et al. 2017 AHA/ACC/HRS guideline for management of patients with ventricular arrhythmias and the prevention of sudden cardiac death: a report of the American College of Cardiology/American Heart Association Task Force on Clinical Practice Guidelines and the Heart Rhythm Society. J Am Coll Cardiol 2018;72(14):e91–220.

2. Stevenson William G, Wilber David J, Andrea Natale, et al. Irrigated radiofrequency catheter ablation guided by electroanatomic mapping for recurrent ventricular tachycardia after myocardial infarction. Circulation 2008;118(25):2773–82.

3. Marchlinski FE, Haffajee CI, Beshai JF, et al. Long-term success of irrigated radiofrequency catheter ablation of sustained ventricular tachycardia: post-approval THERMOCOOL VT trial. J Am Coll Cardiol 2016;67(6):674–83.

4. Kuck K-H, Schaumann A, Eckardt L, et al. Catheter ablation of stable ventricular tachycardia before defibrillator implantation in patients with coronary heart disease (VTACH): a multicentre randomised controlled trial. Lancet 2010;375(9708):31–40.

5. Stevenson WG. Ventricular tachycardia after myocardial infarction: from arrhythmia surgery to catheter ablation. J Cardiovasc Electrophysiol 1995;6(10):942–50.

6. Svenson RH, Littmann L, Gallagher JJ, et al. Termination of ventricular tachycardia with epicardial laser photocoagulation: a clinical comparison with patients undergoing successful endocardial photocoagulation alone. J Am Coll Cardiol 1990;15(1):163–70.

7. Littmann L, Svenson RH, Gallagher JJ, et al. Functional role of the epicardium in postinfarction ventricular tachycardia. Observations derived from computerized epicardial activation mapping, entrainment, and epicardial laser photoablation. Circulation 1991;83(5):1577–91.

8. Bhaskaran A, Nayyar S, Porta-Sanchez A, et al. Direct and indirect mapping of intramural space in

ventricular tachycardia. Heart Rhythm 2019. https://doi.org/10.1016/j.hrthm.2019.10.017.

9. Barkagan M, Leshem E, Shapira-Daniels A, et al. Histopathological characterization of radiofrequency ablation in ventricular scar tissue. JACC Clin Electrophysiol 2019;5(8):920–31.

10. Sarkozy A, Michifumi T, Tedrow Usha B, et al. Epicardial ablation of ventricular tachycardia in ischemic heart disease. Circ Arrhythm Electrophysiol 2013;6(6):1115–22.

11. Di Biase L, Santangeli P, Burkhardt DJ, et al. Endo-epicardial homogenization of the scar versus limited substrate ablation for the treatment of electrical storms in patients with ischemic cardiomyopathy. J Am Coll Cardiol 2012;60(2):132–41.

12. Tung R, Michowitz Y, Yu R, et al. Epicardial ablation of ventricular tachycardia: an institutional experience of safety and efficacy. Heart Rhythm 2013; 10(4):490–8.

13. Acosta J, Fernández-Armenta J, Penela D, et al. Infarct transmurality as a criterion for first-line endo-epicardial substrate-guided ventricular tachycardia ablation in ischemic cardiomyopathy. Heart Rhythm 2016;13(1):85–95.

14. Martinek M, Stevenson WG, Inada K, et al. QRS characteristics fail to reliably identify ventricular tachycardias that require epicardial ablation in ischemic heart disease. J Cardiovasc Electrophysiol 2012;23(2):188–93.

15. Piers SRD, Tao Q, de Riva Silva M, et al. CMR-based identification of critical isthmus sites of ischemic and nonischemic ventricular tachycardia. JACC Cardiovasc Imaging 2014;7(8):774–84.

16. Romero J, Cerrud-Rodriguez RC, Di Biase L, et al. Combined endocardial-epicardial versus endocardial catheter ablation alone for ventricular tachycardia in structural heart disease: a systematic review and meta-analysis. JACC Clin Electrophysiol 2019;5(1):13–24.

17. Rao HB, Yu R, Chitnis N, et al. Ventricular tachycardia ablation in the presence of left ventricular thrombus: safety and efficacy. J Cardiovasc Electrophysiol 2016;27(4):453–9.

18. Berte B, Yamashita S, Sacher F, et al. Epicardial only mapping and ablation of ventricular tachycardia: a case series. Europace 2016;18(2):267–73.

19. Killu AM, Ebrille E, Asirvatham SJ, et al. Percutaneous epicardial access for mapping and ablation is feasible in patients with prior cardiac surgery, including coronary bypass surgery. Circ Arrhythm Electrophysiol 2015;8(1):94–101.

20. Tschabrunn CM, Haqqani HM, Cooper JM, et al. Percutaneous epicardial ventricular tachycardia ablation after noncoronary cardiac surgery or pericarditis. Heart Rhythm 2013;10(2):165–9.

21. Jincun G, Zhou F, Huang W, et al. Outside-in subepicardial dissection during percutaneous epicardial ventricular tachycardia ablation. Circ Arrhythm Electrophysiol 2016;9(10):e004499.

22. Li A, Hayase J, Do D, et al. Hybrid surgical vs percutaneous access epicardial ventricular tachycardia ablation. Heart Rhythm 2018;15(4):512–9.

23. Soejima K, Couper G, Cooper JM, et al. Subxiphoid surgical approach for epicardial catheter-based mapping and ablation in patients with prior cardiac surgery or difficult pericardial access. Circulation 2004;110(10):1197–201.

24. Nakamura T, Davogustto GE, Schaeffer B, et al. Complications and anticoagulation strategies for percutaneous epicardial ablation procedures. Circ Arrhythm Electrophysiol 2018;11(11):e006714.

Epicardial Ablation in Nonischemic Ventricular Tachyardia

Mouhannad M. Sadek, MD[a], Daniele Muser, MD[b],
Pasquale Santangeli, MD, PhD[b], Francis E. Marchlinski, MD[b],*

KEYWORDS

- Nonischemic cardiomyopathy • Ventricular tachycardia ablation • Epicardial ablation

KEY POINTS

- Ventricular arrhythmias in the setting of nonischemic cardiomyopathy (NICM) tend to originate from the His-Purkinje system, septal substrate, or endocardial/epicardial paravalvular substrate.
- Clues to the presence of epicardial substrate include the 12-lead electrocardiogram morphology of the QRS complex during ventricular arrhythmia and sinus rhythm, scar location on MRI, and unipolar endocardial voltage abnormalities.
- Epicardial access and ablation can be performed safely with attention to epicardial structures, such as the coronary arteries, phrenic nerve, and epicardial fat.
- Approximately one- to two-thirds of patients with NICM require epicardial ablation. Arrhythmia-free survival is approximately 69% with a substantial reduction in burden in the remaining patients.

INTRODUCTION

Ventricular arrhythmias (VAs) in patients with non-ischemic cardiomyopathy (NICM) can present as ventricular premature depolarizations (VPDs), monomorphic ventricular tachycardia (VT), and polymorphic VT/ventricular fibrillation. The clinical presentation of VAs depends on hemodynamic stability during the arrhythmia, and includes palpitations, syncope, and death.

Although implantable cardioverter-defibrillators (ICDs) are the mainstay of therapy to prevent sudden cardiac death, VAs can lead to syncope and ICD shocks, and can also be responsible for nonresponse to cardiac resynchronization therapy. In rare cases of NICM and frequent VPDs, the possibility of VPD-induced cardiomyopathy should be explored.[1–3] Catheter ablation has evolved as an important management strategy for VAs. However, in the setting of NICM, epicardial mapping and ablation has been shown to be an important adjunctive measure to endocardial ablation.[4] This article reviews the indications, technique, and evidence for epicardial ablation in the setting of NICM. Specific disease states, such as hypertrophic cardiomyopathy (HCM), arrhythmogenic right ventricular dysplasia (ARVD), valvular cardiomyopathy, and cardiac sarcoidosis, may also have indications for epicardial ablation (with different success rates), and are not addressed in detail in this review.[5]

INDICATIONS FOR EPICARDIAL ABLATION

The location of the substrate responsible for VAs is dependent on underlying cause. Patients with ischemic cardiomyopathy (ICM) have mainly endocardial substrate and endocardial ablation is usually sufficient, except in inaccessible areas

[a] Arrhythmia Service, Division of Cardiology, The Ottawa Hospital-General Campus, Box 703, 501 Smyth Road, Ottawa, Ontario K1H 8L6, Canada; [b] Cardiac Electrophysiology, Cardiovascular Division, Hospital of the University of Pennsylvania, 9 Founders Pavilion – Cardiology, 3400 Spruce Street, Philadelphia, PA 19104, USA
* Corresponding author.
E-mail address: FRANCIS.MARCHLINSKI@PENNMEDICINE.UPENN.EDU

Card Electrophysiol Clin 12 (2020) 321–328
https://doi.org/10.1016/j.ccep.2020.05.004
1877-9182/20/© 2020 Elsevier Inc. All rights reserved.

such as below the papillary muscle.[6] In contrast, other disease states, such as ARVD, apical HCM, cardiac sarcoidosis, Chagas disease, and NICM, have a propensity for epicardial substrate.[7–9]

In patients with NICM, VAs tend to originate from either the His-Purkinje system (manifesting as bundle branch reentry) or scar substrate. Bundle branch reentrant VT typically manifests as monomorphic VT with left bundle branch block morphology. Occasionally right bundle branch block VT is observed, particularly when programmed stimulation is performed from the left ventricle, and a reversed pattern of activation in the Purkinje network manifests. Catheter ablation targeting the right bundle branch is curative.[10]

Patients with NICM tend to have either septal substrate or endocardial/epicardial perivalvular substrate. Typically, only patients with epicardial or subepicardial substrate require epicardial VT ablation. Patients with septal substrate have a higher rate of post-procedural VT recurrence, likely caused by the presence of intramural circuitry.[11] The 12-lead electrocardiogram morphology of the VA may help guide as to a septal substrate versus an endocardial/epicardial substrate away from the septum. Overlap may occur and mapping provides important confirmatory information. Hints at the presence of an epicardial substrate can come from the 12-lead morphology of the VT showing delayed activation or slurring in the initial portion of the VT QRS and the presence of Q waves during VT when not anticipated, particularly in lead I.[12] In addition, findings on electrocardiogram during sinus rhythm, such as lateral lead QRS fragmentation, absence of inferior Q waves, and an S/R ratio greater than or equal to 0.25 in lead V6, all favor a basal-lateral scar caused by NICM rather than a prior myocardial infarction, and suggest an epicardial basal-lateral substrate.[13] In patients in whom an NICM has been confirmed, an r in V1 and s in V6 greater than or equal to 0.15 mV on the sinus rhythm tracing predict the presence of a basal-lateral epicardial substrate with 0.86 sensitivity and 0.88 specificity (**Fig. 1**).[14]

Scar imaging with cardiac MRI may also help in the identification of epicardial substrate by identifying epicardial regions of gadolinium uptake. In such cases, procedural planning with the intent of epicardial access is important for VT elimination (**Fig. 2**).

Finally, unipolar voltage mapping (as referenced between the endocardial ablation catheter and Wilson central terminal) performed during endocardial voltage acquisition can also help to identify potential areas of midmyocardial or epicardial scar. We use a cutoff of 8.3 mV (left ventricle) and 5.5 mV (right ventricle free wall) for defining normal unipolar voltage.[15,16] When an area of unipolar abnormality is seen overlying normal bipolar voltage, midmyocardial or epicardial scar is suspected (**Fig. 3**). Care must be taken to ensure proper tissue contact when assessing for voltage abnormalities. If hypertrophy is present, the unipolar voltage slider bar needs to be adjusted higher to attempt to ghost in an area of unipolar abnormality, which suggests an area of layered epicardial bipolar abnormality consistent with scar (see **Fig. 2**)

EPICARDIAL ACCESS IN PATIENTS WITH NONISCHEMIC CARDIOMYOPATHY

Epicardial access technique is described in elsewhere; however, a specific issue relating to NICM is the access approach. Typically, access is obtained distant to the desired site of ablation to allow for better catheter control and reduce the likelihood of losing epicardial access. In the setting of ARVD an inferior approach may be preferred, whereas for targeting a basal-lateral scar in the setting of NICM, either an anterior or inferior approach may be undertaken (**Fig. 4**). In addition, an anterior approach may be more feasible in obese patients because less soft tissue needs to be penetrated before accessing the epicardium. Both approaches can be performed with low risk when care regarding appropriate technique is addressed.

EPICARDIAL ABLATION TECHNIQUE
Mapping Strategies

Different strategies are used in mapping and ablating VT from the epicardium, and the optimal strategy may appropriately vary for each case. In the setting of hemodynamically tolerated VT, entrainment mapping is used to identify critical channels for reentrant VT. Pacing is performed during VT from sites showing low-voltage and abnormal electrograms in sinus rhythm and diastolic activity during VT.[17] In the setting of VT that is not hemodynamically tolerated, the use of hemodynamic support devices, such as a left ventricular assist device or extracorporeal membrane oxygenation, can allow for end-organ perfusion while entrainment maneuvers during sustained VT are undertaken to identify the region of interest. However, such devices can increase the complexity of the procedure. In addition, as a consequence of general anesthesia for the purpose of epicardial access, the clinical VT may no longer be inducible. Hence, other strategies aimed

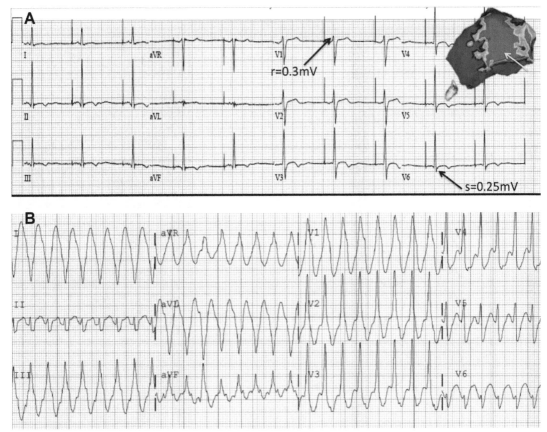

Fig. 1. Electrocardiogram findings in a patient with NICM. During atrial pacing (*A*), the QRS complex shows an r in V1 and s in V6 of ≥0.15 mV (*blue arrows*), corresponding to a 0.86 sensitivity and 0.88 specificity for a basal-lateral epicardial substrate (*yellow arrow*). During ventricular tachycardia (*B*), a QS complex in lead I with initial QRS slurring is also suggestive of a basal-lateral epicardial VT exit site.

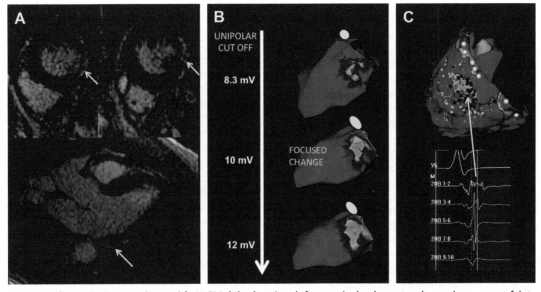

Fig. 2. Cardiac MRI in a patient with NICM (*A*), showing left ventricular hypertrophy and an area of late-gadolinium enhancement (*yellow arrows*) at the basal-lateral left ventricular epicardium. Unipolar voltage mapping is only mildly abnormal, but with adjustment of the upper cutoff from 8.3 mV to 12 mV (*B*), we are able to ghost in an area of unipolar voltage abnormality that corresponds to (*C*) a significant layered epicardial bipolar voltage abnormality and scar (*yellow arrow*).

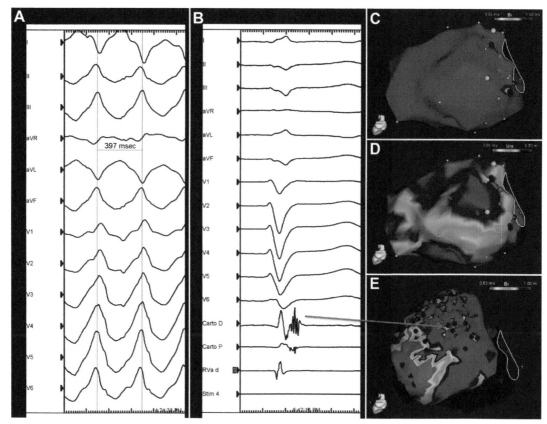

Fig. 3. Clinical ventricular tachycardia with morphology consistent with an epicardial basal anterolateral exit (*A*). Mapping epicardially in the basal anterolateral region shows evidence of a delayed, fractionated potential (*B*). Endocardial mapping reveals normal bipolar (*C*) but abnormal unipolar voltage (*D*), suggestive of midmyocardial or epicardial scar. Epicardial bipolar mapping (*E*) reveals extensive epicardial scar substrate, with significant fractionated potentials basally (*red arrow*) despite "borderline" voltage.

at substrate ablation without the need for mapping during VT are used, such as pace-mapping or substrate-based ablation targeting abnormal, fractionated, split, and late potentials. In such cases, ablation is performed in the setting of normal sinus or paced rhythm targeting the abnormal substrate responsible for the maintenance of VT.[18–21]

There are limits to pace-mapping and substrate-based ablation. The morphology of the paced QRS may vary depending on the area of the myocardium captured, the pacing output, and the pacing coupling interval.[22,23] In addition, the presence of abnormal ventricular electrograms does not necessarily infer involvement in the reentrant circuit.[19] Thus, elimination of all such electrograms translates to potential unnecessary ablation and longer procedural times. Finally, it may be difficult to detect all abnormal substrate, such as intramyocardial circuitry, with resultant VT recurrence in a significant portion of patients.[24]

Avoiding Coronary and Phrenic Nerve Injury

There are specific concerns with respect to epicardial ablation above and beyond that of endocardial ablation. Care must be taken to avoid large coronary vessels by at least 1 cm as assessed by angiography. The ablation catheter is placed at the margin of the planned region of substrate ablation at the time of angiography to define a vessel-free zone. Univue software (Biosense Webster, Diamond Bar, CA) allows for merging angiography with the electroanatomic map to facilitate localization of the coronary anatomy during planned ablation (**Fig. 5**). In addition to defining the coronaries, the course of the phrenic nerve needs to be delineated before ablation by high output pacing. When areas of interest for ablation lie close to the phrenic nerve, the nerve can be displaced either by inflating a large vascular balloon or injecting normal saline into the epicardial space. Pacing of the left phrenic at the left subclavian can be performed during ablation while monitoring for

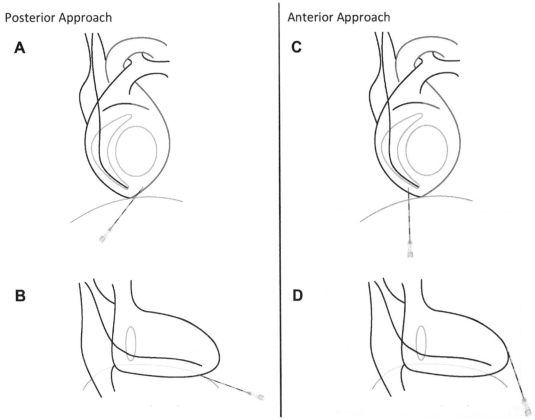

Fig. 4. Epicardial access is performed with the Tuohy needle bevel facing away from the myocardium via a posterior approach (*A, B*) or an anterior approach (*C, D*). With a posterior approach, the needle is advanced at a steep angle leftward of the apex to avoid the coronary vessels. With an anterior approach, the needle is advanced at a shallower angle targeting the anterior right ventricle. Typically, the point of puncture is chosen distant to the desired site of ablation to allow for better catheter control and reduce the likelihood of losing epicardial access.

attenuation in diaphragmatic contraction as an added safety measure when in close proximity but not in direct contact with the phrenic nerve as indexed by ablation catheter pacing.[25]

Other Technical and Mapping Considerations

During mapping and ablation, monitoring for epicardial fluid collection secondary to catheter irrigation is important, with the need for continuous or intermittent drainage. Importantly, because of the presence of dense epicardial fat (>1/2 cm) and coronary vessels, abnormal electrograms in the epicardial surface are defined not just by low voltage (with a cutoff of 1.0 mV), but also by the presence of fractionation, prolonged duration, and late potentials.[4] This is important to distinguish true scar from areas of dense epicardial fat and coronary vessels overlying normal myocardium. Regions of fat are typically localized around large epicardial coronary arteries, the mitral and tricuspid valve annuli,

and apical regions of the right and left ventricle. Signals that are greater than 1.0 mV that exhibit late potentials may also be targeted and are frequently adjacent to low-voltage areas. The abnormal electrograms may only be manifest depending on the direction of the wavefront and are more easily recognized with small multielectrode mapping.[26]

At procedure end, 2 to 3 mg/kg of triamcinolone is administered intrapericardially to reduce inflammation and the possibility of adhesion formation. A pigtail catheter may be left in place in the presence of continued drainage and removed 24 hours following the procedure when drainage abates.

COMPLICATIONS OF EPICARDIAL ACCESS, MAPPING, AND ABLATION

VT ablation procedures have the potential to be complex and prolonged, and patients may experience hemodynamic deterioration. Specific

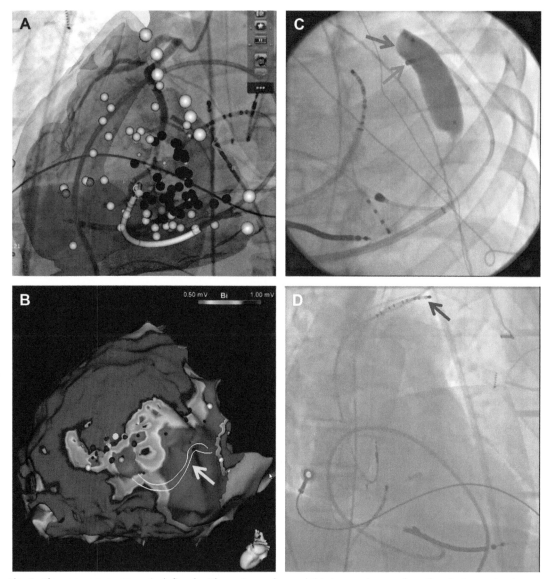

Fig. 5. The coronary anatomy is defined with angiography, and this is superimposed on the electroanatomic map using the Univue module (*A*). The course of the coronary artery transversing the area of interest can also be drawn directly onto the voltage map (*yellow arrow*) to avoid ablation on/near the coronary artery (*B*). In the case of phrenic nerve capture at the site of desired epicardial ablation, inflation of a contrast-filled balloon (*red arrow*) allows for separation of the phrenic nerve from the ablation catheter (*green arrow*)/epicardial surface (*C*). If ablation is performed in close proximity to the phrenic nerve (as indexed by ablation catheter pacing), monitoring phrenic function can be performed during ablation via high-output pacing from the subclavian vein (*blue arrow*) to capture the phrenic nerve while monitoring for attenuation in diaphragmatic contraction (*D*).

patient and procedural characteristics can identify patients who are at a higher periprocedural risk above and beyond that associated with accessing the epicardial space. These include chronic obstructive pulmonary disease, age greater than 60, general anesthesia, ICM, New York Heart Association functional class III-IV heart failure, ejection fraction less than 25%, presentation with VT storm, and diabetes mellitus.[27]

Estimation of risk is important during the consent process, and patients at a higher risk of decompensation may warrant consideration of the anesthesia strategy and potential use of hemodynamic support.

Specific complications related to epicardial access are described elsewhere.[28–30] In case of a complication requiring emergent surgical intervention, it is important to complete epicardial mapping and ablation in the surgical theater, thus allowing for improved patient outcomes.

OUTCOMES OF EPICARDIAL VENTRICULAR TACHYCARDIA ABLATION

There is a significant amount of data supporting the use of catheter ablation in the setting of ICM. The recent Ventricular Tachycardia Ablation versus Escalation of Antiarrhythmic Drugs (VANISH) trial in patients with ICM on antiarrhythmic drug (AAD) therapy showed a reduction in the composite end point of death, VT storm, or appropriate ICD shock in patients receiving ablation versus escalation of AAD therapy.[31] A randomized trial of first-line catheter ablation versus AADs in patients with ICM is currently ongoing (VANISH 2).

In contrast, in patients with NICM, catheter ablation outcomes vary according to the nature of the underlying heart disease, with an overall higher need for epicardial ablation and higher likelihood of VT recurrence.[32–34] Compared with other forms of NICM, VT ablation had better outcomes with dilated cardiomyopathy than valvular cardiomyopathy or HCM, but was less likely to be successful than in patients with ARVD.[5]

Our long-term outcomes after catheter ablation of VT in patients with NICM show a VT-free survival of approximately 69% at 60-month follow-up, with a substantial improvement in VT burden in many of the remaining patients.[35] In patients presenting with electrical storm (defined as the occurrence of >3 episodes of VT/ventricular fibrillation separated by >5 minutes during a 24-hour period resulting in an appropriate ICD therapy), those with NICM (n = 71) undergoing ablation had 93% freedom from electrical storm and 54% had no VT recurrence at a median follow-up for 60 months. This was comparable with patients with ICM.[36] In addition, there was a significant reduction in AAD use in this patient group. VT inducibility at the end of the procedure predicted VT recurrence postablation. Two-thirds of patients required a combined endocardial/epicardial procedure highlighting the important role epicardial ablation plays in eliminating VT in patients with NICM.

FUTURE DIRECTIONS

Future studies assessing the optimum ablation targets, timing of epicardial access, and the incorporation of imaging technology may improve procedural outcomes. Further advances in technology to obtain epicardial access may improve the safety profile and encourage earlier epicardial intervention. Randomized-controlled trials assessing VT ablation in patients with NICM may shed more light on the utility and usefulness of epicardial ablation in this population.

DISCLOSURE

This work was supported in part by the Mark S Marchlinski EP Research and Education Fund.

REFERENCES

1. Bogun F, Crawford T, Reich S, et al. Radiofrequency ablation of frequent, idiopathic premature ventricular complexes: comparison with a control group without intervention. Heart Rhythm 2007;4:863–7.
2. Baman TS, Lange DC, Ilg KJ, et al. Relationship between burden of premature ventricular complexes and left ventricular function. Heart Rhythm 2010;7:865–9.
3. Niwano S, Wakisaka Y, Niwano H, et al. Prognostic significance of frequent premature ventricular contractions originating from the ventricular outflow tract in patients with normal left ventricular function. Heart 2009;95:1230–7.
4. Cano O, Hutchinson M, Lin D, et al. Electroanatomic substrate and ablation outcome for suspected epicardial ventricular tachycardia in left ventricular nonischemic cardiomyopathy. J Am Coll Cardiol 2009;54:799–808.
5. Vaseghi M, Hu TY, Tung R, et al. Outcomes of catheter ablation of ventricular tachycardia based on etiology in nonischemic heart disease: an International Ventricular Tachycardia Ablation Center Collaborative Study. JACC Clin Electrophysiol 2018;4:1141–50.
6. Enriquez A, Briceno D, Tapias C, et al. Ischemic ventricular tachycardia from below the posteromedial papillary muscle, a particular entity: substrate characterization and challenges for catheter ablation. Heart Rhythm 2019;16:1174–81.
7. Garcia FC, Bazan V, Zado ES, et al. Epicardial substrate and outcome with epicardial ablation of ventricular tachycardia in arrhythmogenic right ventricular cardiomyopathy/dysplasia. Circulation 2009;120:366–75.
8. Soto-Becerra R, Bazan V, Bautista W, et al. Ventricular tachycardia in the setting of chagasic cardiomyopathy: use of voltage mapping to characterize endoepicardial nonischemic scar distribution. Circ Arrhythm Electrophysiol 2017;10:e004950.
9. Dukkipati SR, d' Avila A, Soejima K, et al. Long-term outcomes of combined epicardial and endocardial ablation of monomorphic ventricular tachycardia related to hypertrophic cardiomyopathy. Circ Arrhythm Electrophysiol 2011;4:185–94.
10. Balasundaram R, Rao HB, Kalavakolanu S, et al. Catheter ablation of bundle branch reentrant ventricular tachycardia. Heart Rhythm 2008;5:S68–72.

11. Oloriz T, Silberbauer J, Maccabelli G, et al. Catheter ablation of ventricular arrhythmia in nonischemic cardiomyopathy: anteroseptal versus inferolateral scar sub-types. Circ Arrhythm Electrophysiol 2014; 7:414–23.

12. Boyle NG, Shivkumar K. Epicardial interventions in electrophysiology. Circulation 2012;126:1752–69.

13. Betensky BP, Deyell MW, Tzou WS, et al. Sinus rhythm electrocardiogram identification of basal-lateral ischemic versus nonischemic substrate in patients with ventricular tachycardia. J Interv Card Electrophysiol 2012;35:311–21 [discussion: 321].

14. Tzou WS, Zado ES, Lin D, et al. Sinus rhythm ECG criteria associated with basal-lateral ventricular tachycardia substrate in patients with nonischemic cardiomyopathy. J Cardiovasc Electrophysiol 2011; 22:1351–8.

15. Hutchinson MD, Gerstenfeld EP, Desjardins B, et al. Endocardial unipolar voltage mapping to detect epicardial ventricular tachycardia substrate in patients with nonischemic left ventricular cardiomyopathy. Circ Arrhythm Electrophysiol 2011;4:49–55.

16. Polin GM, Haqqani H, Tzou W, et al. Endocardial unipolar voltage mapping to identify epicardial substrate in arrhythmogenic right ventricular cardiomyopathy/dysplasia. Heart Rhythm 2011;8:76–83.

17. Stevenson WG, Friedman PL, Sager PT, et al. Exploring postinfarction reentrant ventricular tachycardia with entrainment mapping. J Am Coll Cardiol 1997;29:1180–9.

18. de Chillou C, Groben L, Magnin-Poull I, et al. Localizing the critical isthmus of postinfarct ventricular tachycardia: the value of pace-mapping during sinus rhythm. Heart Rhythm 2014;11:175–81.

19. Vergara P, Trevisi N, Ricco A, et al. Late potentials abolition as an additional technique for reduction of arrhythmia recurrence in scar related ventricular tachycardia ablation. J Cardiovasc Electrophysiol 2012;23:621–7.

20. Di Biase L, Santangeli P, Burkhardt DJ, et al. Endo-epicardial homogenization of the scar versus limited substrate ablation for the treatment of electrical storms in patients with ischemic cardiomyopathy. J Am Coll Cardiol 2012;60:132–41.

21. Jaïs P, Maury P, Khairy P, et al. Elimination of local abnormal ventricular activities: a new end point for substrate modification in patients with scar-related ventricular tachycardia. Circulation 2012;125:2184–96.

22. Goyal R, Harvey M, Daoud EG, et al. Effect of coupling interval and pacing cycle length on morphology of paced ventricular complexes. Implications for pace mapping. Circulation 1996;94:2843–9.

23. Yamada T, Murakami Y, Yoshida N, et al. Preferential conduction across the ventricular outflow septum in ventricular arrhythmias originating from the aortic sinus cusp. J Am Coll Cardiol 2007;50:884–91.

24. Nayyar S, Wilson L, Ganesan AN, et al. High-density mapping of ventricular scar: a comparison of ventricular tachycardia (VT) supporting channels with channels that Do Not support VT. Circ Arrhythm Electrophysiol 2014;7:90–8.

25. Santangeli P, Marchlinski FE. Left phrenic nerve pacing from the left subclavian vein: novel method to monitor for left phrenic nerve injury during catheter ablation. Circ Arrhythm Electrophysiol 2015;8:241–2.

26. Sadek MM, Schaller RD, Supple GE, et al. Ventricular tachycardia ablation: the right approach for the right patient. Arrhythm Electrophysiol Rev 2014;3:161–7.

27. Santangeli P, Muser D, Zado ES, et al. Acute hemodynamic decompensation during catheter ablation of scar-related ventricular tachycardia: incidence, predictors, and impact on mortality. Circ Arrhythm Electrophysiol 2015;8:68–75.

28. Sosa E, Scanavacca M. Epicardial mapping and ablation techniques to control ventricular tachycardia. J Cardiovasc Electrophysiol 2005;16:449–52.

29. Yamashita S, Sacher F, Mahida S, et al. Role of high-resolution image integration to visualize left phrenic nerve and coronary arteries during epicardial ventricular tachycardia ablation. Circ Arrhythm Electrophysiol 2015;8:371–80.

30. Di Biase L, Burkhardt JD, Pelargonio G, et al. Prevention of phrenic nerve injury during epicardial ablation: comparison of methods for separating the phrenic nerve from the epicardial surface. Heart Rhythm 2009;6:957–61.

31. Sapp JL, Wells GA, Parkash R, et al. Ventricular tachycardia ablation versus escalation of antiarrhythmic drugs. N Engl J Med 2016;375:111–21.

32. Piers SRD, Leong DP, van Huls van Taxis CFB, et al. Outcome of ventricular tachycardia ablation in patients with nonischemic cardiomyopathy: the impact of noninducibility. Circ Arrhythm Electrophysiol 2013;6:513–21.

33. Tokuda M, Tedrow UB, Kojodjojo P, et al. Catheter ablation of ventricular tachycardia in nonischemic heart disease. Circ Arrhythm Electrophysiol 2012;5:992–1000.

34. Shirai Y, Liang JJ, Santangeli P, et al. Comparison of the ventricular tachycardia circuit between patients with ischemic and nonischemic cardiomyopathies. Circ Arrhythm Electrophysiol 2019;12:e007249.

35. Muser D, Santangeli P, Castro SA, et al. Long-term outcome after catheter ablation of ventricular tachycardia in patients with nonischemic dilated cardiomyopathy. Circ Arrhythm Electrophysiol 2016;9:e004328.

36. Muser D, Liang JJ, Pathak RK, et al. Long-term outcomes of catheter ablation of electrical storm in nonischemic dilated cardiomyopathy compared with ischemic cardiomyopathy. JACC Clin Electrophysiol 2017;3:767–78.

Epicardial Ablation of Ventricular Tachycardia in Arrhythmogenic Right Ventricular Cardiomyopathy

Fabrizio R. Assis, MD*, Harikrishna Tandri, MD

KEYWORDS

- Arrhythmogenic right ventricular dysplasia/cardiomyopathy • Ventricular tachycardia
- Catheter ablation • Epicardial ablation • Ventricular tachycardia recurrence

KEY POINTS

- Despite the growing number of patients with arrhythmogenic right ventricular cardiomyopathy (ARVC) undergoing epicardial catheter ablation (CA) and the improving outcomes in the past decade, recurrence is not rare, and CA remains a palliative procedure in this population.
- The efficacy of CA in some genotype-specific forms of the disease, including biventricular disease patterns with significant left ventricular cardiomyopathy (desmoplakin and phospholamban subtypes), has not yet been evaluated.
- Disease progression and the role of substrate expansion in ventricular tachycardia (VT) recurrence are questions still unanswered.
- Ultra-high-density mapping of the scar along with new image integration tools may allow for targeted ablation of conducting channels (scar dechanneling) instead of extensive substrate ablation.
- Although scar-related reentrant VT in late ARVC is well understood, the role of CA in rapid adrenergically mediated arrhythmias in early disease remains unclear.

 Video content accompanies this article at http://www.cardiacep.theclinics.com.

INTRODUCTION

Arrhythmogenic right ventricular cardiomyopathy (ARVC) is an inherited heart muscle disease predominantly caused by mutations in genes encoding desmosomal proteins. The hallmarks of the disease are progressive fibrofatty replacement of the myocardium, right ventricular (RV) enlargement, and malignant ventricular arrhythmias (VAs).[1–4] Although the RV is typically affected, early and primary left ventricular (LV) involvement is now well recognized.[5]

VA in the form of frequent premature ventricular contractions (PVCs) and recurrent ventricular tachycardia (VT) may be seen in all stages of the disease and are associated with the risk of sudden cardiac death.[6] In patients who fail antiarrhythmic medical therapy, catheter ablation (CA) has become an attractive option, as it reduces VT burden and the number of implantable cardioverter-defibrillator (ICD) shocks.[7,8] Despite this, VT recurrence is not uncommon, and repeat ablation procedures are required in a significant number of patients. Over the past decade, remarkable technological advances, as well as a better understanding of the pattern of cardiac involvement, have expanded the role of epicardial ablation strategies, leading to improved long-term

ARVC Program, Division of Cardiology, Johns Hopkins University School of Medicine, Baltimore, MD, USA
* Corresponding author. Division of Cardiology, Johns Hopkins University School of Medicine, 1800 Orleans Street, Zayed Tower 7125U, Baltimore, MD 21287.
E-mail address: fassis1@jhmi.edu

Card Electrophysiol Clin 12 (2020) 329–343
https://doi.org/10.1016/j.ccep.2020.05.005

results and safer risk profiles. In this article, the authors aim to address the overall concepts of epicardial CA in ARVC, focusing on substrate characterization and ablation strategies.

SUBSTRATE OF ARRHYTHMOGENIC RIGHT VENTRICULAR CARDIOMYOPATHY: ARRHYTHMOGENESIS AND DISEASE PHENOTYPE

Myocyte apoptosis, postinflammatory fibrosis, and nonuniform fibrofatty infiltration result in a mosaic of healthy myocytes admixed in electrically inactive areas, forming a complex substrate of electrical heterogeneity.[9,10] As the disease progresses, the substrate expands, and electrical instability may co-exist with ventricular dysfunction and heart failure. Therefore, clinical presentation varies along the course of the disease, with a wide spectrum of manifestations, including a concealed phase (no overt structural disease), early disease (most commonly found and usually associated with VAs and SCD), and either RV or biventricular failure (late disease).[11] In the early stages of the disease, the fibrofatty replacement process is thought to progress from "outside in," that is, from subepicardium to subendocardium, wherein global ventricular function is still preserved, but the risk of SCD is the highest. Herein, the adrenergic drive (sympathetic tone) overcomes the marginal anatomic substrate, and exercise-induced VAs are often described. In late ARVC, further anatomic impairment results in areas of slow conduction and scar-mediated macroreentrant tachycardias, which in turn constitute the main target of CA procedures in this population.

SYMPATHETIC MODULATION AND ARRHYTHMOGENESIS IN ARRHYTHMOGENIC RIGHT VENTRICULAR CARDIOMYOPATHY

The sympathetic nervous system plays an important role in arrhythmogenesis in ARVC.[12] Exercise-induced arrhythmias are often seen, and physical exertion is associated with worse phenotype expression and a higher risk of SCD.[13,14] Not surprisingly, sympathetic modulation by either beta-blocker therapy, the first-line antiarrhythmic therapy in ARVC, or surgical sympathetic denervation in refractory cases is associated with a reduction of VA burden and ICD shocks.[15,16] Mutations of the cardiac ryanodine receptor (RyR2) have been identified in cases of ARVC, suggesting shared mechanisms and triggers with catecholaminergic polymorphic ventricular tachycardia.[17] In late phases of the disease, however, the influence of sympathetic tone in triggering or maintaining VA seems to be reduced due to substrate expansion and predominance of scar-dependent arrhythmias.[18]

Given this catecholamine-sensitive nature of VAs in ARVC, evaluation of patient's arrhythmic response to isoproterenol testing has been described as a sensitive screening strategy in patients with suspected ARVC.[19] Denis and colleagues,[20] in a study with 412 patients, demonstrated that an arrhythmogenic response to infusion of high doses of isoproterenol (45μg/min) was highly sensitive (sensitivity 91.4%; negative predictive value 99.1%), even in early stages of the cardiomyopathy. Also, induction of polymorphic VAs with left bundle branch block morphology during isoproterenol infusion, without any other identified or recognized structural heart disease, strongly suggested ARVC. In fact, early identification of ARVC was recently demonstrated in 6 out of 41 patients who showed a positive adrenergic response but have not fulfilled diagnostic criteria at first evaluation. Despite that, isoproterenol testing has not yet been included as one of the diagnostic task force criteria and, thereby, should be considered with caution.

However, the value of high-dose isoproterenol infusion during the electrophysiologic evaluation of patients with ARVC is well recognized. Philips and colleagues[21] originally reported a high degree of association between the morphology of sustained VTs induced during isoproterenol infusion (20μg/min) and PVCs presented at baseline, wherein mapping and ablation of PVCs eliminated the VTs with the same morphology, all originated from right ventricular outflow tract (RVOT) and RV basal regions (border zones). A high PVC burden during isoproterenol infusion was also associated with shorter VT-free survival after CA, irrespective of the approach used (endocardial or endoepicardial),[22] and, although some centers have incorporated systematic PVC elimination into their ablation protocols, the definite value of this strategy still warrants further investigation.

The downregulation of sympathetic tone during general anesthesia or deep sedation often suppresses adrenergically mediated VAs and may compromise adequate mapping. By virtue of that, noninvasive programmed stimulation (NIPS) during mild sedation, before general anesthesia induction, is often helpful to elucidate the clinical target and has been progressively incorporated as an important step of the electrophysiological assessment in ARVC. A repeat NIPS after ablation (24–48h), before discharge, has also been performed to guide subsequent management of antiarrhythmic therapy, including early reintervention or changes in medical therapy.[23]

SUBSTRATE DISTRIBUTION: PATTERNS OF SCAR AND IMPLICATIONS ON ELECTROANATOMICAL MAPPING

Technological advances in image assessment and electrical characterization of the substrate, as well as a higher sensitivity of diagnostic screening in early ARVC, have provided valuable insights into recognition of scar distribution (patterns) along the course of the disease. The previous concept of scar distribution based on the "Triangle of Dysplasia,"[1] which initially described the typical involvement of RV outflow and inflow tracts and the apex, was updated to a biventricular scar distribution wherein RV basal inferior wall, RV anterior wall, and LV posterolateral wall seem to be preferentially affected.[5,24,25] Cardiac magnetic resonance (CMR) studies also showed no RV apical structural disease in early stages, a finding that was later corroborated by electroanatomical mapping techniques.[5] In addition, early ARVC preferentially affects the basal inferior RV, advancing to the basal anterior segment in moderate disease, and global RV impairment in severe disease (**Fig. 1**). Perivalvar RV is predominantly affected, involving late activated regions in sinus rhythm, which in turn has important implications for CA in ARVC. Epicardial fat infiltration of the LV posterolateral wall is frequently observed in ARVC, especially in mutation-positive patients, whereas impairment of LV function is rare. Importantly, although LV fatty infiltration is a common finding, arrhythmias originated in LV are rarely seen in classic ARVC.

Understanding scar distribution is crucial to CA in ARVC. Affected regions identified by systematic characterization of the electroanatomical substrate match with regions of myocardial loss, reflecting the replacement of electrically active myocardial tissue by electrically silent fibrofatty tissue.[26,27] Low-voltage and fragmented/prolonged duration electrograms, detected within the scar and its borders, and late potentials are typically observed in RV inferobasal regions (perivalvular tricuspid areas) and in different regions of RV anterobasal, anterolateral, and infundibular walls. Isolated scar in the RVOT and apex, as well as interventricular septum involvement, seem to be rare in early ARVC. Additional LV epicardial free wall involvement has also been described and seems to be more frequent than previously recognized.

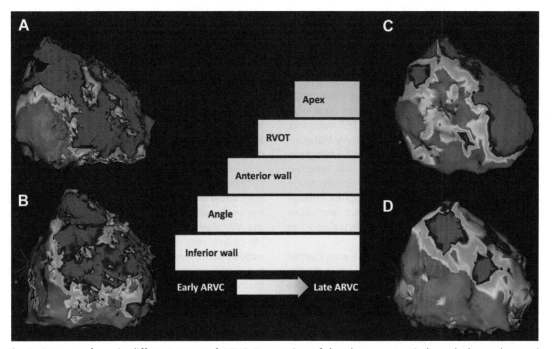

Fig. 1. Patterns of scar in different stages of ARVC. Progression of the electroanatomical scar (voltage abnormalities) on the epicardial RV surface is shown in different patients. Normal epicardium is represented in purple (>1.0 mv), and epicardium scar is represented in red (<0.5 mv). (*A*) In early disease, predominant basal involvement is noted and encompasses the inferior and lateral (angle) walls (peritricuspid region). (*B*) In patients with moderate disease, the scar extends along the inferior wall toward the apex and to the basal anterior wall. (*C*, *D*) In late stages of the disease, the scar extends through lateral and anterior walls, involving the RVOT and, ultimately, the apex. ARVC, arrhythmogenic right ventricular cardiomyopathy; RVOT, right ventricular outflow tract.

In ARVC, the scarring process is heterogeneous and often transmural, and, as it seems to progress from the epicardium toward the endocardium gradually, epicardial electroanatomical substrate usually predominates over endocardial.[9,11] The presence of epicardial electrically abnormal areas extending beyond the underlying endocardial electrical substrate and the identification of large epicardial scar with minimal endocardial involvement in early disease have been consistently reported.[5,7,22,28,29] This is of crucial importance while planning CA and defining ablation targets, as exclusive endocardial mapping may be misleading if one does not recognize the early epicardial involvement in the disease process. By virtue of this centripetal scarring process, intra-myocardial involvement is not rare and may affect procedure outcomes, as technical limitations may obviate successful ablation of such circuits.

THE ROLE OF ENDOCARDIAL MAPPING AND ABLATION IN ARRHYTHMOGENIC RIGHT VENTRICULAR CARDIOMYOPATHY

Despite the growing number of epicardial interventions, the endocardial assessment remains a key step while defining the electroanatomical substrate in ARVC. Systematic voltage mapping of the endocardial surface should be primarily obtained in sinus rhythm, when feasible, and special attention must be drawn to collecting points in the peritricuspid valve region and anterior RVOT. High-density electroanatomical mapping over a larger area results in a more precise delineation of the electrical scar and its surroundings. Adequate contact is critical during RV mapping, as the RV endocardial surface is heavily trabeculated, and voltage abnormalities may be exaggerated due to the inability to reach the wall, which is especially true when mapping with multielectrode catheters. Contiguous bipolar electrogram voltage abnormalities (<1.5 mv) are registered, and areas of low voltage (<0.5 mv) represent dense scar, as validated in the literature.[10,30]

At our center, after delineating the endocardial scar, pace mapping is performed to replicate the morphology of clinical VT from the borders of the defined endocardial scar. Twelve-lead electrocardiogram (ECG) documentation of VT morphology is critical, especially when mapping unstable VTs. Areas of long stimulus to QRS and paced morphology similar to clinical VT are marked as possible participants in the VT circuit. VT can be briefly induced, mapped, and entrained from the scar, even if it is not tolerated, in order to get a glimpse of the participation of the endocardial surface in the VT circuit.

In the early stages of the disease, endocardial scar may be minimal or not even detectable at bipolar voltage mapping. Herein, obtaining a unipolar voltage mapping may provide valuable information regarding both presence and extension of epicardial scar, given the recognized association between unipolar low voltage endocardium areas (<5.5 mv) and epicardial scar.[29,31,32] Failure to obtain a decent pace map match through the endocardial surface also suggests the participation of subepicardial circuit. Nevertheless, it is worth mentioning that the identification of epicardial substrate does not preclude endocardial ablation to be rendered successful, as midmyocardial circuits may be eliminated from the endocardial surface.[33] As a rare disease, most reports come from single-center studies or pooled data from tertiary centers with a high volume of epicardial procedures, and, thereby, the role of endocardial ablation may be underestimated. Hence, some centers have suggested that systematic, upfront epicardial ablation may not be necessary for all patients, especially when considering the risk associated with the procedure.[8,32] Along the same lines, recent clinical studies have reported the role of a stepwise approach for CA of VT in ARVC, wherein only patients who failed a prior endocardial procedure underwent epicardial ablation.[34] In our center, when investigating patients who had their first CA performed locally, although epicardial ablation was performed in over two-thirds of patients, endocardial ablation alone was not associated with worse outcomes or lower VT-free survival rate (Assis et al, 2020).

In that sense, various indicators suggest the existence or participation of a subepicardial circuit. Prior failed endocardial ablation, VT ECG morphology, identification of islands of epicardial scar at cardiac imaging, limited electroanatomical substrate in the endocardium, lack of a good pace map while stimulating potential target areas along the endocardial surface, and failure to eliminate the VT after endocardial mapping and ablation, all collectively favors the value of epicardial assessment. Nevertheless, these findings should not be considered independently, as none of them have been individually linked to better acute- or long-term outcomes.

PERICARDIAL ACCESS

The utilization of percutaneous access into the pericardial space for ablative purposes was originally described by Sosa and colleagues.[35] Since then, as a result of an improved comprehension of the ARVC substrate, the technique has grown as an ablation strategy and has been described in up to two-thirds of procedures reported in the literature.[8]

Preprocedural contrast-enhanced multidetector computed tomography or CMR should be obtained for all patients to define thoracic anatomy and anticipate local anatomic constraints that might complicate or obviate access or even catheter manipulation inside the pericardial space. Of note, anticoagulation must be held before the procedure following drug-specific instructions.

In our institution, we use an anterior approach to obtain epicardial access in all patients undergoing epicardial ablation as previously described (**Fig. 2**).[36] In the supine position, as the heart is heavier than saline and effusion, the pericardial fluid tends to be displaced anteriorly. In a series of 68 patients, Gale and colleagues[37] showed pericardial effusion located solely or predominantly anterior to the RV. We believe that the increased pericardial fluid in the anterior part of RV may

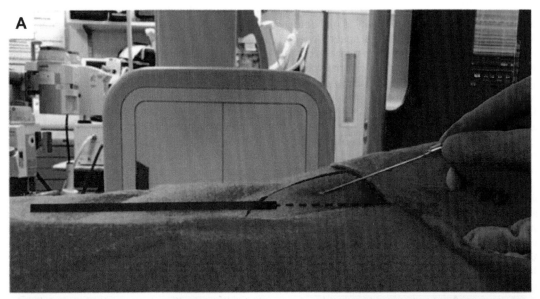

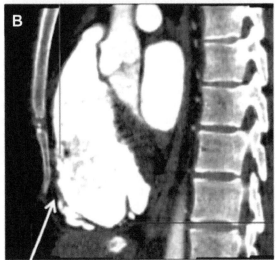

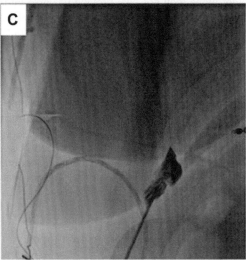

Fig. 2. Anterior epicardial access. (A) An epidural introducer needle is inserted through a small dermatomy, at a 20-degree angle, toward the anterior RV silhouette (*black line* = xiphoid process). As the pericardial fluid tends to be displaced anteriorly in the supine position, the anterior and superficial approach allows for safer access to anterior and basal regions of both ventricles, as it avoids the AV groove and thus reduces the odds of vascular injury. (B) Thoracic computed tomography illustrating the anterior and superficial path to be followed by the needle (*white arrow*). As noted, there is a fair window between the xiphoid process and the diaphragm, wherein the shallow path across thoracoabdominal transition reduces the risk of hepatic or bowel laceration. (C) Contrast is injected to confirm pericardium tenting as the needle approaches the pericardium.

facilitate easier and safer anterior epicardial access. This anterior and superficial approach allows for safer access to anterior and basal regions of both ventricles, as it avoids the AV groove and thus reduces the odds of vascular injury. Also, the shallow path across thoracoabdominal transition reduces the risk of hepatic or bowel laceration.

PERICARDIAL SPACE: ANATOMIC PECULIARITIES

Full understanding of local anatomy is mandatory before manipulating the pericardial space. Awareness of surrounding structures and nuances of the pericardial space is fundamental to avoid complications and optimize ablation results. Access to pericardial space entails a risk of coronary injury due to trauma caused by catheter/sheath manipulation or while ablating nearby sites.

Fat distribution along the epicardial surface must be carefully considered while mapping and ablating epicardially. This is particularly important in ARVC patients, as most VT circuits are located along the basal RV (perivalvar region) and basal lateral wall, which in turn constitute primary sites of epicardial fat distribution. In addition, the presence of fibrofatty replacement resultant from ARVC scarring process further contributes to fat deposition in those same areas. Preprocedural imaging evaluation of fat distribution along potential target areas may not only provide valuable information while interpreting low voltage areas but also affect ablation strategy, as opposite endocardial ablation may be necessary to eliminate some midmyocardial/subepicardial circuits "insulated" from the epicardial side.

In that sense, image integration (computed tomography/CMR and three-dimensional electroanatomical mapping) permits enhanced real-time appreciation of valuable anatomic features during electroanatomical mapping construction and assessment, such as scar distribution, channel delineation, epicardial fat spreading, and coronary artery locations.

EPICARDIAL ELECTROANATOMICAL MAPPING AND ABLATION STRATEGIES

Complex subepicardial and midmyocardial circuits often participate in arrhythmogenesis in ARVC. Segmented and delayed activation within those regions provides the environment for independent VT circuits to occur, wherein the inability to create deep lesions from the endocardial surface is considered one of the central reasons leading to failed endocardial-only ablation,[38] which is particularly demonstrated by the negative relationship between the thickness of the basal wall and efficacy of the ablation lesions.[28]

Electroanatomic mapping of RV endocardium and biventricular epicardium has been increasingly used in most experienced centers. The techniques of epicardial mapping and ablation used in ARVC are not different from those used in other nonischemic cardiomyopathies. Detailed biventricular epicardium mapping allows for an extensive assessment of scar and its borders, wherein voltage greater than 1.0 mv identifies normal myocardium.[39] The unique pattern of scar distribution in the peritricuspid region, especially in the basal inferior RV, results in reentrant circuits and hence superior axis VTs with late precordial transition in V4 and V5. Late potentials well after the QRS are the rule in this region, and detailed pace mapping in this scar is often valuable in determining potential exit sites of reentrant VTs (**Fig. 3**). Multiple VT morphologies often share the same circuit (different exit sites), and channels in the basal scar are commonly involved (**Fig. 4**). Inferior axis VTs are most often related to the epicardial scar in the anterior RVOT. Careful annotation of late potentials and recording the EGMs that represent the AV groove are critical for planning ablation in ARVC. Epicardial scar often extends to the AV groove, and ablation in this region also carries a risk of injury to the right coronary artery. Further, the AV groove hosts a variable but often significant amount of epicardial fat, which may affect mapping quality and ablation results. Some electrogram features can help to differentiate low voltage electrograms associated with sick myocardium from those derived from fat. Longer (>80 ms; specificity 99%) and more fractionated electrograms ($\geq$5 deflections, sensitivity 95%; $\geq$8 deflections, specificity 92%) were able to discriminate myocardial scar, given gross histopathological, especially when found combined. The presence of late potentials was highly specific for scar (99%), whereas bipolar low-voltage signals alone were not able to differentiate epicardial scar from fat. Unipolar voltage maps, however, seem not to be impaired by fat distribution and may be superior to identify scar swathed by fat.[40]

Although techniques of pace mapping and entrainment mapping are similar in ARVC as compared with other cardiomyopathies, the importance of substrate-guided ablation cannot be overemphasized in ARVC. After ablation of critical VT circuits, special attention should be devoted to systematically ablate all late potentials in the epicardial scar. Large isthmuses are often found in moderate-severe ARVC and may impair

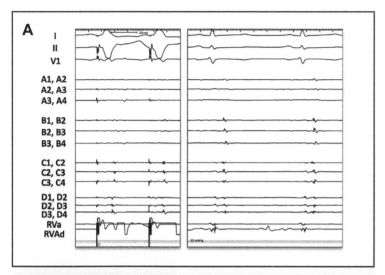

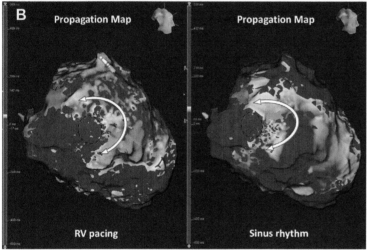

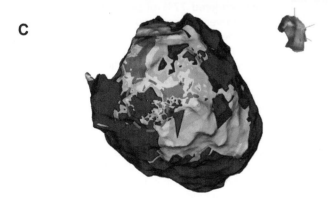

Fig. 3. Electrophysiological assessment of ARVC substrate. (*A*) Late potentials identified during both sinus rhythm and ventricular pacing within the epicardial basal inferolateral RV. (*B*) In the same patient, propagation maps performed during RV pacing and sinus rhythm reveal similar slow conduction regions (*black dashed circle*) along the lower border of the scar (*red dashed circle, C*). See Video 1. ARVC, arrhythmogenic right ventricular cardiomyopathy. RV, right ventricle.

a good pace map match. In this case, linear lesions through isthmus or diastolic pathway, extended to valvular anatomic boundaries, scar, or preserved myocardium, should be performed to achieve efficient substrate modification.

Noninducibility during programmed stimulation after the ablation has been associated with better arrhythmic, particularly when performed under isoproterenol sensibilization.[41–44] Mapping and systematic ablation of PVCs are also undertaken

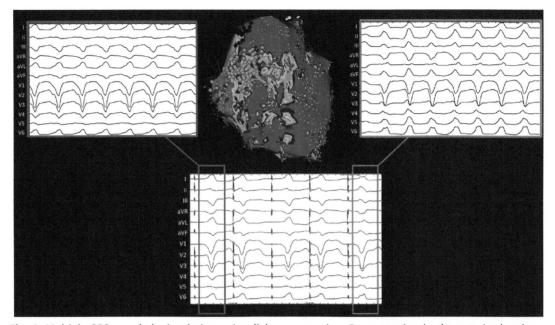

Fig. 4. Multiple QRS morphologies during epicardial pace mapping. Pace mapping in the anterior basal scar elicits different QRS morphologies with variable stimulus to QRS intervals suggesting different exit sites (*bottom*). First and last paced beats match the morphologies of the 2 sustained ventricular tachycardias induced during the study (*top left* and *top right* figures, respectively).

at some centers; however, the effect of this strategy on overall outcomes remains unclear.

COMPLICATIONS

In our experience, the anterior approach to access, map, and ablate the ARVC substrate seems to be safe, and the presence of enlarged RVs was not associated with incremental risk. In a recent study including 100 consecutive epicardial procedures using the anterior approach, among which 69 patients had ARVC, successful epicardial access was obtained in all patients without significant pericardial bleeding (>80 mL), RV puncture, or need for emergent cardiac surgery.[36]

Some degree of pericarditis is uniformly reported after epicardial ablation, and neither its incidence nor the severity seems to differ in ARVC when compared with other cardiomyopathies. In our center, we systematically inject methylprednisolone (125 mg) into the pericardial space at the end of the procedure. Additional antiinflammatory medication and/or colchicine may be required following standard recommendations.[45]

OUTCOMES OF EPICARDIAL ABLATIONS IN ARRHYTHMOGENIC RIGHT VENTRICULAR CARDIOMYOPATHY

Several studies have consistently reported the growing importance of epicardial ablation in

ARVC over the past decade. Although VT-free survival rates after ablation vary across different studies, ranging between 35% and 85% (**Table 1**), a combined endoepicardial approach has been associated with better long-term results, especially in patients who failed a prior endocardial-only ablation. Garcia and colleagues,[28] in a small study including 13 patients who failed endocardial VT ablation, showed that a combined endoepicardial rendered 77% of patients free of VT recurrence over a mean follow-up of 18 months. This was then corroborated by the findings of Bai and colleagues,[22] who investigated the long-term results of CA in 49 ARVC patients and reported a lower VA recurrence rate associated with the combined strategy when compared with endocardial-only ablation (84.6% vs 52.2%; *P*<.001). Our group, in a study of 30 consecutive ARVC patients who underwent an epi-endo ablative strategy, reported long-term VT-free survival of 70% (24 months) with 69% of VT critical circuits located on the epicardial surface.[7] In a recent meta-analysis including 258 patients with ARVC, a combined endoepicardial ablation was associated with lower VT recurrence rates, although it did not affect mortality when compared with endocardial-only procedures.[46]

Although existent data suggest a potential benefit of an early epicardial approach, whether its systematic application as a first-line strategy

Table 1
Acute and long-term results of catheter ablation for ventricular tachycardia in arrhythmogenic right ventricular cardiomyopathy

Study, Year	Patients/ Procedures (n)	Target Surface	Follow-up Duration	Acute Results	Long-Term Results and Observations
Marchlinski et al,[10] 2004	21/19	Endo (1 epi—RBBB VT)	27 ± 22 mo	Complete success: 74%	VT-free survival: 89%
Verma et al,[49] 2005	22/25	Endo	37 mo (25–44 mo)	Complete success: 82%	VT recurrence: 23% (1 y), 27% (2 y), 47% (3 y)
Dalal et al,[47] 2007	24/48	Endo No EAM: 79%	32 ± 36 mo	Complete success: 46% Partial success: 31% Failure: 23%	Cumulative VT-free survival: 75% (1.5m), 50% (5 m) and 25% (14 m) Cumulative incidence of VT recurrence: 64% (1 y), 75% (2 y) and 91% (3 y)
Garcia et al,[28] 2009	13/15	Endo + Epi	18 ± 13mo	Noninducible monomorphic VT: 85% Eliminated all targeted VT: 92%	VT-free survival (last ablation): 77%
Bai et al,[22] 2011	49/49	Endo: 47% Endo + Epi: 53%	3 y (overall) 1224 ± 310 d (endo) 1175 ± 112 d (endo + epi)	No inducibility of ablated VT or monomorphic sustained VT (endpoint): 100%	Freedom from VAs or ICD therapy (Endo): 52.2% Freedom from VAs or ICD therapy (Endo + Epi): 84.6%
Berruezo et al,[50] 2012	11/11	Endo + Epi: scar dechanneling	11 mo (6-24 mo)	Complete success: 100%	VT-free survival: 91% (mid-term follow-up)
Philips et al,[51] 2012	87/175	EAM—69% procedures Endo: 85% Endo + Epi: 9% Epi: 6%	88 ± 66 mo	Clinical VT ablated: 82% Complete acute success: 47% Partial acute success:38% Failure: 15%	VT-free survival (single procedure): 47% (1 y), 31% (2 y), 21% (5 y) and 15% (10 y) VT-free survival (after a single Endo CA): 45% (1 y), 29% (2 y) and 19% (5 y) VT-free survival (after a single Epi CA): 64% (1 y), 45% (2 y) and 45% (5 y)

(continued on next page)

Table 1
(continued)

Study, Year	Patients/ Procedures (n)	Target Surface	Follow-up Duration	Acute Results	Long-Term Results and Observations
Santangeli et al,[8] 2015	62/121	Endo: 37% Endo + Epi (adjuvant): 63%	56 ± 44 mo	Complete success: 77% (44/57) No inducibility also at repeat PVS: 86% (43/50)	VT-free survival: 71%
Philips et al.[7] 2015	30/30	Endo + Epi: 40% Epi: 60%	19.7 ± 11.7 mo	Complete success: 97% Partial success: 3%	VT-free survival: 83% (6m), 76% (12m), 70% (24m)
Wei et al,[52] 2017	48/70	Endo: 74% Endo + Epi: 26%	71.4 ± 45.7 mo	Complete success: 81%	VT-free survival after a single CA: 37.5% VT-free survival after last CA: 56.3% • Acute procedural success was associated with longer VT-free survival
Berruezo et al,[32] 2017	41/41	Endo + Epi (first ablation)	32.2 ± 21.8 mo	Complete success: 90% Partial success: 10%	VT-recurrence (end of follow-up): 26.8% • Left-dominant AC associated with a higher risk of VT recurrence • Bi/Uni-LVA ratio >0.23 was associated with limited epicardial substrate
Mussigbrodt et al,[34] 2017	45/92	Endo: 100% Epi (adjuvant): 49%	31.1 ± 27.4 mo	Complete success: 84%	VT-free survival (endo-only): 56.5% VT-free survival (endo + epi): 59.1% • Inducibility-guided ablation strategy yielded similar long-term results irrespective of the approach (endo or endo + epi)
Laredo et al,[53] 2019	23/24 (ES)	Epi: 17%	3.9 y (1 mo–10 y)	Complete success: 46% Partial success: 46% Undetermined: 8%	ES-free survival:100% (1 y), 85% (5 y) VT-free survival: 77% (1 y), 66% (5 y)
Mathew et al,[54] 2019	47/81	Endo: 56% Epi + Endo: 31% Epi: 13%	50.8 (18.6–99.2 mo)	Complete success: 80% Partial success: 16%	Freedom of VT/VF, heart transplant, death after index CA: 36% (end of follow-up) VT/VF-free survival after multiple CA: 63% (1 y), 45% (5 y) • 36% of patients underwent only endocardial CA

| Mahida et al,[55] 2019 | 75[a]/75 | Endo:47% Epi: 53% | 3 ± 4.2 y | – | VT-free survival after a single CA: 35% (3 y)
VT-free survival after the last CA: 56% (3 y)
VT-free survival after the last CA (at least one Endo-Epi): 71% (3 y)
VT-free survival after the last CA (Endo-only): 47% (3 y)
• No difference in VT-free survival was observed when comparing a single CA vs AAD escalation |

Abbreviations: AC, arrhythmogenic cardiomyopathy; Bi/Uni-LVA, endocardial bipolar/unipolar-LVA; EAM, electroanatomical mapping; Endo, endocardial; Epi, epicardial; ES, electrical storm; PVS, programmed ventricular stimulation.
[a] Number of patients in the study who underwent VT ablation.

yields additional benefit is still to be determined. Berruezo and colleagues investigated the role of a combined endoepicardial ablation as first-line therapy and reported low VT recurrence rates (26.8%) over a mean follow-up of 32 months. Those results, however, did not prevent the investigators from suggesting that an upfront epicardial ablation may not be required for all patients, as they identified a negative correlation between the area of endocardial scar and epicardial substrate.[32] The identification of an electroanatomical scar pattern where a large endocardial substrate, given by the local bipolar low-voltage areas (LVA), co-exists with smaller areas of epicardial scar, given by endocardial unipolar-LVA, may indicate a low yield of additional epicardial mapping and ablation, especially when weighing the inherited risks associated with the procedure. Along the same lines, in a study investigating the role of an adjuvant epicardial CA, a combined approach was only performed in cases of recurrent VT or persistent VT inducibility after endocardial ablation; endoepicardial ablation was required in 63% of patients, with an overall VT-free survival rate of 71% (mean follow-up of 56 months).[8] In our institution, while using a similar strategy, approximately two-thirds of patients underwent epicardial ablation during the first ablation procedure, and no significant difference in VT-free or ICD shocks survival was observed when comparing both strategies (endocardial vs epicardial) (Assis et al, 2020).

It is worth mentioning that, besides the improved short- and long-term VT-free outcomes, VT ablation also reduces the need for antiarrhythmic drugs and ICD interventions. Although redo procedures are not rare, the value of multiple procedures is still debatable. Although early studies have failed to prove the existence of a cumulative benefit on VT-free survival rates associated with repeat procedures,[7,47] recent data seem to suggest a further reduction of VA burden after subsequent ablations.[48]

PERSPECTIVES

Despite the growing number of patients with ARVC undergoing epicardial CA and the improving outcomes in the past decade, recurrence is not rare, and CA remains a palliative procedure in this population. The efficacy of CA in some genotype-specific forms of the disease, including biventricular disease patterns with significant LV cardiomyopathy (desmoplakin and phospholamban subtypes), has not yet been evaluated. Disease progression and the role of substrate expansion in VT recurrence are questions still unanswered. Ultra-high-density mapping of the scar along with new image integration tools may allow for targeted ablation of conducting channels (scar dechanneling) instead of extensive substrate ablation.

Although scar-related reentrant VT in late ARVC is well understood, the role of catheter ablation in rapid adrenergically mediated arrhythmias in early disease remains unclear. Inability to induce the VT in the electrophysiology laboratory and lack of a defined substrate in the early phase limit the utility of ablative strategies. The excess of catecholamine-/exercise-mediated arrhythmias, the sensitivity of the arrhythmias to isoproterenol infusion, and the favorable response to beta-blockers highlight the sympathetic dysregulation encountered in ARVC. Neuraxial modulation with bilateral cardiac sympathetic denervation (BCSD) has shown to be beneficial in patients with structural heart disease and refractory VT, and this seems to be extensible to ARVC patients. In our experience, BCSD significantly reduced the VT burden, the number of ICD shocks, and the need for antiarrhythmic medications in patients who failed a prior VT ablation procedure. This is especially true in young patients with rapid adrenergically mediated VAs and a high burden of polymorphic PVCs. Nevertheless, further investigation is necessary to define the optimal timing of BCSD and whether different stages of the disease equally benefit from the procedure.

DISCLOSURE STATEMENT

The Johns Hopkins ARVC Program is supported by the Leonie-Wild Foundation, the Leyla Erkan Family Fund for ARVD Research, the Dr. Satish, Rupal, and Robin Shah ARVD Fund at Johns Hopkins, the Bogle Foundation, the Healing Hearts Foundation, the Campanella family, the Patrick J. Harrison Family, the Peter French Memorial Foundation, and the Wilmerding Endowments. The authors also wish to acknowledge funding from the Dr. Francis P. Chiaramonte Private Foundation and Fondation Leducq.

ACKNOWLEDGMENTS

The authors wish to acknowledge Dr Mohammadali Habibi for his valuable contribution to some of the images presented in the text.

SUPPLEMENTARY DATA

Supplementary data related to this article can be found online at https://doi.org/10.1016/j.ccep. 2020.05.005.

REFERENCES

1. Marcus FI, Fontaine GH, Guiraudon G, et al. Right ventricular dysplasia: a report of 24 adult cases. Circulation 1982;65:384–98.
2. Nava A, Thiene G, Canciani B, et al. Familial occurrence of right ventricular dysplasia: a study involving nine families. J Am Coll Cardiol 1988;12:1222–8.
3. Corrado D, Thiene G. Arrhythmogenic right ventricular cardiomyopathy/dysplasia: clinical impact of molecular genetic studies. Circulation 2006;113(13):1634–7.
4. Basso C, Corrado D, Marcus FI, et al. Arrhythmogenic right ventricular cardiomyopathy. Lancet 2009;373:1289–300.
5. Te Riele AS, James CA, Philips B, et al. Mutation-positive arrhythmogenic right ventricular dysplasia/cardiomyopathy: the triangle of dysplasia displaced. J Cardiovasc Electrophysiol 2013;24:1311–20.
6. Calkins H, Corrado D, Marcus F. Risk stratification in arrhythmogenic right ventricular cardiomyopathy. Circulation 2017;136:2068–82.
7. Philips B, te Riele AS, Sawant A, et al. Outcomes and ventricular tachycardia recurrence characteristics after epicardial ablation of ventricular tachycardia in arrhythmogenic right ventricular dysplasia/cardiomyopathy. Heart Rhythm 2015;12:716–25.
8. Santangeli P, Zado ES, Supple GE, et al. Long-term outcome with catheter ablation of ventricular tachycardia in patients with arrhythmogenic right ventricular cardiomyopathy. Circ Arrhythm Electrophysiol 2015;8:1413–21.
9. Basso C, Thiene G, Corrado D, et al. Arrhythmogenic right ventricular cardiomyopathy: dysplasia, dystrophy, or myocarditis? Circulation 1996;94:983–91.
10. Marchlinski FE, Zado E, Dixit S, et al. Electroanatomic substrate and outcome of catheter ablative therapy for ventricular tachycardia in setting of right ventricular cardiomyopathy. Circulation 2004;110:2293–8.
11. Corrado D, Basso C, Thiene G, et al. Spectrum of clinicopathologic manifestations of arrhythmogenic right ventricular cardiomyopathy/dysplasia: a multicenter study. J Am Coll Cardiol 1997;30:1512–20.
12. Wichter T, Hindricks G, Lerch H, et al. Regional myocardial sympathetic dysinnervation in arrhythmogenic right ventricular cardiomyopathy. An analysis using 123I-meta-iodobenzylguanidine scintigraphy. Circulation 1994;89:667–83.
13. Corrado D, Basso C, Rizzoli G, et al. Does sports activity enhance the risk of sudden death in adolescents and young adults? J Am Coll Cardiol 2003;42:1959–63.
14. James CA, Bhonsale A, Tichnell C, et al. Exercise increases age-related penetrance and arrhythmic risk in arrhythmogenic right ventricular dysplasia/cardiomyopathy-associated desmosomal mutation carriers. J Am Coll Cardiol 2013;62:1290–7.
15. Corrado D, Wichter T, Link MS, et al. Treatment of arrhythmogenic right ventricular cardiomyopathy/dysplasia: an international task force consensus statement. Eur Heart J 2015;36:3227–37.
16. Assis FR, Krishnan A, Zhou X, et al. Cardiac sympathectomy for refractory ventricular tachycardia in arrhythmogenic right ventricular cardiomyopathy. Heart Rhythm 2019;16(7):1003–10.
17. Tiso N, Stephan DA, Nava A, et al. Identification of mutations in the cardiac ryanodine receptor gene in families affected with arrhythmogenic right ventricular cardiomyopathy type 2 (ARVD2). Hum Mol Genet 2001;10:189–94.
18. Assis FR, Camm CF, Te Riele ASJM, et al. Nocturnal premature ventricular contraction burden as a marker of disease severity in arrhythmogenic right ventricular cardiomyopathy. JACC Clin Electrophysiol 2017;3:1607–8.
19. Haissaguerre M, Montserrat P, Le PM, et al. Value of the isoprenaline test in arrhythmogenic heart diseases. Arch Mal Coeur Vaiss 1989;82:1845–53.
20. Denis A, Sacher F, Derval N, et al. Diagnostic value of isoproterenol testing in arrhythmogenic right ventricular cardiomyopathy. Circ Arrhythm Electrophysiol 2014;7:590–7.
21. Philips B, Madhavan S, James C, et al. High prevalence of catecholamine-facilitated focal ventricular tachycardia in patients with arrhythmogenic right ventricular dysplasia/cardiomyopathy. Circ Arrhythm Electrophysiol 2013;6:160–6.
22. Bai R, Di Biase L, Shivkumar K, et al. Ablation of ventricular arrhythmias in arrhythmogenic right ventricular dysplasia/cardiomyopathy: arrhythmia-free survival after endo-epicardial substrate based mapping and ablation. Circ Arrhythm Electrophysiol 2011;4:478–85.
23. Frankel DS, Mountantonakis SE, Zado ES, et al. Noninvasive programmed ventricular stimulation early after ventricular tachycardia ablation to predict risk of late recurrence. J Am Coll Cardiol 2012;59:1529–35.
24. Sen-Chowdhry S, Syrris P, Ward D, et al. Clinical and genetic characterization of families with arrhythmogenic right ventricular dysplasia/cardiomyopathy provides novel insights into patterns of disease expression. Circulation 2007;115:1710–20.
25. Bauce B, Basso C, Rampazzo A, et al. Clinical profile of four families with arrhythmogenic right ventricular cardiomyopathy caused by dominant desmoplakin mutations. Eur Heart J 2005;26:1666–75.
26. Boulos M, Lashevsky I, Reisner S, et al. Electroanatomic mapping of arrhythmogenic right ventricular dysplasia. J Am Coll Cardiol 2001;38:2020–7.
27. Thiene G, Basso C, Calabrese F, et al. Pathology and pathogenesis of arrhythmogenic right ventricular cardiomyopathy. Herz 2000;25:210–5.

28. Garcia FC, Bazan V, Zado ES, et al. Epicardial substrate and outcome with epicardial ablation of ventricular tachycardia in arrhythmogenic right ventricular cardiomyopathy/dysplasia. Circulation 2009;120:366–75.

29. Polin GM, Haqqani H, Tzou W, et al. Endocardial unipolar voltage mapping to identify epicardial substrate in arrhythmogenic right ventricular cardiomyopathy/dysplasia. Heart Rhythm 2011;8:76–83.

30. Hsia HH, Callans DJ, Marchlinski FE. Characterization of endocardial electrophysiological substrate in patients with nonischemic cardiomyopathy and monomorphic ventricular tachycardia. Circulation 2003;108:704–10.

31. Tschabrunn CM, Santangeli P, Frankel DS, et al. Isolated epicardial electrogram abnormalities in arrhythmogenic right ventricular cardiomyopathy (ARVC): implications for diagnosis and treatment. Circulation 2019;140:A15876.

32. Berruezo A, Acosta J, Fernandez-Armenta J, et al. Safety, long-term outcomes and predictors of recurrence after first-line combined endoepicardial ventricular tachycardia substrate ablation in arrhythmogenic cardiomyopathy. Impact of arrhythmic substrate distribution pattern. A prospective multicentre study. Europace 2017;19:607–16.

33. Sellal JM, Magnin-Poull I, Battaglia A, et al. First simultaneous endocardial and epicardial mapping of a ventricular tachycardia in an ARVD/C patient. JACC Clin Electrophysiol 2018;4:1265–7.

34. Mussigbrodt A, Efimova E, Knopp H, et al. Should all patients with arrhythmogenic right ventricular dysplasia/cardiomyopathy undergo epicardial catheter ablation? J Interv Card Electrophysiol 2017;48:193–9.

35. Sosa E, Scanavacca M, d'Avila A, et al. A new technique to perform epicardial mapping in the electrophysiology laboratory. J Cardiovasc Electrophysiol 1996;7:531–6.

36. Keramati AR, DeMazumder D, Misra S, et al. Anterior pericardial access to facilitate electrophysiology study and catheter ablation of ventricular arrhythmias: a single tertiary center experience. J Cardiovasc Electrophysiol 2017;28:1189–95.

37. Gale M, Kiwak M, Gale D. Pericardial fluid distribution: CT analysis. Radiology 1987;162:171–4.

38. Haqqani HM, Tschabrunn CM, Betensky BP, et al. Layered activation of epicardial scar in arrhythmogenic right ventricular dysplasia: possible substrate for confined epicardial circuits. Circ Arrhythm Electrophysiol 2012;5:796–803.

39. Cano O, Hutchinson M, Lin D, et al. Electroanatomic substrate and ablation outcome for suspected epicardial ventricular tachycardia in left ventricular nonischemic cardiomyopathy. J Am Coll Cardiol 2009;54:799–808.

40. van Taxis CFvH, Wijnmaalen AP, Piers SR, et al. Real-time integration of MDCT-derived coronary anatomy and epicardial fat: impact on epicardial electroanatomic mapping and ablation for ventricular arrhythmias. JACC Cardiovasc Imaging 2013;6:42–52.

41. Calkins H, Epstein A, Packer D, et al. Catheter ablation of ventricular tachycardia in patients with structural heart disease using cooled radiofrequency energy: results of a prospective multicenter study. J Am Coll Cardiol 2000;35:1905–14.

42. Kottkamp H, Hindricks G, Chen X, et al. Radiofrequency catheter ablation of sustained ventricular tachycardia in idiopathic dilated cardiomyopathy. Circulation 1995;92:1159–68.

43. Soejima K, Stevenson WG, Sapp JL, et al. Endocardial and epicardial radiofrequency ablation of ventricular tachycardia associated with dilated cardiomyopathy: the importance of low-voltage scars. J Am Coll Cardiol 2004;43:1834–42.

44. Stevenson WG, Wilber DJ, Natale A, et al. Irrigated radiofrequency catheter ablation guided by electroanatomic mapping for recurrent ventricular tachycardia after myocardial infarction: the multicenter thermocool ventricular tachycardia ablation trial. Circulation 2008;118:2773–82.

45. Boyle NG, Shivkumar K. Epicardial interventions in electrophysiology. Circulation 2012;126:1752–69.

46. Cardoso R, Assis FR, D'Avila A. Endo-epicardial vs. endocardial only catheter ablation of ventricular tachycardia: a meta-analysis. J Cardiovasc Electrophysiol 2019;30(9):1537–48.

47. Dalal D, Jain R, Tandri H, et al. Long-term efficacy of catheter ablation of ventricular tachycardia in patients with arrhythmogenic right ventricular dysplasia/cardiomyopathy. J Am Coll Cardiol 2007;50:432–40.

48. Tzou WS, Tung R, Frankel DS, et al. Outcomes after repeat ablation of ventricular tachycardia in structural heart disease: an analysis from the International VT Ablation Center Collaborative Group. Heart Rhythm 2017;14:991–7.

49. Verma A, Kilicaslan F, Schweikert RA, et al. Short- and long-term success of substrate-based mapping and ablation of ventricular tachycardia in arrhythmogenic right ventricular dysplasia. Circulation 2005;111:3209–16.

50. Berruezo A, Fernández-Armenta J, Mont L, et al. Combined endocardial and epicardial catheter ablation in arrhythmogenic right ventricular dysplasia incorporating scar dechanneling technique. Circ Arrhythm Electrophysiol 2012;5:111–21.

51. Philips B, Madhavan S, James C, et al. Outcomes of catheter ablation of ventricular tachycardia in arrhythmogenic right ventricular dysplasia/cardiomyopathy. Circ Arrhythm Electrophysiol 2012;5:499–505.

52. Wei W, Liao H, Xue Y, et al. Long-term outcomes of radio-frequency catheter ablation on ventricular tachycardias due to arrhythmogenic right ventricular cardiomyopathy: a single center experience. PLoS One 2017;12:e0169863.

53. Laredo M, Oliveira Da Silva L, Extramiana F, et al. Catheter ablation of electrical storm in patients with arrhythmogenic right ventricular cardiomyopathy. Heart Rhythm 2019;17(1):41–8.

54. Mathew S, Saguner AM, Schenker N, et al. Catheter ablation of ventricular tachycardia in patients with arrhythmogenic right ventricular cardiomyopathy/ dysplasia: a sequential approach. J Am Heart Assoc 2019;8:e010365.

55. Mahida S, Venlet J, Saguner AM, et al. Ablation compared with drug therapy for recurrent ventricular tachycardia in arrhythmogenic right ventricular cardiomyopathy: results from a multicenter study. Heart Rhythm 2019;16:536–43.

Epicardial Ablation in Brugada Syndrome

Pier D. Lambiase, PhD, FRCP, FHRS[a,b,*], Rui Providência, MD, PhD[a,c]

KEYWORDS

- Arrhythmia • Channelopathies • Sudden cardiac death • Repolarization abnormalities
- Depolarization abnormalities • Ventricular fibrillation • Mapping • substrate • Triggers

KEY POINTS

- Catheter ablation in experienced centers should be offered to patients with Brugada syndrome and recurrent ventricular fibrillation episodes.
- Obtaining epicardial access and ablating areas of low-voltage fractionated potentials with ajmaline, flecainide, or procainamide provocation in the epicardial anterior RV and RVOT is required to eliminate these sites.
- This procedure achieved initially good results with 75% to 100% of patients being free from arrhythmia relapse during an average 2- to 3-year follow-up.
- Future studies are required to refine the end point and role of ablation in primary prevention of VF in Brugada syndrome.

 Video content accompanies this article at http://www.cardiacep.theclinics.com.

INTRODUCTION

Brugada syndrome (BrS) is an inherited cardiac condition characterized by a typical electrocardiogram (ECG) signature of coved-type ST-segment elevation in the right precordial leads and ventricular arrhythmias leading to sudden cardiac death, in the absence of unequivocal structural heart disease.[1]

The 2017 North American guidelines recommend that an implantable cardioverter defibrillator (ICD) is offered to patients with spontaneous type 1 Brugada ECG with sustained ventricular arrhythmias or a recent history of syncope presumed caused by ventricular arrhythmias/cardiac arrest and expected meaningful survival of greater than 1 year (class of recommendation I, level of evidence B obtained from nonrandomized trials).[2] The 2015 European Society of Cardiology guidelines also recommended an ICD for patients with a diagnosis of BrS who were survivors of cardiac arrest or had documentation of sustained ventricular tachycardia (class of recommendation I, level of evidence C). Consideration should also be given to patients with spontaneous type 1 ECG and history of syncope (class of recommendation IIa, level of evidence C), or those developing ventricular fibrillation (VF) during programmed ventricular stimulation (class of recommendation IIb, level of evidence C).[3]

In small case series some authors have suggested quinidine as an alternative to the ICD in selected patients,[4,5] or as an option for the prevention of arrhythmic storms.[6] Accordingly, guidelines suggest its use in patients with BrS with malignant arrhythmias who either are not candidates for or decline an ICD, and ICD recipients with recurring events.[2,3]

[a] St Bartholomew's Hospital, Barts Heart Centre, Barts Health NHS Trust, West Smithfield, London EC1A 7BE, UK; [b] Institute of Cardiovascular Science, University College of London, London, UK; [c] Institute of Health Informatics, University College of London, London, UK
* Corresponding author. St Bartholomew's Hospital, Barts Heart Centre, Barts Health NHS Trust, West Smithfield, London EC1A 7BE, UK.
E-mail address: p.lambiase@ucl.ac.uk

Card Electrophysiol Clin 12 (2020) 345–356
https://doi.org/10.1016/j.ccep.2020.04.006

Recent data have demonstrated that catheter ablation is an emerging treatment modality in this patient population. In the recent Expert Consensus on catheter ablation of ventricular arrhythmias, ablation is given a class IIa recommendation (level of evidence B from nonrandomized trials) for patients experiencing recurrent sustained arrhythmia episodes or ICD therapies.[7] The recent North American guidelines for the management of ventricular arrhythmias and prevention of sudden cardiac death assign catheter ablation a class I recommendation (level of evidence B from nonrandomized trials) to the following subsets of patients: patients with BrS and spontaneous type 1 ECG and symptomatic ventricular arrhythmias who are either not candidates to or decline an ICD, and patients with BrS implanted with an ICD and experiencing recurrent ventricular arrhythmia episodes.[2]

In the following review we discuss this treatment option and its evidence base in more detail.

ELECTROPHYSIOLOGIC MECHANISMS IN BRUGADA SYNDROME

The mechanism of the Brugada pattern ECG is still a focus of much debate being broadly categorized into the "depolarization" and "repolarization" hypotheses, respectively. The former explains the ECG pattern based on a phasic difference in depolarization of the right ventricular outflow tract (RVOT) and RV body with the delay between the two promoting a voltage gradient between these sites leading to the coved ST-segment elevation. There is certainly evidence to support this from endocardial mapping studies that have demonstrated marked conduction delays in the RVOT of patients with BrS.[8,9]

The alternative repolarization hypothesis arises from mechanistic studies in the canine wedge preparation that showed that pharmacologically induced action potential duration differences in the epicardium and endocardium result in a transmural repolarization gradient. These gradients are exaggerated by the spike and dome shaped epicardial action potential that is shorter in duration than the endocardial action potential. Epicardial mapping studies have demonstrated that this action potential shortening does exist in humans and promotes the transmural gradients that can induce the Brugada pattern ECG.[10,11] However, for these gradients to be maintained and not eliminated by electrotonic coupling, it is recognized that structural abnormalities in the form of fibrosis enables these gradients to persist and indeed recent data from myocardial biopsies in patients with BrS support this demonstrating the presence of fibrosis and connexin downregulation, which promotes cellular electrical uncoupling.[12] Indeed, these structural changes promote current-load mismatch delaying endoepicardial activation and lead to ST-segment elevation on the ECG in its own right without having to invoke epicardial action potential shortening in the mechanism. Epicardial mapping studies have demonstrated fractionated electrograms, which support discontinuous conduction,[13] although Antzelevitch and Patocskai[14] propose these are explained by localized phase 2 reentry also reproducing a fractionated bipolar signal. That ajmaline promotes more fractionation in the diseased epicardium in patients with BrS strongly supports the depolarization hypothesis with structural abnormalities causing endoepicardial conduction delay. These controversies could be resolved by epi-endocardial mapping studies assessing the effects of pacing and ajmaline on the conduction-repolarization characteristics of the RVOT endocardium and epicardium.[15]

TRIGGER ABLATION USING AN ENDOCARDIAL APPROACH

Haïssaguerre and colleagues[16] were the first to map and ablate VF triggers in patients with BrS with good results leading to changes in VF-inducibility status, and prevention of VF relapse. These three patients with BrS had frequent isolated or repetitive premature beats, which could be mapped to the endocardium of the RVOT or to the anterior RV Purkinje network. However, the occurrence of these triggers is unpredictable and rarely occur spontaneously, which makes this approach applicable only to a small subset of patients.

More recent work from the Bordeaux group has shown that the low-voltage fractionated potentials found in the epicardium could be eliminated in two patients through long periods of endocardial ablation (22–30 minutes of radiofrequency ablation with 30–35 W).[17] In the third case, additional epicardial ablation was required. The same group used the multipolar radiofrequency ablation catheter (nMARQ, Biosense-Webster, Diamond Bar, CA) with 25 W for a mean of 10 minutes, and achieved isolation of the RVOT, elimination of the type 1 Brugada pattern, disappearance of epicardial potentials, and freedom from VF relapse at 2 years follow-up in a series of three patients.[18]

Talib and colleagues[19] have developed a stepwise endocardial ablation approach for treating patients with drug-refractory VF/electrical storm. The first step involved identification and ablation of VF triggers that is ventricular ectopics, and then performing endocardial mapping and ablation of VF substrates. These consisted of ventricular electrograms exhibiting abnormal low-voltage and fractionation. The authors were able to achieve moderate success with freedom from VF relapse in 14 out of 21 patients during a 5-year follow-up.

EPICARDIAL APPROACH: MAPPING THE EPICARDIAL SUBSTRATE

A new epicardial mapping technique was developed in the 1990s by Sosa and colleagues,[20] in Brazil. This group was dealing with the endemic and challenging substrate of Chagas' cardiomyopathy with recurrent ventricular tachycardia despite endocardial ablation. It took nearly 20 years since the description by Sosa and colleagues, but the introduction of the subxiphoid approach to enter the pericardial space was one of the critical steps to make BrS ablation with acceptable efficacy a reality.

Nademanee and colleagues[21] changed the paradigm of catheter ablation for BrS after their landmark 2011 publication. In a series of nine patients with BrS and recurrent ICD therapies for VF, the authors identified unique regions of abnormal low voltage, prolonged electrogram duration, and fractionated late potentials clustering exclusively in the anterior aspect of the RVOT epicardium. **Fig. 1**A provides an example of these potentials and **Fig. 1**B their epicardial distribution in relation to a voltage map. The authors classified this as the substrate for BrS ECG

changes and arrhythmogenicity and concluded that this was proof that the electrophysiologic mechanism in this disease was delayed depolarization. All electrograms in the corresponding endocardial sites were normal. As a proof of this concept, ablation of these sites rendered seven of these patients noninducible (VF was inducible in all before ablation) and normalized the type 1 Brugada ECG pattern in eight cases. Additionally no recurrent events were observed during a 20-month follow-up and all patients, but one, were free from antiarrhythmic drugs.

Brugada and colleagues[22] developed an ablation protocol including drug-challenge with flecainide to unmask the functional substrate of BrS. An increase in the area of low-voltage fractionated components after administering the drug was observed for every patient. After ablation, drug-challenge was used once again to confirm noninducibility of type 1 BrS pattern and hence acute procedural success. In cases where the type 1 pattern was still present further mapping and ablation was performed until the type 1 pattern could not be induced.

With this approach, the authors acutely eradicated the type 1 Brugada pattern in all patients, and the ECG remained normal after median follow-up of 5 months. All patients had ventricular arrhythmias inducible before ablation, but after elimination of the type 1 pattern this was no longer possible despite aggressive ventricular stimulation. During follow-up ICD interrogation showed no arrhythmic events. Subsequently, this group of authors adopted an ajmaline-based approach

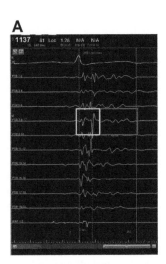
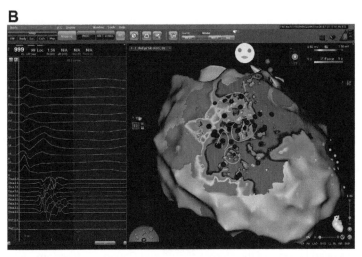

Fig. 1. (*A*) Example of typical epicardial RVOT potentials in patients with Brugada syndrome with high-density mapping (Pentaray, Biosense-Webster). The *yellow box* highlights prolonged depolarization, and the *red box* illustrates what is interpreted as repolarization changes. Complex, fractionated, low-voltage signals observed throughout. (*B*) Distribution of prolonged electrograms in relation to a CARTO epicardial voltage map. The *black dots* represent the sites of the prolonged potentials (See Video 1 for ripple map of activation).

and a CARTO-algorithm allowing them to create potential duration maps in a semiautomated manner to map the area of BrS substrate in 135 patients and confirmed the previously reported preliminary results.[23]

Pappone and colleagues[24] have studied the association of substrate and VF inducibility in a series of 191 patients. They observed that the extension/area of BrS substrate is independently associated with arrhythmia inducibility. The authors identified 4.0 cm^2 as the area cutoff associated with VF inducibility, and suggested that assessing the area of substrate (using ajmaline to induce type 1 pattern if not present at baseline) is used to identify high-risk patients missed by standard clinical criteria.

Ablation may eliminate the typical type 1 Brugada ECG and obliterate the RVOT transmural gradient by two mechanisms: removal of the epicardial layer of shortened action potential cells, or creation of a transmural lesion to obliterate the entire segment of abnormal tissue. In theory the latter would be expected to promote depolarization delay between the RV body and RVOT and exaggerate the Brugada ECG unless a significant area of delay is treated to neutralize it electrophysiologically or the endoepicardial site of current-load mismatch to prevent ST-segment elevation is removed.

CLINICAL EXPERIENCE

We identified nine case series including five or more patients receiving epicardial ablation.[21–23,25–30] All included young populations with mean ages ranging from 37 to 48 years (Table 1). Cohorts were composed mostly, or exclusively, of men, and nearly all patients had had ICDs. Brugada and Pappone ablated more than 50% of patients without previous ICD therapies or documented spontaneously occurring VF before ablation.[22,23]

With regards to ablation protocol, minor differences were observed between the different groups of experts (Table 2). All groups except two[28,30] routinely tested for VF inducibility at the start of the procedure. Substrate ablation was performed exclusively in all but two case series.[26,29] Drug challenge during the procedure was performed in most cohorts, but drugs used for induction of the functional substrate varied: class Ic, ajmaline[23,28–30] and flecainide.[22,26] A class Ia drug, procainamide, was used in some of the studies,[25,27,29] and Chung and colleagues[26] described the use of instilled warm water for the same purpose.

Most groups mapped the epicardium using 3.5-mm nonirrigated catheters. Use of the Pentaray (Biosense-Webster) was reported by two groups,[26,30] the Decanav (Biosense-Webster) was also used in two case series,[29,30] one group reported use of a circular mapping catheter.[29] No consensus was observed in the used ablation settings with power ranging from 30 to 50 W. Ablation duration for each lesion was not commonly reported, and varied from 30 to 120 seconds. Similarly, duration of radiofrequency varied widely even in the same study, going from slightly more than 5 minutes in some cases to beyond 30 minutes in others, which is explained by the differences in the functional substrate area observed in this population (Fig. 2). In most studies ablation was performed exclusively in the epicardium, usually in the anterior RVOT area. Nademanee and colleagues[29] observed that in patients with early repolarization syndrome and BrS, substrate was also frequently present (in nearly 90%) in the RV inferior wall. A minority of patients required additional endocardial ablation (see Table 2).

Three-dimensional mapping was used in all cases, with CARTO 3 being the most frequently used. A minority of cases were performed with Ensite NavX (Abbott).[27,28] Our group has experience ablating one patient using the Rhythmia (Boston Scientific, Marlborough, MA) system,[31] but no further experience has yet been reported.

Most groups perform point-by-point mapping with annotation/tagging of areas of interest. A specific and noncommercially available algorithm for automatic measurement of potential duration, allowing their marking on CARTO (Biosense-Webster) (ie, a potential duration map) was used by Pappone and colleagues.[23] Our group has observed that Ripple Mapping (Biosense-Webster) can be used to identify and delineate the areas of long and low-voltage fractionated electrograms in the RVOT epicardium (Fig. 3, Video 1).[30] Retrospective use of this approach identified other important sites of fractionation that were missed for ablation in a patient who later relapsed.[32]

The acute procedural end point for all cases was elimination of the functional fractionated electrogram drug-induced substrate area and disappearance of the type 1 BrS pattern. Most studies performed a drug challenge at the end to confirm noninducibility of type 1 pattern after substrate ablation. All studies except one tested for VF inducibility postablation.[29]

Mid-term ablation results were good with freedom from ventricular arrhythmia relapse (73%–100%) and type 1 Brugada pattern in most patients (64%–100%), and a minority of patients requiring antiarrhythmic drugs postablation (0%–33%).

Table 1
Clinical experience: epicardial approach for ablation of Brugada syndrome, baselines

Study ID	N, % of Men	Mean Age	Region/Countries	ICD	ICD Therapies or Documented VF Before Ablation	SCN5A Mutation	Spontaneous Type 1 BrS ECG	Use of Quinidine	Other Antiarrhythmic Agents
Nademanee et al,[21] 2011	9 100%	39	Thailand	100%	100%	NS	78%	0%	Amiodarone in 100%
Brugada et al,[22] 2015	14 100%	37	Italy	100%	43%	29%	86%	NS	NS
Zhang et al,[25] 2016	11 100%	48	China, United States	73%	82%	40%	82%	NS	NS
Chung et al,[26] 2017	15 100%	41	Taiwan	NA	100%	20%	53%	NS	NS
Pappone et al,[23] 2017	135 78.5%	39–40	Italy	100%	47%	24%	23%	NS	NS
Shelke et al,[27] 2018	5 80%	29	India	100%	100%	NS	100%	40%	Cilostazol in 100%
Haanschoten et al,[28] 2019	6 83%	43	Netherlands	100%	100%	67%	100%	83%	NS
Nademanee et al,[29] 2019	32 100%	39	Thailand, United States, Japan, France, United Kingdom	100%	92%	19%	64%	27%	NS
Providencia et al,[30] 2019	8 75%	44	Brazil, France, Portugal, United Kingdom	88%	75%	NS	75%	50%	No

Abbreviations: NA, not applicable; NS, not statistically significant.

Table 2
Clinical experience: epicardial approach for ablation of Brugada syndrome, procedural data

Study ID	Ablation of Triggers/Substrate	Ablation Site Epic.	Ablation Site Endo.	Drug Challenge During Procedure	Power Settings (W) and Ablation Catheter	Time per Ablation Lesion (s)	Ablation Time (min)	Mapping System
Nademanee et al,[21] 2011	Substrate	Anterior RVOT (+++) RV	None (all electrograms were normal in the endocardium)	NS	30–50 NaviStar-ThermoCool 3.5-mm tip NaviStar-ThermoCool	NS	6–32	CARTO XP EP Navigation System
Brugada et al,[22] 2015	Substrate	Anterior RV free wall Anterior RVOT	None	Flecainide	Max 40 W NaviStar-ThermoCool 3.5-mm tip NaviStar-ThermoCool	30–60	11–35	CARTO 3
Zhang et al,[25] 2016	Substrate	Anterior RVOT	9%	Propafenone Procainamide	Up to 50 W 3.5-mm tip NaviStar-ThermoCool	NS	NS	CARTO 3
Chung et al,[26] 2017	Substrate + triggers	RVOT	Triggers: 13% LV papillary muscle 20% RVOT	Flecainide Warm water	Max of 40 W in the endocardium and 30 W in the epicardium NaviStar 3.5-mm tip NaviStar ThermoCool or Pentaray	120	Mean, 27.5	CARTO 3
Pappone et al,[23] 2017	Substrate	Anterior RVOT	None	Ajmaline	35–45 Navistar-ThermoCool SF	NS	12–31	CARTO 3 With potential duration mapping software

Study	Strategy	Ablation site	Ablation distribution	Drug challenge	RF settings / catheter				Mapping system
Shelke et al,[27] 2018	Substrate	Anterior RVOT 80% (20% epicardial ablation only)	Ablation in 80%: 60% anterior wall, 20% posterior wall, 20% septum (20% endocardial ablation only)	Procainamide in 60%	Epic: 30 W, 43°C at 2 mL/min Endo: 30 W, 43°C at 30 mL/min Thermocool Celsius Therapy Cool Path	NS	NS	NS	Ensite Navx mapping system CARTO 3 system
Haanschoten et al,[28] 2019	Substrate	Anterior RVOT	17% requiring posteroseptal RVOT ablation	Ajmaline	NS NaviStar, ThermoCool or Smart Touch, or Tacticath	NS	NS	NS	Ensite Navx mapping system CARTO 3 system
Nademanee et al,[29] 2019	Substrate + triggers	Anterior RVOT/RV 100% Inferior RV 85% Post-Lat LV 3%	Triggers: LV-Purkinge system 6% LV-posterior wall 3%	United Kingdom, France, and Thailand: ajmaline United States and Japan: pilsicainide and procainamide	20–50 W ≥5 g Thermocool Celsius, Thermocool SmartTouch, Lasso, Decanav	NS	12–45	NS	CARTO 3
Providencia et al,[30] 2019	Substrate	Anterior RVOT	13% RVOT	Ajmaline in 13%	30–40 Thermocool SmartTouch, Pentaray, Decanav	NS	13–53	NS	CARTO (+ ripple mapping)

Abbreviations: LV, left ventricle; RV, right ventricle; NS, not statistically significant.

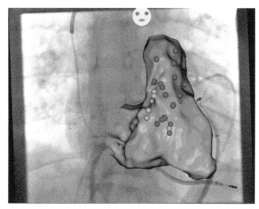

Fig. 2. Extensive epicardial ablation performed in a patient with Brugada syndrome. Visitag (CARTO) lesions in *pink* and *red* projected on the endocardial anatomic map corresponding to a surface area of 27.5 cm² of ablation.

POTENTIAL CAVEATS OF THE EPICARDIAL APPROACH

Since its original description by Sosa and colleagues,[20] the epicardial approach for ablation of arrhythmias has been adopted worldwide in experienced centers. Even though the risk of and severity of complications reported in the literature is not negligible, in this cohort of patients, ablated in experienced centers, side effects were minor and non–life threatening (pericardial complications in a minority of patients) (**Table 3**). The most severe side effect occurred because of ajmaline use to unmask the functional substrate in the RVOT, which in a patient led to electromechanical dissociation and hemodynamic collapse successfully reverted after a short period of resuscitation.[28]

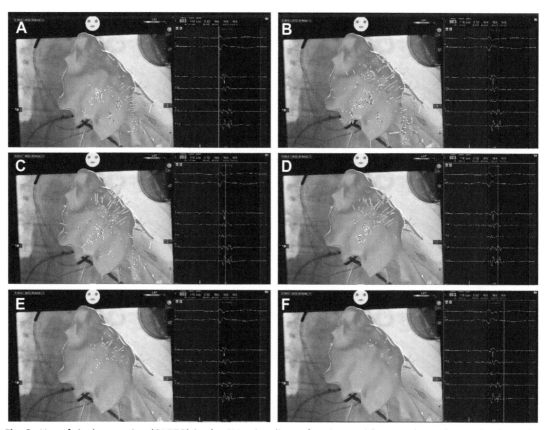

Fig. 3. Use of ripple mapping (CARTO) in the RV epicardium of patients with Brugada syndrome. (*A–F*) Ripples observed during depolarization and repolarization. On the right side of each panel, one can observe the low-voltage, prolonged duration potentials acquired with Decanav catheter (Biosense-Webster) in the epicardium. These are seen during the depolarization (*A–C*) and repolarization phases on the ECG (*D–E*). Unlike in a normal activation/voltage map, where a certain point is only assigned with one timing/voltage decided or chosen on annotation, ripple mapping does not require annotation and choses information for that given special point throughout the cardiac cycle, allowing easy identification and marking of the areas with typical BrS potentials.

Table 3
Clinical experience: epicardial approach for ablation of Brugada syndrome, outcomes

Study ID	VF Inducibility Preablation	VF Inducibility Postablation	Drug Challenge Postablation	Mean Follow-up Duration (mo)	Freedom from Type 1 Brugada Pattern Relapse	Freedom from VT/VF Relapse	Need of AADs After Ablation	Complications
Nademanee et al,[21] 2011	100%	22%	None	20	89%	100%	11%	Mild pericarditis (n = 2)
Brugada et al,[22] 2015	100%	0%	Flecainide	10	100%	100%	NS	Pericarditis (n = 1)
Zhang et al,[25] 2016	100% (n = 9)	0%	Propafenone (n = 9)	25	100%	73%[a]	0%	Pericarditis (n = 2)
Chung et al,[26] 2017	100% (n = 11)	0%	Warm water instillation	3–6	63.6% (n = 11)	93%	0%	None
Pappone et al,[23] 2017	100%	0%	Ajmaline	10	98.5%	99.3%	0%	Pericardial effusion (n = 5)
Shelke et al,[27] 2018	40%	0%	NS	46	100%	80%	NS	Pericarditis (n = 1)
Haanschoten et al,[28] 2019	Not performed	0% (attempted in 4)	Ajmaline	43	67%	83%	33%	Electromechanical dissociation and hemodynamic collapse after ajmaline (n = 1)
Nademanee et al,[29] 2019	73%	15%	NS	27	3%	91%	0%	Hemopericardium (n = 1)
Providencia et al,[30] 2019	Not performed	Not performed	Ajmaline in 50%	22	87.5%	87.5%	0%	Hemopericardium (n = 1)

Abbreviation: AAD, antiarrhythmic drug; NS, not statistically significant; VT, ventricular tachycardia.
[a] One patient refused an ICD and died suddenly 1 y after ablation.

FUTURE PROSPECTS

The role of prophylactic ablation is still a matter of discussion. There is currently an ongoing trial for addressing that matter, the Ablation in Brugada Syndrome for Prevention of VF (BRAVE) trial.[33] This trial plans to enroll 200 patients with BrS implanted with ICD or with an ICD therapy within the last 5 years, and randomize them to ablation versus conventional care, with a follow-up of 3 years. The estimated completion date is July of 2021.

The early repolarization pattern has been associated with idiopathic VF and there are emerging data that the sites of VF drivers correspond to regions of fractionation in the epicardium causing J-point elevation through similar mechanism to the Brugada pattern ECG.[29] In a recent study, Nademanee and colleagues[29] demonstrated that there are two groups of idiopathic VF substrates linked to the early repolarization syndrome/J-wave syndrome: one with late depolarization abnormality as the underlying mechanism of high-amplitude J-wave elevation that predominantly resides in the RVOT and RV inferolateral epicardium (group 1), and the other with pure early repolarization syndrome devoid of VF substrates but with VF triggers that are associated with Purkinje sites (group 2). Ablation was effective in treating symptomatic patients with early repolarization syndrome/J-wave syndrome with frequent VF episodes. In this study the sites of abnormal fractionated electrograms were eliminated by ablation of the epicardial sites using the same ablation settings as in Brugada substrates described previously. Using ECG imaging they demonstrated that late depolarization areas colocalize with VF drivers.

A Brugada pattern ECG was present in most patients in category 1 (33 patients), who were then classified as group 1A. The remaining seven patients in group 1, category 1B, did not have a Brugada type 1 ECG pattern, and the late depolarization abnormalities were located mostly in the RV inferior wall. Ablation results in this series of patients with early repolarization were good, with only 3 of the 33 patients with Brugada ECG receiving ablation presenting with VF relapse, and all of the five patients in group 1B and six in group 2 receiving ablation remaining free from sustained ventricular arrhythmias.

SUMMARY

- Catheter ablation is useful for reducing the arrhythmia burden in patients with BrS with recurring episodes of VF. The BRAVE trial (NCT02704416) will examine the role of prophylactic ablation in Brugada patients.

- Even though the epicardial approach has been associated with severe complications, no fatal event or major complications were observed in our review of the literature, which included highly experienced centers.
- A drug challenge with class Ic agents is frequently required for mapping the full-extent of the target area.
- Controversy still exists regarding the procedural end point of catheter ablation of BrS, but complete eradication and ablation of the functional substrate should be achieved. Ideally this should lead to the disappearance of the type 1 ECG pattern.
- Debate still exists regarding eradication of the type 1 Brugada pattern and achieving VF non-inducibility at the end of the procedure and their meaning. However, our literature search showed that patients where these acute end points were achieved can still experience VF relapse during follow-up.[29]

DISCLOSURE

P.D. Lambiase receives educational grants and speaker fees from Abbott Medical, Boston Scientific, and Medtronic. He is supported by UCLH Biomedicine NIHR and Barts BRC.

SUPPLEMENTARY DATA

Supplementary data related to this article can be found online at https://doi.org/10.1016/j.ccep. 2020.04.006.

REFERENCES

1. Brugada P, Brugada J. Right bundle branch block, persistent ST segment elevation and sudden cardiac death: a distinct clinical and electrocardiographic syndrome. A multicenter report. J Am Coll Cardiol 1992;20:1391–6.
2. Al-Khatib SM, Stevenson WG, Ackerman MJ, et al. 2017 AHA/ACC/HRS guideline for management of patients with ventricular arrhythmias and the prevention of sudden cardiac death. Circulation 2018;138: e272–391.
3. Priori SG, Blomström-Lundqvist C, Mazzanti A, et al. 2015 ESC guidelines for the management of patients with ventricular arrhythmias and the prevention of sudden cardiac death: the task force for the management of patients with ventricular arrhythmias and the prevention of sudden cardiac death of the European Society of Cardiology (ESC) Endorsed by: Association for European Paediatric and Congenital Cardiology (AEPC). Europace 2015;17: 1601–87.

4. Belhassen B, Rahkovich M, Michowitz Y, et al. Management of Brugada syndrome: thirty-three-year experience using electrophysiologically guided therapy with class 1A antiarrhythmic drugs. Circ Arrhythm Electrophysiol 2015;8:1393–402.

5. Bouzeman A, Traulle S, Messali A, et al. Long-term follow-up of asymptomatic Brugada patients with inducible ventricular fibrillation under hydroquinidine. Europace 2014;16:572–7.

6. Márquez MF, Bonny A, Hernández-Castillo E, et al. Long-term efficacy of low doses of quinidine on malignant arrhythmias in Brugada syndrome with an implantable cardioverter-defibrillator: a case series and literature review. Heart Rhythm 2012;9: 1995–2000.

7. Cronin EM, Bogun FM, Maury P, et al. 2019 HRS/EHRA/APHRS/LAHRS expert consensus statement on catheter ablation of ventricular arrhythmias. Heart Rhythm 2019;21(8):1143–4.

8. Lambiase PD, Ahmed AK, Ciaccio EJ, et al. High-density substrate mapping in Brugada syndrome: combined role of conduction and repolarization heterogeneities in arrhythmogenesis. Circulation 2009; 120(106–17):1–4.

9. Postema PG, van Dessel PF, de Bakker JM, et al. Slow and discontinuous conduction conspire in Brugada syndrome: a right ventricular mapping and stimulation study. Circ Arrhythm Electrophysiol 2008;1:379–86.

10. Nagase S, Kusano KF, Morita H, et al. Epicardial electrogram of the right ventricular outflow tract in patients with the Brugada syndrome: using the epicardial lead. J Am Coll Cardiol 2002;39:1992–5.

11. Bhar-Amato J, Finlay M, Santos D, et al. Pharmacological modulation of right ventricular endocardial-epicardial gradients in Brugada syndrome. Circ Arrhythm Electrophysiol 2018;11:e006330.

12. Nademanee K, Raju H, de Noronha SV, et al. Fibrosis, connexin-43, and conduction abnormalities in the Brugada syndrome. J Am Coll Cardiol 2015; 66:1976–86.

13. Zhang J, Sacher F, Hoffmayer K, et al. Cardiac electrophysiological substrate underlying the ECG phenotype and electrogram abnormalities in Brugada syndrome patients. Circulation 2015;131: 1950–9.

14. Antzelevitch C, Patocskai B. Brugada syndrome: clinical, genetic, molecular, cellular, and ionic aspects. Curr Probl Cardiol 2016;41:7–57.

15. Sacher F, Jesel L, Jais P, et al. Insight into the mechanism of Brugada syndrome: epicardial substrate and modification during ajmaline testing. Heart Rhythm 2014;11:732–4.

16. Haïssaguerre M, Extramiana F, Hocini M, et al. Mapping and ablation of ventricular fibrillation associated with long-QT and Brugada syndromes. Circulation 2003;108:925–8.

17. Sacher F, Derval N, Denis A, et al. Endocardial Brugada syndrome ablation to eliminate epicardial substrate. Heart Rhythm 2015;12(Suppl):S135–6.

18. Hocini M, Denis A, Shah A, et al. Elimination of Brugada syndrome phenotype by endocardial ablation using novel multipolar RF ablation catheter. Heart Rhythm 2016;13(Suppl):S94.

19. Talib AK, Takagi M, Shimane A, et al. Efficacy of endocardial ablation of drug-resistant ventricular fibrillation in Brugada syndrome. Circ Arrhythm Electrophysiol 2018;11:e005631.

20. Sosa E, Scanavacca M, d'Avila A, et al. A new technique to perform epicardial mapping in the electrophysiology laboratory. J Cardiovasc Electrophysiol 1996;7:531–6.

21. Nademanee K, Veerakul G, Chandanamattha P, et al. Prevention of ventricular fibrillation episodes in Brugada syndrome by catheter ablation over the anterior right ventricular outflow tract epicardium. Circulation 2011;123:1270–9.

22. Brugada J, Pappone C, Berruezo A, et al. Brugada syndrome phenotype elimination by epicardial substrate ablation. Circ Arrhythm Electrophysiol 2015; 8:1373–81.

23. Pappone C, Brugada J, Vicedomini G, et al. Electrical substrate elimination in 135 consecutive patients with Brugada syndrome. Circ Arrhythm Electrophysiol 2017;10:e005053.

24. Pappone C, Ciconte G, Manguso F, et al. Assessing the malignant ventricular arrhythmic substrate in patients with Brugada syndrome. J Am Coll Cardiol 2018;71:1631–46.

25. Zhang P, Tung R, Zhang Z, et al. Characterization of the epicardial substrate for catheter ablation of Brugada syndrome. Heart Rhythm 2016;13:2151–8.

26. Chung FP, Raharjo SB, Lin YJ, et al. A novel method to enhance phenotype, epicardial functional substrates, and ventricular tachyarrhythmias in Brugada syndrome. Heart Rhythm 2017;14:508–17.

27. Shelke A, Tachil A, Saggu D, et al. Catheter ablation for electrical storm in Brugada syndrome: results of substrate based ablation. Indian Heart J 2018;70: 296–302.

28. Haanschoten DM, Elvan A, Postema PG, et al. Catheter ablation in highly symptomatic Brugada patients: a Dutch case series. Clin Res Cardiol 2019. https://doi.org/10.1007/s00392-019-01540-9.

29. Nademanee K, Haissaguerre M, Hocini M, et al. Mapping and ablation of ventricular fibrillation associated with early repolarization syndrome. Circulation 2019;140:1477–90.

30. Providencia R, Cavaco D, Waintraub X, et al. Ripple-mapping for the identification of ablation targets in Brugada syndrome. (under review).

31. Providência R, Carmo P, Moscoso Costa F, et al. Brugada syndrome is associated with scar and endocardial involvement: Insights from high-

density mapping with the Rhythmia™ mapping system. Rev Port Cardiol 2017;36:773.e1-4.

32. Providencia R, Cavaco D, Carmo P, et al. Ripple-mapping for the detection of long duration action potential areas in patients with Brugada syndrome. BioRxiv 2018. https://doi.org/10.1101/263145.

33. A randomized, Multi-center study of epicardial ablation in Brugada syndrome patients to prevent arrhythmia recurrence. Ablation in Brugada syndrome for the prevention of VF (BRAVE). Available at: https://clinicaltrials.gov/ct2/show/NCT02704416. Assessed November 1, 2019.

Epicardial Ablation of Supraventricular Tachycardias

Martin Aguilar, MD[a], Usha B. Tedrow, MD, MSc[a,b,c,d],*

KEYWORDS

• Supraventricular tachycardia • Catheter ablation • Epicardial access

KEY POINTS

• Epicardial mapping and ablation is uncommonly required for successful catheter ablation of supraventricular tachycardia.
• Accessory pathways may require epicardial mapping and ablation when pathways involve the musculature of the coronary sinus or have appendage-to-ventricle connections.
• The coronary sinus gives off a middle cardiac vein branch that passes perpendicularly to the posterior left ventricular coronary artery in many patients. Ablation in this region can produce coronary occlusion if the operator is not careful.
• It is important to understand the anatomic relationship of the phrenic nerve, coronary sinus, as well as right and left atria, when approaching atrial tachycardias.

INTRODUCTION

Supraventricular arrhythmias (SVTs) are the most common arrhythmias encountered in clinical practice with an estimated incidence of 35/100,000 person-years in the general population.[1] SVT subtypes have well-characterized age- and sex-specific distributions.[2–4] Early in the experience of electrophysiology as a field, epicardial surgical mapping played a major role in the advancement of our understanding of the pathophysiology of cardiac arrhythmias and was also the treatment-of-choice for patients with SVTs refractory to medical therapy.[5–7] Advancements in catheter-based techniques have long since supplanted surgical mapping/ablation as first-line invasive treatment. Today, SVTs are among the most common arrhythmias treated in the cardiac electrophysiology laboratory. The proportion of patients treated with catheter ablation is highly variable and modulated by arrhythmia risk, patient age, symptoms, and comorbidities. As a representative example, half the study population received ablation in a contemporary series of patients with the Wolff-Parkinson-White syndrome.[8] Endocardial catheter ablation for SVT is an appealing strategy because it is a potentially curative treatment with a procedural success rate in excess of 95% in experienced centers.[9] The risk of major complication during SVT ablation, such as vascular complications (bleeding and thrombosis), heart block, cardiac tamponade and, rarely, injury to the coronary arteries and/or phrenic nerves, is as low as 0.8% in contemporary series.[10] Despite the excellent safety and efficacy profile of endocardial procedures, a minority of patients with SVT will have unsuccessful ablation. The reasons for failure vary according to the arrhythmia location and mechanism as well as individual operator concern

[a] Cardiovascular Division, Brigham and Women's Hospital, 75 Francis Street, Boston, MA 02115, USA;
[b] Harvard Medical School; [c] Clinical Cardiac Electrophysiology Fellowship; [d] Ventricular Arrhythmia Program
* Corresponding author. Cardiovascular Division, Brigham and Women's Hospital, Harvard Medical School, 75 Francis Street, Boston, MA 02115.
E-mail address: utedrow@bwh.harvard.edu
Twitter: @utedrow (U.B.T.)

Card Electrophysiol Clin 12 (2020) 357–369
https://doi.org/10.1016/j.ccep.2020.05.001

regarding damage to adjacent structures, such as the phrenic nerve or coronary arteries. Percutaneous epicardial access with mapping and ablation is a valuable treatment strategy for patients with SVT refractory to endocardial ablation and may allow safe therapy for patients with higher risk arrhythmia locations.

ANATOMIC CONSIDERATIONS SPECIFIC TO EPICARDIAL ABLATION OF SUPRAVENTRICULAR ARRHYTHMIA

Percutaneous epicardial access was first used for ablation of ventricular tachycardia in patients with Chagas disease and is now commonly used in ischemic and nonischemic cardiomyopathies.[11] The anatomy and techniques for access of the epicardial space are reviewed in detail in an accompanying article. Some anatomic considerations specific to epicardial ablation of SVT are discussed here.

In the absence of pericardial adhesions, the ventricular epicardium forms a continuous and uninterrupted virtual space between the visceral and parietal layers of the pericardium. Conversely the atrial epicardial space is interrupted by reflections (the oblique and transverse sinuses) of the pericardium onto neighboring thoracic structures, limiting the free movement of mapping/ablation catheters. The oblique sinus reflects inferoposteriorly on the inferior pulmonary veins, the anterior aspect of the descending aorta, and the inferior vena cava; it can be identified on transthoracic echocardiogram as the space between the posterior left atrium (LA) and the aorta on the parasternal long-axis view (versus posterior to the aorta in the case of a left pleural effusion).[12] The transverse sinus connects the superior pulmonary veins and reflects on the LA roof and ascending aorta. The pericardial reflections restrict access to the posterior LA, which is not covered by pericardium.

Critical structures may also be close to desirable sites for ablation. The right phrenic nerve (RPN) borders the superior vena cava (SVC)-right atrial (RA) junction and is in close proximity to the right superior pulmonary vein as it courses inferiorly to contact the right hemidiaphragm. The left phrenic nerve (LPN) borders the left lateral aspect of the aortic arch and pulmonary trunk before coursing in close proximity to the left atrial appendage (LAA) and over the lateral left ventricle (LV). The left circumflex coronary courses along the left atrioventricular groove and may bear a close relationship with the LAA and the LPN. The posterior left ventricular branch of the right coronary artery courses along the posterior interventricular septum and often is in close proximity to the

coronary sinus (CS) and/or its proximal tributaries. The coronary vasculature is therefore susceptible to injury with ablation in the CS or from the epicardium. Epicardial ablation may be paradoxically unsuccessful as these structures may be covered by variable amounts of epicardial fat, limiting energy delivery.

The optimal approach (anterior versus posterior versus lateral) for epicardial access depends on the anatomic location of the substrate of interest for mapping/ablation. The anterior approach may be better suited to access the RA appendage (RAA) and anterior/anterolateral tricuspid annulus. Conversely, posteroseptal and CS accessory pathways (APs) may be more readily accessible from a posterior approach. In the absence of pericardial adhesions, the LAA may be reached from either the anterior or the posterior approach, although the anterior approach has been favored for percutaneous epicardial LAA occlusion. The anterior approach is increasingly used for most epicardial access and, in the absence of adhesions, can reach all the areas necessary for SVT ablation.

EPICARDIAL ABLATION OF ACCESSORY PATHWAYS

The first surgical division of an AP was performed by Sealy and colleagues[5] in 1968 in a patient with a right-lateral bypass tract refractory to medical therapy. However, catheter ablation with radiofrequency energy has emerged as a safe and highly effective treatment and has supplanted surgery since the late 1980s as first-line therapy for symptomatic or high-risk APs. However, a minority of patients will have unsuccessful endocardial procedures. In a series of 619 patients referred for AP ablation, 51 (8%) had prolonged or failed endocardial ablation.[13] The most common reasons for failure were (1) catheter-related (inability to position the catheter at the target site or unstable catheter position), (2) errors in pathway localization, or (3) an epicardial location of the AP (5 of 51 patients [8% of failures]).[13] Sacher and colleagues[14] reported a similar incidence of epicardial APs (8 [8%] of 89 patients) in a more contemporary series of patients with previous failed endocardial ablation. The CS and its tributaries can provide transvenous access to a limited portion of the epicardium. In addition, patients with CS diverticula or an enlarged CS may harbor muscular AP connections.[15] Haissaguerre and colleagues[7] first described a series of 8 patients with left-sided APs and failed endocardial ablation who were successfully ablated from the CS with no major complication. Several series have since replicated these findings[16-20] and CS ablation is now a commonly used strategy when annular endocardial sites fail. In addition to concerns about potential coronary injury, the coronary venous circulation is anatomically constrained and does not give access to large portions of the epicardial surface, and percutaneous epicardial access can be required for successful ablation.[21] Not all AP locations have the same propensity for requiring epicardial access for successful ablation; almost all the reported cases mapped and/or ablated from the epicardial space are (1) posteroseptal APs and (2) atrial appendage-to-ventricle APs.

Posteroseptal Accessory Pathways

Posteroseptal APs course in the posterior atrioventricular sulcus or crux of the heart, an anatomically complex region formed by the continuation of the tricuspid and mitral AV annuli.[22] Electrocardiographically, posteroseptal APs are characterized by a negative delta wave in leads II and III, with the former being highly associated with subepicardial tracts (100% specific and sensitive in 1 report, **Fig. 1**C).[23] In a seminal series, posteroseptal APs represented 43 (26%) of 177 AP variants in symptomatic patients, and most (40 [93%] of 43 APs) were successfully ablated from the endocardium.[24] Nevertheless, these represent the most common AP variant associated with challenging or failed endocardial ablation. This may be, at least in part, related to the potential for complex myocardial sleeve-like connections surrounding the CS and its branches, which may electrically connect the adjacent atrial and ventricular myocardium. These connections can occur in a location that is anatomically displaced from the valve annuli, making successful mapping and ablation quite challenging. These sleeve-like connections occur most commonly in the region of the middle cardiac vein, but can occur in more distal branches as well (**Fig. 1**A).[15] Importantly, most CS APs are not associated with a CS diverticulum, hence, a normal CS anatomy does not exclude the presence of such an AP.[15] Attention must be paid however to the course of the coronary arteries when mapping near the middle cardiac vein or in CS diverticula (**Fig. 1**B). The posterior left ventricular coronary artery often crosses the middle cardiac vein in a perpendicular fashion and is very susceptible to injury from radiofrequency energy.

In 2001, Sapp and colleagues[25] were the first to report on their attempt at percutaneous epicardial ablation of a rapidly conducting posteroseptal AP in a 60-year-old man with preexcited atrial fibrillation (AF) and failed endocardial ablation. Acute procedural success with epicardial ablation was achieved but AP conduction recovered within hours. The procedure was complicated by intraperitoneal bleeding requiring blood transfusion; the patient ultimately underwent successful surgical division of his AP. Saad and colleagues[26] mapped an epicardial posteroseptal AP in a 46-year-old woman with preexcited AF and failed endocardial ablation. However, epicardial ablation was limited by impedance rises; successful ablation was achieved by treating around the neck of a large CS diverticulum endocardially. Finally, the first truly successful epicardial ablation of a posteroseptal AP was reported in 2004 by de Paola and colleagues[27] in a 57-year-old man with preexcited AF and failed endocardial ablation; the APs was interrupted with a single epicardial lesion without complication. Other case reports of successful epicardial ablation for posterolateral APs have been published.[28-30]

Since these original single-case reports, many case series have been published. Schweikert and colleagues reported a series of 18 patients referred after failed endocardial SVT ablation in which epicardial mapping/ablation was performed. Of the 18 patients, 5 had posteroseptal APs (2 right posterolateral, 2 left posteroseptal, 1 left posterolateral) of which 2 (40%) were found to have earliest activation in the epicardium.[31] However, none could be ablated from the epicardium and all had successful endocardial ablation; no complications from epicardial access were reported.[32] Subsequently, Valderrabano and colleagues[33] reported a series of 32 patients referred for failed AP ablation; epicardial mapping was performed in 6 (18%) patients. Of the 6 patients, 2 (33%) were successfully ablated from the epicardium (right free wall and right posteroseptal APs), whereas the other 4 (66%) were successfully ablated from the endocardial after refining the location of the AP with epicardial mapping. Finally, Scanavacca and colleagues[34] reported the largest series of epicardial mapping/ablation in 21 patients with previous failed AP ablation, most (90%) of which were posteroseptal APs. Overall, earliest activation was found to be in the epicardium in 6 (29%) patients, in the endocardium in 9 (43%) patients, and equally early on the epicardium versus endocardium in 3 (14%) patients; an early site could not be identified in 3 (14%) patients. Of the 6 patients with earliest activation in the epicardium, all (100%) underwent successful epicardial ablation. Two (66%) of the 3 patients with equal epi- versus endocardial activation had successful epicardial-guided endocardial ablation. Four (19%) patients required surgical interruption of their APs. Non-

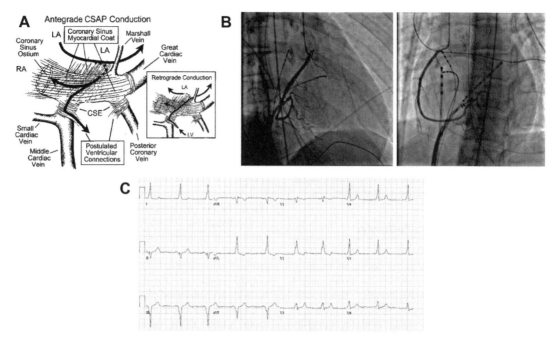

Fig. 1. (*A*) Proposed anatomic basis of CS atrioventricular connections. The CS and its proximal tributaries are surrounded by electrically active muscular sleeves, the CS extensions (CSE), connecting the atrial and ventricular myocardium.[15] (*B*) Anatomic relationship between the posteroseptal coronary arterial and venous circulation. Right anterior oblique coronary artery (RAO) (*left*) and left anterior oblique coronary artery (LAO) (*right*) fluoroscopic projections of the right coronary artery with a decapolar catheter in the middle cardiac vein (MCV) and the ablation catheter at the site of successful ablation for a posteroseptal accessory pathway. Note the close proximity of the site of earliest activation, the MCV, and the posterior left ventricular coronary artery. (*C*) A 12-lead ECG example of a posteroseptal accessory pathway preexcitation pattern. Note the negative deflections in leads II and III in this example. The AP was ablated within the MCV. ([*A*] *From* Sun Y, Arruda M, Otomo K, Beckman K, Nakagawa H, Calame J, et al. Coronary sinus-ventricular accessory connections producing posteroseptal and left posterior accessory pathways: incidence and electrophysiological identification. Circulation. 2002;106(11):1362-7; with permission.)

posteroseptal AP locations were never associated with early activation in the epicardium.

In summary, we have identified 6 single-case reports of which 4 (66%) reported successful epicardial ablation.[25,26,28–30] In the case series, a total of 32 APs were reported, with 8 (25%) successful epicardial ablations; these are summarized in **Fig. 2**.[32–34] The discrepancy between the yield of epicardial ablation between case reports and case series may be in part related to publication bias. The complication rate was low with a total of 5 epicardial access-related complications (13%; 1 hemoperitoneum, 1 hemopericardium, and 3 case of pericarditis) in the 38 reported patients, all of which were treated conservatively.[25,34] This seems to be an acceptable tradeoff for patients who would otherwise have required open-chest surgery.

The above-cited yield of epicardial ablation of approximately 25% likely underestimates the usefulness of epicardial access. In many cases, endocardial ablation was successful only after mapping the epicardium, so-called epicardial-guided endocardial ablation. The main benefit of epicardial mapping for endocardial ablation in these cases is likely related to a better localization of the AP. In fact, erroneous AP localization with endocardial mapping is a common reason for failure.[13] The value of epicardial-guided endocardial ablation has been well documented in patients with ventricular arrhythmias.[31] Furthermore, the presence of a catheter buttressing the AP from the epicardial side may allow for better endocardial contact and more effective energy delivery. Finally, there is experimental evidence that metallic objects in the vicinity of the ablation catheter act as heat sinks.[35] Hence, the presence of a mapping catheter in the epicardial space may potentiate current delivery to the AP. Some of these cases may also have been aided by smaller multielectrode catheters allowing for more detailed evaluation of the region of AP insertion.

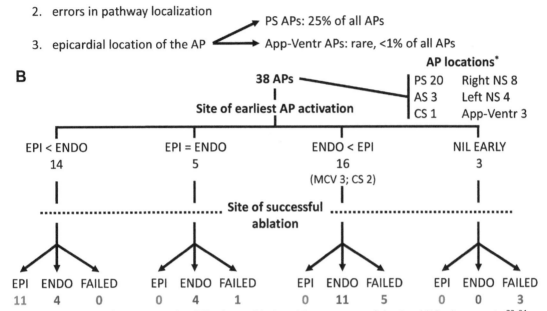

A
Reasons for prolonged/failed endocardial ablation (~8% of APs)

1. catheter-related
   a. inability to position the catheter at the target site
   b. unstable catheter position

2. errors in pathway localization

   PS APs: 25% of all APs

3. epicardial location of the AP

   App-Ventr APs: rare, <1% of all APs

AP locations*

B   **38 APs**

PS 20	Right NS 8
AS 3	Left NS 4
CS 1	App-Ventr 3

Site of earliest AP activation

EPI < ENDO	EPI = ENDO	ENDO < EPI	NIL EARLY
14	5	16	3
		(MCV 3; CS 2)	

Site of successful ablation

EPI	ENDO	FAILED	EPI	ENDO	FAILED	EPI	ENDO	FAILED	EPI	ENDO	FAILED
11	4	0	0	4	1	0	11	5	0	0	3

Fig. 2. (*A*) Summary of the reasons for difficult AP ablation. (*B*) Aggregate of the 3 published case series[32–34] on difficult/failed AP ablation summarizing the sites of successful ablation is relationship to the sites earliest AP activation. *some APs had more than 1 reported location. App-Ventr, appendage-to-ventricle; AS, anteroseptal; CS, coronary sinus; ENDO, endocardial; EPI, epicardial; MCV, middle cardiac vein; NS, nonseptal; PS, posteroseptal; some APs had more than 1 reported location.

One may potentially have expected a higher success rate of epicardial ablation for epicardial posteroseptal APs. However, the crux of the heart is covered by abundant amounts of epicardial fat, effectively shielding the myocardium from the ablation catheter. Moreover, part of the coronary arterial circulation courses in the posteroseptum such that there is a potential risk of coronary artery injury during ablation in this region. In 1 series, ablation within 2 mm of a coronary artery was associated with a 50% risk of coronary injury, whereas no patient with ablation at greater than 5 mm had evidence of coronary injury.[36] Intraprocedural imaging of the coronary arteries should be considered when ablation in the CS/posteroseptal epicardium is planned. In cases in whom the proximity of the target ablation site to an artery is prohibitive, cryoablation may also be considered. Efficacy of cryoablation in adults is likely lower than radiofrequency ablation, with more acute pathway recovery and unidirectional block. More data are also needed regarding the long-term safety of cryoablation performed very close to coronary arteries.

Atria Appendage-to-Ventricle Accessory Pathways

Atrial appendage-to-ventricle APs are a rare form of AP variants representing less than 1% of all APs. These APs course along the epicardium, some distance from the AV annulus, making for an AP variant for which endocardial ablation may be challenging. The first 2 reported cases of atrial appendage-to-ventricle connections were in patients with congenital tricuspid atresia in whom the Fontan RA-to-right ventricle (RV) surgical anastomosis created an iatrogenic bypass tract; interestingly, both patients were successfully treated with endocardial catheter ablation.[37,38] Milstein and colleagues[39] were the first to report a noniatrogenic RAA-to-RV AP in a 42-year-old patient with orthodromic reentrant tachycardia and failed endocardial ablation requiring surgery. Intraoperatively a discrete bridge of tissue connecting the base of the RAA to the RV was identified and successfully severed. Mah and colleagues[40] described a series of 3 young patients (1 LAA-to-LV AP; 2 biatrial appendage-to-ventricle APs) with unsuccessful endocardial ablation who also required surgery. Contrary to the observations of Milstein and colleagues, these patients were found to have their atrial appendages diffusely adherent to the ventricular epicardium and extensive surgical dissection was required in all cases.

Many groups have reported a total of 6 cases with successful endocardial catheter ablation for R/LAA-to-R/LV APs[41–45]; epicardial mapping was performed in 3 of the 6 cases but ablation from the epicardium was unsuccessful.[44,45] Despite acutely effective endocardial ablation, a common limitation noted in the published experience is that power delivery is often limited by impedance increases from low blood flow velocities and complex trabeculations in the appendage. In 1 case, exchanging from a 4- to an 8-mm catheter allowed for successfully endocardial ablation,[41] whereas in another case several lower-energy applications interrupted AP conduction.[42] We have identified 4 cases of atrial appendage-to-ventricular AP successfully ablated from the epicardium, all of which were right-sided and presented with manifest pre-excitation.[21,32] Overall, of the 10 reported cases of atrial appendage-to-ventricle APs, 6 had epicardial mapping, of which 2 had unsuccessful epicardial ablation (all LAA-to-LV APs) and 4 had successful epicardial ablation (all RAA-to-RV APs); 6 APs were successfully ablated from the endocardium.

Anatomic factors likely account for some of the reported failures of epicardial ablation for atrial appendage-to-ventricle APs. First, some have reported that the appendage and respective ventricle can be diffusely adherent, making catheter ablation challenging.[21] Second, the significant variability in the anatomy of the atrial appendage, especially the LAA, such that part of the appendage may actually cover the atrioventricular groove and protect the AP from an epicardial ablation catheter. Finally, the left circumflex coronary artery and LPN course in close proximity to potential ablation sites on the LAA. In summary, atrial appendage-to-ventricular APs are rare and many can be successfully treated from the endocardium. Epicardial ablation remains a useful strategy in patients with failed endocardial procedures.

EPICARDIAL ABLATION OF ATRIAL TACHYCARDIAS

Atrial tachycardias (ATs) are a heterogeneous group of arrhythmias. Most ATs can be successfully treated with endocardial ablation in the thin-walled atria. Nevertheless, epicardial access may be useful in the subset of patients with failed endocardial procedures. LAA ATs and inappropriate sinus tachycardia (IST) are the 2 AT variants for which epicardial mapping and ablation has been reported in the contemporary literature.

Left Atrial Appendage Tachycardias

The LAA is a relatively unusual site for focal ATs: only found in 7 (3%) of 232 AT variants in a series of patients with symptomatic AT.[46] Electrocardiographically, the P wave morphology is positive in the inferior leads and positive or biphasic in V1; the finding of negative P waves in leads I and aVL has been shown to have good sensitivity (92.3%) and specificity (97.3%) for an LAA origin (**Fig. 3**).[47,48] The mechanism of LAA ATs tends to be automatic, being elicited by isoproterenol, rather than reentrant.[46] We have identified a total of 14 cases of LAA ATs with successful endocardial ablation in the published literature; 2 had recurrences and no complications were reported (**Fig. 4**).[30,46,48] These ATs present site-specific challenges to endocardial ablation similar to those described above for LAA-to-LV APs, which include reduced LAA flows limiting effective energy delivery to the tissue and proximity to the LPN and left circumflex coronary artery. Furthermore, the LAA is a trabeculated and thin-walled structure making catheter manipulation challenging and associated with an increased risk of perforation.[49]

A total of 3 cases of LAA ATs requiring epicardial mapping and/or ablation have been reported.[50,51] All 3 patients were young (age 14–27 years) with incessant tachycardia and multiple failed endocardial procedures. In 2 patients, the site of earliest activation was mapped to the epicardium (anterolateral LAA and tip of LAA); both had successful epicardial radiofrequency ablation. In 1 patient, the LAA roof endocardium was found to have a slightly earlier activation than the epicardium and the AT was successfully ablated from the endocardium. The authors, however, note that epicardium mapping was key in refining the earliest site and providing counterpressure from the epicardium for optimal endocardial tissue contact.[51] No recurrence or complications were reported. In summary, LAA ATs are a rare AT variant for which endocardial ablation is often effective; epicardial access can assist in endocardial ablation or serve as an alternative ablation approach in patients in whom an endocardial approach was unsuccessful.

Inappropriate Sinus Tachycardia

Endocardial sinus node modification is a therapeutic option for patients with IST refractory to medical therapy. IST is another AT variant for which

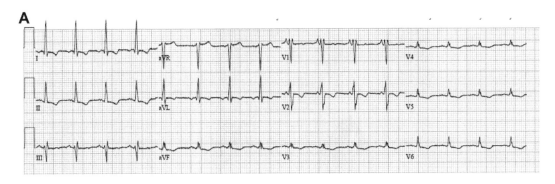

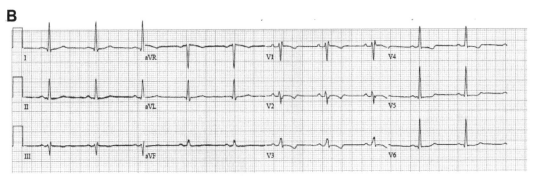

Fig. 3. Surface electrocardiogram of a 54-year-old woman with iron overload cardiomyopathy and incessant LAA tachycardia (*A*) and in sinus rhythm (*B*). Contrast the normal P wave axis in sinus rhythm with the negative P waves in I and aVL during tachycardia, compatible with the LAA origin.

epicardial mapping/activation has been described. However, the sinus node is a subepicardial structure located in a relatively thick part of the RA such that endocardial ablation may be ineffective. Koplan and colleagues[47] reported a highly symptomatic patient with IST refractory to medical therapy and unsuccessful endocardial sinus node modification. Epicardial access was obtained through a subxiphoid approach and the phrenic nerve course was identified with high-output pacing; epicardial radiofrequency sinus node modification was achieved without complication. The patient recurred and required a repeat endocardial procedure. In their series, Schweikert and colleagues[32] reported on 4 cases of IST for which epicardial mapping was performed. Of these 4 patients, 2 had the site of earliest activation mapped to the epicardium and only 1 was successfully ablated on the epicardial surface. Of the 3 patients undergoing endocardial ablation, 2 recurred, highlighting the challenges in ablation for IST. Limitations of epicardial ablation for IST include the added risk associated with epicardial access, and the risk of RPN injury and of SVC syndrome. In addition, novel targeted medications, such as ivabradine that block the sinus node "funny" current specifically targeting pacemaking cells may prove to render this therapy

unnecessary. In summary, the yield of epicardial access for IST ablation appears low but may be offered in patients with debilitating symptoms refractory to medical therapy and endocardial ablation.

Ligament of Marshall-Related Tachycardias

There has been a growing recognition of the role played by the ligament of Marshall (LOM) in atrial arrhythmogenesis. The LOM has been found to harbor AF-triggering ATs, to be involved in pulmonary vein reconnection after AF ablation, post-AF ablation tachycardias, and/or sustain reentrant arrhythmias and focal and/or reentrant tachyarrhythmias.[52] The LOM connections can be challenging to ablate from the endocardium because of their epicardial course. For example, extensions of the LOM can be responsible for failed endocardial ablation of mitral annular flutter; ablation at adjacent sites in the CS is commonly used in this scenario. A recent series, including 60 LOM-related ATs (31 macro-reentrant and 29 focal) in patients post-AF ablation found that most could be successfully ablated from the endocardium (81.6%), whereas a minority (15%) required ethanol ablation into the vein of Marshall.[53] Circuits were most commonly found at the LOM-LA junction

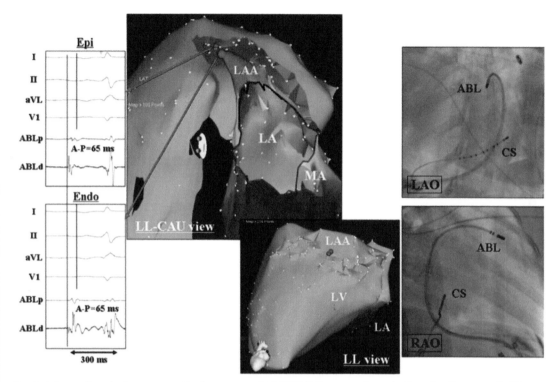

Fig. 4. Intracardiac electrograms, activation map and LAO/RAO fluoroscopic projections for the case of a 27-year-old woman with tachycardia-induced cardiomyopathy from a LAA tachycardia. Ablation at the earliest endocardial site of activation was unsuccessful. The tachycardia was successfully ablated with radiofrequency energy from the epicardium with percutaneous pericardial access. (*From* Yamada T, McElderry HT, Allison JS, Kay GN. Focal atrial tachycardia originating from the epicardial left atrial appendage. Heart Rhythm. 2008;5(5):766-7; with permission.)

(93.1%). The LOM be part a variety of different circuits, including mitral flutter as well as a number of circuits involving the left pulmonary veins; detailed electroanatomic mapping can help in delineating the areas to target for ablation.[54] A recent series of 35 patients demonstrated the feasibility and potential benefits of percutaneous epicardial ablation in the area of the LOM for patients with recurrent atrial arrhythmias after repeated endocardial AF ablation attempts.[55] More research on the role and optimal therapeutic approach to LOM-related arrhythmias is needed.

EPICARDIAL ABLATION AND THE PHRENIC NERVE

Epicardial access is associated with number of potential complications; these are reviewed in detail in an accompanying paper. As alluded to above, epicardial ablation for SVT has site-specific potential complications related to surrounding anatomic structures. The phrenic nerves can be in close proximity to target ablation sites. The RPN descends from the neck on the right of

the mediastinum and courses on the posterior surface of the right atrium in close proximity to the SVC and right superior pulmonary vein (RSPV) before reaching the right hemidiaphragm. RPN injury has been reported with ablation for AF, crista terminalis ATs, RA-SVC junction ATs, RSPV ATs, and IST. The LPN courses over the roof of the LAA before descending to the inferolateral LV and contacting the left hemidiaphragm. LPN injury has been described during ablation for AF, LA ATs, and left-sided AP. The risk of phrenic nerve injury is potentially greater with epicardial ablation because of the proximity to the ablation catheter (**Fig. 5**).

A routinely used strategy to prevent phrenic nerve injury is to delineate the course of the nerve with pacing. However, this does not resolve situations where the target ablation site is in close proximity to the phrenic nerve. Many strategies for phrenic nerve preservation have been described, including air and saline insufflation into the pericardial space, all with limited success (**Fig. 6**).[56] Lee and colleagues[57] reported on 4 patients with right-sided ATs (2 SVC/RA junction; 2 crista

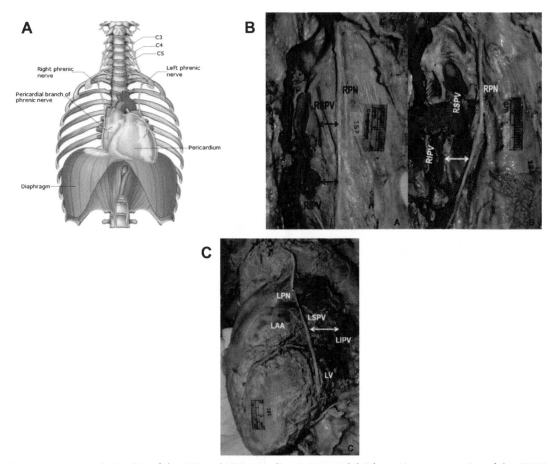

Fig. 5. Anatomic relationship of the RPN and LPN to cardiac structures. (*A*) Schematic representation of the C3/C4/C5 tributaries to the RPN and LPN and their intrathoracic course. The RPN borders the SVC-RA junction and is in close proximity to the right superior pulmonary veins as it courses inferiorly to contact the right hemidiaphragm. The LPN borders the left lateral aspect of the aortic arch and pulmonary trunk before coursing in close proximity to the LAA and over the lateral LV. (*B*) Cadaver specimen showing the relationship of the RPN to the right pulmonary veins. (*C*) Cadaver specimen showing the relationship of the LPN to LAA, left pulmonary veins and LV.[60] (*From* Randhawa A, Sahni D, Aggarwal A, Rohit MK, Sehgal S, Reddy YM. Study of spatial relationship of phrenic nerves with cardiac structures relevant to electrophysiologic interventions. Pacing Clin Electrophysiol. 2014;37(11):1477-84; with permission.)

terminalis) in whom endocardial ablation was limited by proximity to the RPN. Three of the 4 patients had successful endocardial ablation assisted by epicardial displacement of the phrenic nerve by a steerable sheath/catheter combination and/or an angioplasty balloon without reported procedural complication. Kumar and colleagues[58] reported their experience with epicardial phrenic nerve displacement in 13 patients also using a steerable sheath/catheter combination and/or a balloon to displace the phrenic. In all but 1 of the 8 atrial cases (6 high crista terminalis; 1 low crista terminalis; 1 SVC triggered AF), previous ablation had been unsuccessful because of proximity to the phrenic nerve. Acute procedural success was achieved in all patients after phrenic displacement

without periprocedural or follow-up evidence of phrenic injury. One patient developed pericardial bleeding after epicardial access which was successfully managed conservatively. There were several technical challenges identified in this study, including challenging maneuverability of the displacement apparatus, the use of more than 1 displacement modality in several patients, the need for more than 1 epicardial access in some patients, and distortion of the atrial anatomy requiring electroanatomic remapping. Moreover, the level of patient sedation (conscious sedation versus general anesthesia) has to factor patient comfort and inducibility of the clinical arrhythmia. A similar technique was used to protect the RPN during endocardial sinus node modification for

A

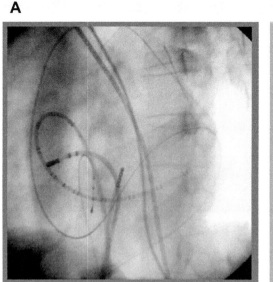

B

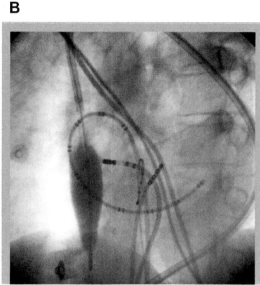

Fig. 6. Shown here is an example of a mid-crista atrial tachycardia that was mapped to an area of phrenic nerve stimulation. Percutaneous epicardial access was obtained (*A*) and a peripheral interventional balloon was used to displace the phrenic nerve away from the epicardial surface of the RA to allow safe endocardial catheter ablation (*B*).

IST.[59] We did not find cases of left phrenic displacement for epicardial ablation of SVT, although theoretically it could be required for displacement of the phrenic nerve away from the tip of the LAA. In summary, epicardial access for displacement of the phrenic nerve is feasible for patients in whom proximity to the phrenic nerve is an impediment to successful ablation.

SUMMARY

SVTs are common and routine catheter ablation success rates are high. The need for epicardial access and ablation exists in a minority of refractory cases involving unusual APs or ATs. Most SVTs are associated with good prognosis. However, APs can be associated with risk of sudden death and incessant ATs can lead to cardiomyopathy and heart failure. It is always important to balance the risks and benefits of epicardial access and ablation with the risk of the targeted arrhythmia, to achieve the optimal outcome for the patient. That said, epicardial access and ablation can be a critically important adjunct to successful mapping and safe ablation of these complex arrhythmias.

DISCLOSURE

Dr U.B. Tedrow has received honoraria from Biosense Webster, Abbott Medical, and Medtronic. She has also received consulting fees from

Thermedical Inc. Dr. Aguilar: George Mines Travelling Fellowship from the Canadian Heart Rhythm Society.

REFERENCES

1. Orejarena LA, Vidaillet H Jr, DeStefano F, et al. Paroxysmal supraventricular tachycardia in the general population. J Am Coll Cardiol 1998;31(1):150–7.
2. Clair WK, Wilkinson WE, McCarthy EA, et al. Spontaneous occurrence of symptomatic paroxysmal atrial fibrillation and paroxysmal supraventricular tachycardia in untreated patients. Circulation 1993;87(4):1114–22.
3. Rodriguez LM, de Chillou C, Schlapfer J, et al. Age at onset and gender of patients with different types of supraventricular tachycardias. Am J Cardiol 1992;70(13):1213–5.
4. Porter MJ, Morton JB, Denman R, et al. Influence of age and gender on the mechanism of supraventricular tachycardia. Heart Rhythm 2004; 1(4):393–6.
5. Cobb FR, Blumenschein SD, Sealy WC, et al. Successful surgical interruption of the bundle of Kent in a patient with Wolff-Parkinson-White syndrome. Circulation 1968;38(6):1018–29.
6. Guiraudon G, Fontaine G, Frank R, et al. Encircling endocardial ventriculotomy: a new surgical treatment for life-threatening ventricular tachycardias resistant to medical treatment following myocardial infarction. Ann Thorac Surg 1978;26(5): 438–44.

7. Haissaguerre M, Gaita F, Fischer B, et al. Radiofrequency catheter ablation of left lateral accessory pathways via the coronary sinus. Circulation 1992; 86(5):1464–8. https://doi.org/10.1161/01.cir.86.5.1464.

8. Lu CW, Wu MH, Chen HC, et al. Epidemiological profile of Wolff-Parkinson-White syndrome in a general population younger than 50 years of age in an era of radiofrequency catheter ablation. Int J Cardiol 2014;174(3):530–4.

9. Calkins H, Yong P, Miller JM, et al. Catheter ablation of accessory pathways, atrioventricular nodal reentrant tachycardia, and the atrioventricular junction: final results of a prospective, multicenter clinical trial. The Atakr Multicenter Investigators Group. Circulation 1999;99(2):262–70.

10. Bohnen M, Stevenson WG, Tedrow UB, et al. Incidence and predictors of major complications from contemporary catheter ablation to treat cardiac arrhythmias. Heart Rhythm 2011;8(11):1661–6.

11. Sosa E, Scanavacca M, d'Avila A, et al. A new technique to perform epicardial mapping in the electrophysiology laboratory. J Cardiovasc Electrophysiol 1996;7(6):531–6.

12. Penmasta S, Silbiger JJ. The transverse and oblique sinuses of the pericardium: anatomic and echocardiographic insights. Echocardiography 2019;36(1):170–6.

13. Morady F, Strickberger A, Man KC, et al. Reasons for prolonged or failed attempts at radiofrequency catheter ablation of accessory pathways. J Am Coll Cardiol 1996;27(3):683–9.

14. Sacher F, Wright M, Tedrow UB, et al. Wolff-Parkinson-White ablation after a prior failure: a 7-year multicentre experience. Europace 2010;12(6):835–41.

15. Sun Y, Arruda M, Otomo K, et al. Coronary sinus-ventricular accessory connections producing posteroseptal and left posterior accessory pathways: incidence and electrophysiological identification. Circulation 2002;106(11):1362–7.

16. Langberg JJ, Man KC, Vorperian VR, et al. Recognition and catheter ablation of subepicardial accessory pathways. J Am Coll Cardiol 1993;22(4):1100–4.

17. Kuck K, Schluter M, Chiladakis I. Accessory pathways anatomically related to the coronary sinus. Circulation 1992;8b(suppl 11):1–782.

18. Wang X, McClelland J, Beckman K, et al. Left free-wall accessory pathways which require ablation from the coronary sinus—unique coronary sinus electrogram pattern. Circulation 1992;86(4):581.

19. Beukema WP, Van Dessel PF, Van Hemel NM, et al. Radiofrequency catheter ablation of accessory pathways associated with a coronary sinus diverticulum. Eur Heart J 1994;15(10):1415–8.

20. Kleinman D, Winters SL. Successful catheter ablation of an inferoseptal accessory pathway within the coronary sinus in a patient with a previously unsuccessful attempt at surgical interruption. Coronary sinus ablation for Wolff-Parkinson-White syndrome. J Electrocardiol 1996;29(1):55–60.

21. Lam C, Schweikert R, Kanagaratnam L, et al. Radiofrequency ablation of a right atrial appendage-ventricular accessory pathway by transcutaneous epicardial instrumentation. J Cardiovasc Electrophysiol 2000;11(10):1170–3.

22. Anderson RH, Ho SY. Structure and location of accessory muscular atrioventricular connections. J Cardiovasc Electrophysiol 1999;10(8):1119–23.

23. Arruda MS, McClelland JH, Wang X, et al. Development and validation of an ECG algorithm for identifying accessory pathway ablation site in Wolff-Parkinson-White syndrome. J Cardiovasc Electrophysiol 1998;9(1):2–12.

24. Jackman WM, Wang XZ, Friday KJ, et al. Catheter ablation of accessory atrioventricular pathways (Wolff-Parkinson-White syndrome) by radiofrequency current. N Engl J Med 1991;324(23):1605–11.

25. Sapp J, Soejima K, Couper GS, et al. Electrophysiology and anatomic characterization of an epicardial accessory pathway. J Cardiovasc Electrophysiol 2001;12(12):1411–4.

26. Saad EB, Marrouche NF, Cole CR, et al. Simultaneous epicardial and endocardial mapping of a left-sided posteroseptal accessory pathway associated with a large coronary sinus diverticulum: successful ablation by transection of the diverticulum's neck. Pacing Clin Electrophysiol 2002;25(10):1524–6.

27. de Paola AA, Leite LR, Mesas CE. Nonsurgical transthoracic epicardial ablation for the treatment of a resistant posteroseptal accessory pathway. Pacing Clin Electrophysiol 2004;27(2):259–61.

28. Ho I, d'Avila A, Ruskin J, et al. Images in cardiovascular medicine. Percutaneous epicardial mapping and ablation of a posteroseptal accessory pathway. Circulation 2007;115(16):e418–21.

29. Scharf C, Dang L. Epicardial Wolff-Parkinson-White ablation. Eur Heart J 2013;34(35):2738.

30. Faustino M, Bellotti H, Hardy C, et al. Percutaneous epicardial access as an alternative approach for catheter ablation of a posteroseptal accessory pathway related to the coronary venous system. J Cardiovasc Electrophysiol 2016;27(6):754–6.

31. Schweikert RA, Saliba WI, Tomassoni G. Percutaneous pericardial instrumentation for endo-epicardial mapping of previously failed ablations. Circulation 2003;108(11):1329–35. https://doi.org/10.1161/01.CIR.0000087407.53326.31.

32. Schweikert RA, Saliba WI, Tomassoni G, et al. Percutaneous pericardial instrumentation for endo-epicardial mapping of previously failed ablations. Circulation 2003;108(11):1329–35.

33. Valderrabano M, Cesario DA, Ji S, et al. Percutaneous epicardial mapping during ablation of difficult accessory pathways as an alternative to cardiac surgery. Heart Rhythm 2004;1(3):311–6.

34. Scanavacca MI, Sternick EB, Pisani C, et al. Accessory atrioventricular pathways refractory to catheter ablation: role of percutaneous epicardial approach. Circ Arrhythm Electrophysiol 2015;8(1):128–36.

35. Nguyen DT, Barham W, Zheng L, et al. Effect of radiofrequency energy delivery in proximity to metallic medical device components. Heart Rhythm 2015; 12(10):2162–9.

36. Stavrakis S, Jackman WM, Nakagawa H, et al. Risk of coronary artery injury with radiofrequency ablation and cryoablation of epicardial posteroseptal accessory pathways within the coronary venous system. Circ Arrhythm Electrophysiol 2014;7(1): 113–9.

37. Case CL, Schaffer MS, Dhala AA, et al. Radiofrequency catheter ablation of an accessory atrioventricular connection in a Fontan patient. Pacing Clin Electrophysiol 1993;16(7 Pt 1):1434–6.

38. Rosenthal E, Bostock J, Gill J. Iatrogenic atrioventricular bypass tract following a Fontan operation for tricuspid atresia. Heart 1997;77(3):283–5.

39. Milstein S, Dunnigan A, Tang C, et al. Right atrial appendage to right ventricle accessory atrioventricular connection: a case report. Pacing Clin Electrophysiol 1997;20(7):1877–80.

40. Mah D, Miyake C, Clegg R, et al. Epicardial left atrial appendage and biatrial appendage accessory pathways. Heart Rhythm 2010;7(12):1740–5.

41. Soejima K, Mitamura H, Miyazaki T, et al. Catheter ablation of accessory atrioventricular connection between right atrial appendage to right ventricle: a case report. J Cardiovasc Electrophysiol 1998;9(5): 523–8.

42. Goya M, Takahashi A, Nakagawa H, et al. A case of catheter ablation of accessory atrioventricular connection between the right atrial appendage and right ventricle guided by a three-dimensional electroanatomic mapping system. J Cardiovasc Electrophysiol 1999;10(8):1112–8.

43. Shah MJ, Garabedian H, Garoutte MC, et al. Catheter ablation of a right atrial appendage to the right ventricle connection in a neonate. Pacing Clin Electrophysiol 2001;24(9 Pt 1):1427–9.

44. Di Biase L, Schweikert RA, Saliba WI, et al. Left atrial appendage tip: an unusual site of successful ablation after failed endocardial and epicardial mapping and ablation. J Cardiovasc Electrophysiol 2010; 21(2):203–6.

45. Servatius H, Rostock T, Hoffmann BA, et al. Catheter ablation of an atrioventricular bypass tract connecting a funnel-shaped bilobular left atrial appendage with the ventricular free wall. Heart Rhythm 2009; 6(7):1075–6.

46. Wang YL, Li XB, Quan X, et al. Focal atrial tachycardia originating from the left atrial appendage: electrocardiographic and electrophysiologic characterization and long-term outcomes of radiofrequency ablation. J Cardiovasc Electrophysiol 2007; 18(5):459–64.

47. Koplan BA, Parkash R, Couper G, et al. Combined epicardial-endocardial approach to ablation of inappropriate sinus tachycardia. J Cardiovasc Electrophysiol 2004;15(2):237–40.

48. Yamada T, Murakami Y, Yoshida Y, et al. Electrophysiologic and electrocardiographic characteristics and radiofrequency catheter ablation of focal atrial tachycardia originating from the left atrial appendage. Heart Rhythm 2007;4(10): 1284–91.

49. Hillock RJ, Singarayar S, Kalman JM, et al. Tale of two tails: the tip of the atrial appendages is an unusual site for focal atrial tachycardia. Heart Rhythm 2006;3(4):467–9.

50. Phillips KP, Natale A, Sterba R, et al. Percutaneous pericardial instrumentation for catheter ablation of focal atrial tachycardias arising from the left atrial appendage. J Cardiovasc Electrophysiol 2008; 19(4):430–3.

51. Yamada T, McElderry HT, Allison JS, et al. Focal atrial tachycardia originating from the epicardial left atrial appendage. Heart Rhythm 2008;5(5): 766–7.

52. Chugh A, Gurm HS, Krishnasamy K, et al. Spectrum of atrial arrhythmias using the ligament of Marshall in patients with atrial fibrillation. Heart Rhythm 2018; 15(1):17–24.

53. Vlachos K, Denis A, Takigawa M, et al. The role of Marshall bundle epicardial connections in atrial tachycardias after atrial fibrillation ablation. Heart Rhythm 2019;16(9):1341–7.

54. Kawamura I, Fukamizu S, Arai M, et al. Characteristics of Marshall bundle-related atrial tachycardias using an ultrahigh-resolution mapping system. J Interv Card Electrophysiol 2019;55(2):161–9.

55. Yu L, Liu Q, Jiang RH, et al. Adjunctive percutaneous ablation targeting epicardial arrhythmogenic structures in patients of atrial fibrillation with recurrence after multiple procedures. J Cardiovasc Electrophysiol 2019;31(2):401–9.

56. Di Biase L, Burkhardt JD, Pelargonio G, et al. Prevention of phrenic nerve injury during epicardial ablation: comparison of methods for separating the phrenic nerve from the epicardial surface. Heart Rhythm 2009;6(7):957–61.

57. Lee JC, Steven D, Roberts-Thomson KC, et al. Atrial tachycardias adjacent to the phrenic nerve: recognition, potential problems, and solutions. Heart Rhythm 2009;6(8):1186–91.

58. Kumar S, Barbhaiya CR, Baldinger SH, et al. Epicardial phrenic nerve displacement during catheter

ablation of atrial and ventricular arrhythmias: procedural experience and outcomes. Circ Arrhythm Electrophysiol 2015;8(4):896–904. https://doi.org/10.1161/CIRCEP.115.002818.

59. Rubenstein JC, Kim MH, Jacobson JT. A novel method for sinus node modification and phrenic nerve protection in resistant cases. J Cardiovasc Electrophysiol 2009;20(6):689–91.

60. Randhawa A, Sahni D, Aggarwal A, et al. Study of spatial relationship of phrenic nerves with cardiac structures relevant to electrophysiologic interventions. Pacing Clin Electrophysiol 2014;37(11):1477–84.

Percutaneous Epicardial Ablation of Atrial Fibrillation

Roderick Tung, MD

KEYWORDS

• Ablation • Epicardial • Atrial fibrillation

KEY POINTS

- The observations afforded by epicardial mapping have not only increased the appreciation of distinct epicardial structures in the left atrium but also underscore the need to address the substrate transmurally.
- Although epicardial access and ablation has attendant risks, comparative studies with hybrid surgical approaches are lacking.
- In the search to find unifying mechanisms of atrial fibrillation, a conceptual shift that emphasizes the substrate in 3 dimensions, with the epicardium distinct from the endocardium, holds promise for future investigation and evolving therapeutic tools.

BACKGROUND

The cornerstone of atrial fibrillation (AF) therapy with catheter ablation is predicated on the achievement of pulmonary vein isolation (PVI). Electrical disconnection of the pulmonary vein creates conduction block in and out of the vein, whereby exit block impairs a pulmonary vein focus from triggering AF.[1] However, reconnection of pulmonary vein conduction is common in patients both with and without recurrences of AF.[2,3] Additional linear ablation has not been shown to improve outcomes,[4] and a unifying mechanism outside of the pulmonary veins has not been identified. Alternative approaches to direct therapy outside of the pulmonary veins (complex electrograms,[5] low-voltage areas,[6] posterior wall,[7] and rotational activity identified by unipolar phase mapping[8]) have not been shown to be consistently beneficial. Therefore, over the past 2 decades, there has been considerable focus on improving the durability of PVI with attention to biophysical parameters and contact force.[9,10]

RATIONALE

The success rate of endocardial ablation for AF is highly variable and incomplete in its current state. The principles for defining a potential cure for AF are rooted in (1) identification of a reproducible and common electrophysiologic mechanism, (2) an understanding of underlying mechanisms (triggers and substrate) specific to different phenotypes, (3) the creation of durable and transmural lesions to ensure what was done, was done, and remains done. In many ways, the more than 30-year quest to understand a unifying mechanism for AF is based on deductive reasoning, in which the field has attempted to eliminate 1 target or region in order to understand its mechanistic impact.

Failure of current ablation strategies such as PVI is thought to be caused by gaps in ablation lines.[11] Although gaps during ablation are typically conceptualized in a planar and two-dimensional construct, the creation of nontransmural lesions introduces the reality of three-dimensional (3D) gaps, at greater depth. As such, the main

Department of Medicine, Section of Cardiology, The University of Chicago Medicine, Center for Arrhythmia Care, Pritzker School of Medicine, 5841 South Maryland Avenue MC 6080, Chicago, IL 60637, USA
E-mail address: rodericktung@uchicago.edu

Card Electrophysiol Clin 12 (2020) 371–381
https://doi.org/10.1016/j.ccep.2020.06.005
1877-9182/20/© 2020 Elsevier Inc. All rights reserved.

differentiator between surgical and catheter-based approaches lies in the approach to achieve transmural ablation (outside-in vs inside-out approach). Hybrid approaches have been systematically shown to achieve higher freedom from AF recurrence than endocardial catheter ablation.[12–14] The interpretation of these data is that there is an urgent need to achieve transmural and durable ablation therapy using a percutaneous approach. Infusion of ethanol in the vein of Marshall has been used in order to achieve transmural treatment in the region of the left atrium (LA) ridge between the appendage and left-side pulmonary veins and inferior mitral isthmus, a complex anatomic area known to have thicker tissue with epicardial fibers.[15,16] New technologies on the horizon with pulsed field ablation (electroporation) and larger-footprint catheter designs hold promise to shorten the duration of energy application and increase the durability of lesions.[17,18] However, until multicenter prospective data are available, there are important and valuable insights that can be gained from simultaneous epicardial and endocardial mapping of AF.

Mechanistically, asynchronous conduction between the epicardium and endocardium may increase vulnerability to reentrant wave fronts and AF perpetuation.[19–21] Dissociation of these surfaces of the atrium as a functional bilayer has been proposed as well as intramural reentry with focal breakthroughs.[22] This article provides a review of the current state of the art with epicardial mapping of AF with regard to:

1. Anatomy of the epicardial LA/pericardial space with attention to critical epicardial structures that may be functionally relevant to the pathogenesis of AF
2. Existing data and experience with a percutaneous approach to epicardial mapping during AF ablation
3. Novel insights afforded by exploring the epicardial space with high-density mapping

ANATOMY ACCESSIBLE VIA PERCUTANEOUS APPROACH

Using the technique pioneered by Sosa and colleagues[23] for ventricular tachycardia ablation in Chagas disease, a posterior approach is preferred for direct access into the oblique sinus (**Fig. 1**). The puncture is performed before systemic heparinization and transseptal access, and a steerable sheath is used to facilitate catheter manipulation into and within the oblique sinus. Mapping at the mitral annulus is unimpeded, but, within the posterior wall, the U-shaped pericardial reflections limits

the catheter from crossing the dome, roof, and carina on both sides (**Fig. 2**). With regard to the pulmonary veins, antra around the inferior veins are more exposed via epicardial approach, although pericardial reflections surround the pulmonary veins.

The epicardial correlate for the endocardial ridge between the left atrial appendage (LAA) and left superior pulmonary vein (LSPV) is a sulcus epicardially, and an ablation catheter freely advances within the sulcus and over the epicardial LAA. Additional advancement of a catheter gains access to the anterior wall of the LA toward the Bachmann's region. The ascending aorta lies anterior to the septal portion of the anterior wall.

EPICARDIAL STRUCTURES AND FIBERS

Although the LA is predominantly a thin-walled structure, there are highly conserved regions that consist of specialized epicardial bundles[24,25] that can serve as 3D bridges for activation, even in the setting of endocardial block. The areas are anatomically thicker relative to the thin-walled LA and present challenges to achieving transmural ablation. To best highlight these structures, this article outlines the challenges associated with creation of mitral block for perimitral flutter:

1. Anterior line: Bachmann's region
2. Superolateral line: vein/ligament of Marshall
3. Inferior line: coronary sinus

The primary interatrial connections are (1) Bachmann's region, (2) fossa ovalis, (3) coronary sinus.[26] In addition, the intercaval bundle is an epicardial network that shunts activation from the right atrium posterior to the septum across the Waterston groove toward the posterior wall, ending in the anterior carina of the right-sided veins. Conduction via the intercaval bundles is a common cause of failure to isolate the right-sided veins with wide antral circumferential ablation, and ablation within the carina is often required to isolate the conduction via these epicardial fibers.[27] It is important to emphasize that most pulmonary venous muscle sleeves are epicardial in origin and have greater redundancy at the carina.[28] Ablation from the earliest right atrial insertion site can achieve a similar result but requires activation mapping during left atrial pacing to assess the location.[29,30]

Bachmann's region

The Bachmann's region is critical to maintaining interatrial synchronization and runs anterior to the superior vena cava across the septum to the

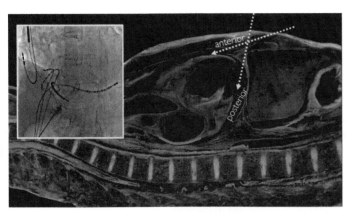

Fig. 1. Percutaneous access to pericardial space via posterior approach allows access into the oblique sinus (*pink*) for mapping for the epicardial posterior wall. Fluoroscopic view in LAO for percutaneous contrast-guided puncture of the pericardium (*Insert*).

anterior wall of the LA, where it then bifurcates anterior to the LAA and extends toward the ridge where the vein or ligament of Marshall extends.[24] The region of the Bachmann's region is thick, and ablation from the anterior mitral annulus toward the right superior pulmonary vein must cross this structure. With high-resolution mapping, there are clear demonstrations of endocardial block across anterior mitral lines with continuation of flutter epicardially across the Bachmann's region, which makes the right atrium a critical part of the circuit.[31] These biatrial flutters do not necessitate ablation from the right atrium but highlight the need to create a transmural mitral line of block. In our experience, additional ablation across the endocardial line of block seldom achieves the

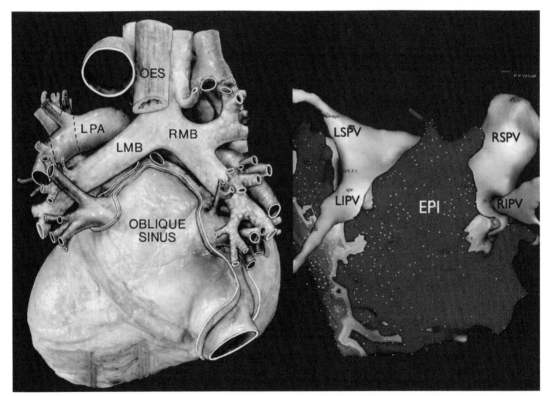

Fig. 2. Anatomy of the pericardial space with pericardial reflections that form a dome around the epicardial posterior wall. Access to the anterior wall and roof requires a course anterior to the left-sided veins. EPI, epicardial; LIPV, left inferior pulmonary vein; LMB, left main bronchus; LPA, left pulmonary artery; LSPV, left superior pulmonary vein, OES, esophagus; RIPV, right inferior pulmonary vein; RMB, right main bronchus; RSPV, right superior pulmonary vein.

end point, but the creation of a separate line for mitral block is more successful.

Percutaneous epicardial mapping allows access over the anterior wall through the sulcus between the LAA and LSPV (endocardial ridge). Piorkowski and colleagues[32] were the first to show the need for epicardial ablation in this region to achieve transmural and durable block. In a recent case report, the authors highlighted the anatomic basis for multiple attempts to create block across an anterior mitral line, where entrainment and termination of flutter in the epicardial region of the Bachmann's region were achieved during epicardial ablation (**Fig. 3**). Although confirmation of direct recordings of the Bachmann's region can only be achieved with direct visualization, the region of interest correlates with this well-recognized anatomic location.

Coronary sinus and vein of Marshall

When creating an inferior mitral line connecting the left inferior pulmonary vein and coronary sinus, the mitral annulus represents the thicker portion of

myocardium, which is resistant to transmural block. Further, the coronary sinus serves as a heat sink, with a large-caliber vein that cools the surrounding myocardium during ablation. Temporary occlusion of coronary venous blood flow has been proposed to facilitate mitral block to minimize concomitant cooling.[33] In addition, the coronary sinus musculature is distinct from both the endocardial and epicardial LA, and can serve as an activation bridge during inferior mitral ablation.[34] Ablation within the coronary sinus is frequently required to achieve inferior block, and, in spite of this approach, block may still be challenging to achieve.[35,36]

A superolateral line connecting the left carina of the upper vein to the annulus at the level of the LAA has been proposed to create mitral block with higher efficacy than inferior lesion sets.[37] However, the vein or ligament of Marshall courses in this region and may also serve as an epicardial barrier to achieving transmural block (**Fig. 4**). For this reason, ethanol infusion within the vein has been proposed to expedite the achievement of mitral block this region.[38] The necessity for alcohol

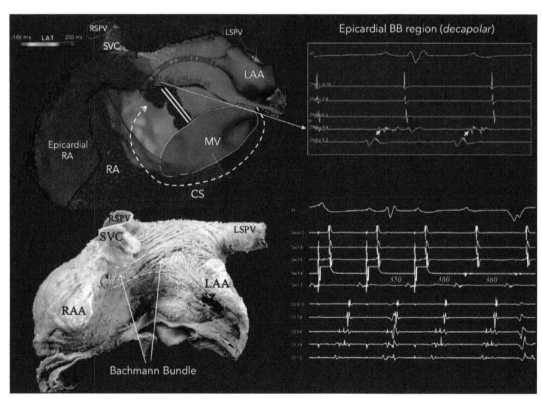

Fig. 3. Epicardial mapping in the Bachmann's region reveals epicardial flutter activation bridging more than a region with endocardial block. Concealed entrainment is demonstrated from a long fractionated epicardial signal. Correlative anatomy shows the region of Bachmann's region accessed with a decapolar catheter advanced anterior to the left-sided veins. BB, Bachmann bundle; MV, mitral valve; RA, right atrium. (*Courtesy of* José-Ángel Cabrera, MD, PhD, Madrid, Spain.)

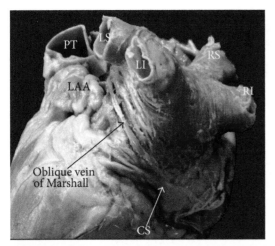

Fig. 4. Anatomy of the ridge between the LAA and left-sided veins with the course of the vein of Marshall. Endocardial ablation may fail to achieve transmural lesion extending toward this critical structure. CS, coronary sinus; LAA, left atrial appendage; LI, left inferior; LS, left superior; PT, pulmonary trunk; RI, right inferior; RS, right superior. (*Courtesy of* José-Ángel Cabrera, MD, PhD, Madrid, Spain.)

highlights the limitation of endocardial ablation to penetrate both intramurally and epicardially. Direct epicardial ablation within the sulcus may be an important adjunct to endocardial ridge ablation. Further, percutaneous epicardial ablation has been shown to be highly efficacious to complete inferior mitral block.[39,40]

Recent mapping studies with automated high-resolution mapping (Rhythmia, Boston Scientific, Natick, MA) have shown discontinuous activation patterns during flutter that are highly suggestive of the existence of epicardial bridging through the aforementioned structures. Activation gaps during complete endocardial high-density mapping indicate activation that is present beyond the surface recording virtual electrode. Recent case reports with recordings within the vein of Marshall show the critical nature of this epicardial structure.[41,42]

Septopulmonary bundle

The septopulmonary bundles run vertically along the posterior wall of the LA from the LA dome and roof extending toward the pulmonary venous component of the poster wall toward the inferior mitral annulus.[24,25] Posterior isolation with a box lesion set can be particularly challenging in some cases because of epicardial bridging via the thicker septopulmonary bundles, where extensive endocardial ablation may still yield a focal breakthrough pattern in the middle of the box lesion set (**Fig. 5**). For this reason, extensive ablation throughout the posterior wall has been advocated in order to optimize durable electrical isolation.[43] Although the fiber orientation of the septopulmonary bundle is variable between patients, recent high-resolution MRI with diffusion tensor imaging shows the basis for these distinct preferential epicardial connections.[25]

Epicardial ablation via percutaneous approach is not as safe because of close proximity to the esophagus. In selected cases, an intrapericardial balloon can be used to displace and protect the esophagus during both endocardial and epicardial ablation.[40] However, high-density epicardial mapping can be used to inform a more precise endocardial target across from the insertion of the septopulmonary bundle. Recent hybrid approaches with linear ablation tools (convergent procedure) hold promise to achieve higher rates of durable transmural posterior wall isolation but require surgical access and coordinated multispecialty care.[13,44]

INITIAL EXPERIENCE WITH CATHETER-BASED MAPPING AND ABLATION

To the best of our knowledge, the first reported experience of epicardial ablation of AF via percutaneous access was by Pak and colleagues[45] These investigators used this adjunctive approach to isolate veins that were resistant to endocardial ablation and show rapid isolation with focal epicardial targeted ablation. This proof-of-concept study highlights the importance of 3D gaps. Reddy and colleagues[46] were the first to show nonuniform epicardial activation running superiorly over the posterior wall after a failed box isolation attempt from the endocardium.

Piorkowski and colleagues[32] presented the largest experience to date, in which 80 patients underwent a combined epicardial-endocardial approach. They performed linear lesion sets prompted by low-voltage substrate and showed the need for epicardial ablation to complete these lines of block in 38%. In a selected cohort with prior failed ablation with isolated veins, this study introduces a paradigm shift when approaching patients with multiple failed endocardial ablations. Similarly, the authors began investigating the potential utility of a percutaneous approach in patients with refractory AF in 2014.[40] Examining a patient population refractory to previous ablation, we assessed whether discordance and asynchrony could be observed with high-density epicardial and endocardial mapping. In 22% of the cohort, nontransmural low-voltage regions

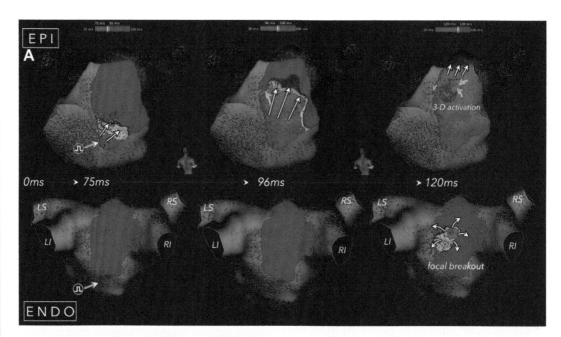

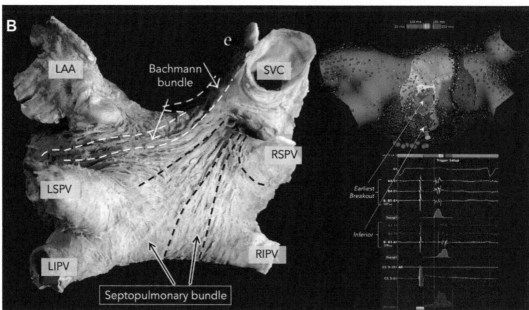

Fig. 5. (*A*) Epicardial activation of the posterior wall via the septopulmonary bundles in spite of a box isolation attempt results in epicardial bridging with a focal endocardial breakout pattern. (*B*) Correlative anatomy shows the orientation of septopulmonary bundle fibers and local electrograms, and confirms that earliest activation is in the middle of the posterior wall rather than inferior to the breakout, where the epicardial bridging occurs. SVC, superior vena cava.

were delineated on the posterior wall, providing direct evidence of substrates with nonuniform transmurality (**Fig. 6**). In 3 patients, epicardial pulmonary vein conduction was shown with pacing despite endocardial exit block (**Fig. 7**). Mitral flutter refractory to traditional endocardial approaches was eliminated in 2 patients during the first

radiofrequency application from the epicardial inferior mitral annulus region.

Perhaps one of the most important insights derived from this observational cohort was a single bipolar recording with a high-density minibasket catheter (Orion, Boston Scientific) showing complete epicardial-endocardial dissociation during

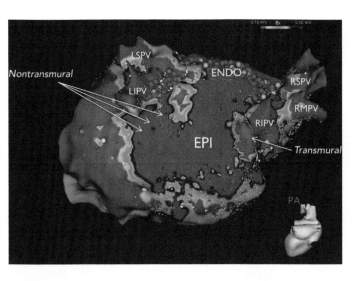

Fig. 6. Example of nontransmural ablation with epicardial sparing inferior to the left-side pulmonary vein. In contrast, the right inferior pulmonary vein shows transmurally uniform low voltage. RMPV, right middle pulmonary vein.

AF and flutter (**Fig. 8**). The epicardium persisted in fibrillation despite a slower conduction into the coronary sinus and higher degree of multilevel block into the endocardial posterior wall. Glover and colleagues[47] previously showed nonuniform findings on the epicardium during surgical exposure relative to the endocardium. These recordings confirm the intraoperative findings of De

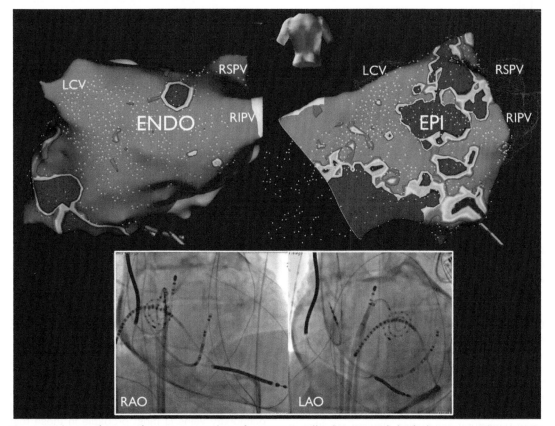

Fig. 7. Evidence of nonuniform transmurality of posterior wall substrate with high-density mapping. Despite diffuse endocardial low voltage across the posterior wall, there is sparing on the epicardial surface. Two high-density catheters are shown on right anterior oblique (RAO) and left anterior oblique (LAO) fluoroscopic views, circular endocardial and linear epicardial. LCV, left common vein.

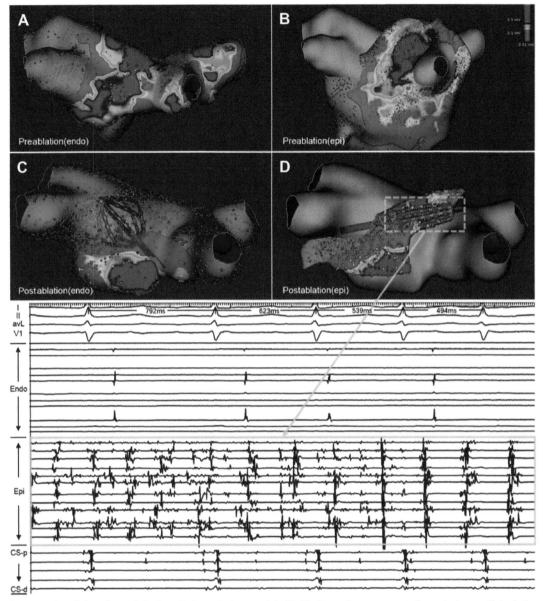

Fig. 8. Epicardial-endocardial dissociation during atrial fibrillation after attempted posterior wall isolation (*lower*). Although the endocardium appears isolated relative to pre-ablation map (*A* and *C*), localized fibrillatory activity is recorded from the epicardium (*B* and *D*).

Groot and colleagues,[47] who showed evidence of epicardial-endocardial asynchronous conduction with a clamp preparation. A 2-layer hypothesis is critical to the understanding of AF perpetuation, because dissociation may be sufficient to sustained reentry across the atrial wall.[21,22] More recent observations during incremental pacing show transmural conduction slowing resulting in higher curvature, which may promote localized 3D reentrant wave fronts or scroll waves.[48]

CURRENT CLINICAL APPROACH AND FUTURE DIRECTIONS

At present, the authors offer the therapeutic option of an adjunctive percutaneous approach to all patients that have failed multiple ablations (>2 prior ablations.) Because reconnection of pulmonary veins is most probable in those that failed a single procedure, patients who continue to have AF despite pulmonary veins most likely have non–pulmonary vein triggers or nontransmural ablation lesions. In those with failed mitral isthmus lines, the creation of a different endocardial lesion set is most practical before considering epicardial ablation. In our experience, the higher the number of previous failures, the higher the pretest probability of finding critical epicardial substrate.

There is guarded optimism that newer ablation strategies such as electroporation and large-footprint catheters will render the need to access the epicardial space obsolete.[17,18] The observations afforded by epicardial mapping have not only increased the appreciation of distinct epicardial structures in the LA but also underscore the need to address the substrate transmurally. Although epicardial access and ablation has attendant risks, comparative studies with hybrid surgical approaches are lacking. In the search to find unifying mechanisms of AF, a conceptual shift that emphasizes the substrate in 3 dimensions, with the epicardium distinct from the endocardium, holds promise for future investigation and evolving therapeutic tools.

DISCLOSURE

None.
Funding: none.

REFERENCES

1. Haissaguerre M, Jais P, Shah DC, et al. Spontaneous initiation of atrial fibrillation by ectopic beats originating in the pulmonary veins. N Engl J Med 1998;339:659–66.

2. Jiang RH, Po SS, Tung R, et al. Incidence of pulmonary vein conduction recovery in patients without clinical recurrence after ablation of paroxysmal atrial fibrillation: mechanistic implications. Heart Rhythm 2014;11:969–76.

3. Callans DJ, Gerstenfeld EP, Dixit S, et al. Efficacy of repeat pulmonary vein isolation procedures in patients with recurrent atrial fibrillation. J Cardiovasc Electrophysiol 2004;15:1050–5.

4. Verma A, Jiang CY, Betts TR, et al. Approaches to catheter ablation for persistent atrial fibrillation. N Engl J Med 2015;372:1812–22.

5. Oral H, Chugh A, Yoshida K, et al. A randomized assessment of the incremental role of ablation of complex fractionated atrial electrograms after antral pulmonary vein isolation for long-lasting persistent atrial fibrillation. J Am Coll Cardiol 2009;53:782–9.

6. Yang B, Jiang C, Lin Y, et al. STABLE-SR (electrophysiological substrate ablation in the left atrium during sinus rhythm) for the treatment of nonparoxysmal atrial fibrillation: a prospective, multicenter randomized clinical trial. Circ Arrhythm Electrophysiol 2017;10:e005405.

7. Tamborero D, Mont L, Berruezo A, et al. Left atrial posterior wall isolation does not improve the outcome of circumferential pulmonary vein ablation for atrial fibrillation: a prospective randomized study. Circ Arrhythm Electrophysiol 2009;2:35–40.

8. Narayan SM, Krummen DE, Shivkumar K, et al. Treatment of atrial fibrillation by the ablation of localized sources: CONFIRM (Conventional Ablation for Atrial Fibrillation With or Without Focal Impulse and Rotor Modulation) trial. J Am Coll Cardiol 2012;60: 628–36.

9. Natale A, Reddy VY, Monir G, et al. Paroxysmal AF catheter ablation with a contact force sensing catheter: results of the prospective, multicenter SMART-AF trial. J Am Coll Cardiol 2014;64:647–56.

10. Reddy VY, Dukkipati SR, Neuzil P, et al. Randomized, controlled trial of the safety and effectiveness of a contact force-sensing irrigated catheter for ablation of paroxysmal atrial fibrillation: results of the TactiCath contact force ablation catheter study for atrial fibrillation (TOCCASTAR) study. Circulation 2015;132:907–15.

11. Kuck KH, Hoffmann BA, Ernst S, et al. Impact of complete versus incomplete circumferential lines around the pulmonary veins during catheter ablation of paroxysmal atrial fibrillation: results from the gap-atrial fibrillation-german atrial fibrillation competence network 1 trial. Circ Arrhythm Electrophysiol 2016;9: e003337.

12. Tahir K, Kiser A, Caranasos T, et al. Hybrid epicardial-endocardial approach to atrial fibrillation ablation. Curr Treat Options Cardiovasc Med 2018; 20:25.

13. Gehi AK, Mounsey JP, Pursell I, et al. Hybrid epicardial-endocardial ablation using a pericardioscopic technique for the treatment of atrial fibrillation. Heart Rhythm 2013;10:22–8.

14. Kress DC, Erickson L, Choudhuri I, et al. Comparative effectiveness of hybrid ablation versus endocardial catheter ablation alone in patients with persistent atrial fibrillation. JACC Clin Electrophysiol 2017;3:341–9.

15. Baez-Escudero JL, Morales PF, Dave AS, et al. Ethanol infusion in the vein of Marshall facilitates mitral isthmus ablation. Heart Rhythm 2012;9: 1207–15.

16. Pambrun T, Denis A, Duchateau J, et al. MARSHALL bundles elimination, Pulmonary veins isolation and Lines completion for ANatomical ablation of persistent atrial fibrillation: MARSHALL-PLAN case series. J Cardiovasc Electrophysiol 2019;30:7–15.

17. Reddy VY, Neuzil P, Koruth JS, et al. Pulsed field ablation for pulmonary vein isolation in atrial fibrillation. J Am Coll Cardiol 2019;74:315–26.

18. Reddy VY, Anter E, Rackauskas G, et al. A lattice-tip focal ablation catheter that toggles between radio-frequency and pulsed field energy to treat atrial fibrillation: a first-in-human trial. Circ Arrhythm Electrophysiol 2020. https://doi.org/10.1161/CIRCEP.120.008718.

19. de Groot N, van der Does L, Yaksh A, et al. Direct proof of endo-epicardial asynchrony of the atrial wall during atrial fibrillation in humans. Circ Arrhythm Electrophysiol 2016;9:e003648.

20. Gharaviri A, Verheule S, Eckstein J, et al. How disruption of endo-epicardial electrical connections enhances endo-epicardial conduction during atrial fibrillation. Europace 2017;19:308–18.

21. Eckstein J, Zeemering S, Linz D, et al. Transmural conduction is the predominant mechanism of break-through during atrial fibrillation: evidence from simultaneous endo-epicardial high-density activation mapping. Circ Arrhythm Electrophysiol 2013;6:334–41.

22. Hansen BJ, Zhao J, Csepe TA, et al. Atrial fibrillation driven by micro-anatomic intramural re-entry re-vealed by simultaneous sub-epicardial and sub-endocardial optical mapping in explanted human hearts. Eur Heart J 2015;36:2390–401.

23. Sosa E, Scanavacca M, d'Avila A, et al. A new tech-nique to perform epicardial mapping in the electro-physiology laboratory. J Cardiovasc Electrophysiol 1996;7:531–6.

24. Sanchez-Quintana D, Lopez-Minguez JR, Macias Y, et al. Left atrial anatomy relevant to catheter abla-tion. Cardiol Res Pract 2014;2014:289720.

25. Pashakhanloo F, Herzka DA, Ashikaga H, et al. My-ofiber architecture of the human atria as revealed by submillimeter diffusion tensor imaging. Circ Ar-rhythm Electrophysiol 2016;9:e004133.

26. Platonov PG, Mitrofanova LB, Chireikin LV, et al. Morphology of inter-atrial conduction routes in pa-tients with atrial fibrillation. Europace 2002;4:183–92.

27. Yoshida K, Baba M, Shinoda Y, et al. Epicardial connection between the right-sided pulmonary venous carina and the right atrium in patients with atrial fibrillation: a possible mechanism for preclu-sion of pulmonary vein isolation without carina abla-tion. Heart Rhythm 2019;16:671–8.

28. Perez-Castellano N, Villacastin J, Salinas J, et al. Epicardial connections between the pulmonary veins and left atrium: relevance for atrial fibrillation ablation. J Cardiovasc Electrophysiol 2011;22:149–59.

29. Patel PJ, D'Souza B, Saha P, et al. Electroana-tomic mapping of the intercaval bundle in atrial fibrillation. Circ Arrhythm Electrophysiol 2014;7:1262–7.

30. Miyazaki S, Hasegawa K, Mukai M, et al. Epicardial connections via posterior interatrial bundles during atrial tachycardia. J Cardiovasc Electrophysiol 2019;30:438–9.

31. Kitamura T, Martin R, Denis A, et al. Characteristics of single-loop macroreentrant biatrial tachycardia diagnosed by ultrahigh-resolution mapping sys-tem. Circ Arrhythm Electrophysiol 2018;11:e005558.

32. Piorkowski C, Kronborg M, Hourdain J, et al. Endo-/epicardial catheter ablation of atrial fibrillation: feasi-bility, outcome, and insights into arrhythmia mecha-nisms. Circ Arrhythm Electrophysiol 2018;11:e005748.

33. Reddy VY, Ruskin JN, D'Avila A. Balloon occlusion of the coronary sinus to facilitate mitral isthmus abla-tion. J Cardiovasc Electrophysiol 2008;19:651.

34. Miyazaki S, Shah AJ, Haissaguerre M. Recurrent perimitral tachycardia using epicardial coronary si-nus connection to bypass endocardial conduction block at the mitral isthmus. Circ Arrhythm Electro-physiol 2011;4:e39–41.

35. Hocini M, Shah AJ, Nault I, et al. Mitral isthmus abla-tion with and without temporary spot occlusion of the coronary sinus: a randomized clinical comparison of acute outcomes. J Cardiovasc Electrophysiol 2012;23:489–96.

36. Jais P, Hocini M, Hsu LF, et al. Technique and results of linear ablation at the mitral isthmus. Circulation 2004;110:2996–3002.

37. Maurer T, Metzner A, Ho SY, et al. Catheter ablation of the superolateral mitral isthmus line: a novel approach to reduce the need for epicardial ablation. Circ Arrhythm Electrophysiol 2017;10:e005191.

38. Valderrabano M, Liu X, Sasaridis C, et al. Ethanol infusion in the vein of Marshall: adjunctive effects during ablation of atrial fibrillation. Heart Rhythm 2009;6:1552–8.

39. Berruezo A, Bisbal F, Fernandez-Armenta J, et al. Transthoracic epicardial ablation of mitral isthmus for treatment of recurrent perimitral flutter. Heart Rhythm 2014;11:26–33.

40. Jiang R, Buch E, Gima J, et al. Feasibility of percu-taneous epicardial mapping and ablation for re-fractory atrial fibrillation: insights into substrate and lesion transmurality. Heart Rhythm 2019;16:1151–9.

41. Thompson N, Kitamura T, Martin R, et al. Demonstra-tion of persistent conduction across the mitral isthmus via the vein of marshall with high-density activation mapping. Circ Arrhythm Electrophysiol 2017;10:e005152.

42. Hasegawa K, Miyazaki S, Kaseno K, et al. Ultrahigh resolution activation mapping of a left atrial macro-reentrant tachycardia using a Marshall bundle epicardial connection. J Cardiovasc Electrophysiol 2019;30:442–3.

43. Bai R, Di Biase L, Mohanty P, et al. Proven isolation of the pulmonary vein antrum with or without left

atrial posterior wall isolation in patients with persistent atrial fibrillation. Heart Rhythm 2016;13:132–40.

44. Khan Z, Hamandi M, Khan H, et al. Convergent epicardial-endocardial ablation for treatment of long-standing persistent atrial fibrillation: a review of literature. J Card Surg 2020. https://doi.org/10.1111/jocs.14562.

45. Pak HN, Hwang C, Lim HE, et al. Hybrid epicardial and endocardial ablation of persistent or permanent atrial fibrillation: a new approach for difficult cases. J Cardiovasc Electrophysiol 2007;18:917–23.

46. Reddy VY, Neuzil P, D'Avila A, et al. Isolating the posterior left atrium and pulmonary veins with a "box" lesion set: use of epicardial ablation to complete electrical isolation. J Cardiovasc Electrophysiol 2008;19:326–9.

47. Glover BM, Hong KL, Baranchuk A, et al. Preserved left atrial epicardial conduction in regions of endocardial "isolation". JACC Clin Electrophysiol 2018;4:557–8.

48. Parameswaran R, Teuwen CP, Watts T, et al. Functional atrial endocardial-epicardial dissociation in patients with structural heart disease undergoing cardiac surgery. JACC Clin Electrophysiol 2020;6:34–44.

Hybrid Surgical Ablation for Ventricular Arrhythmias

Anthony Li, MBBS, MD[a],*, Justin Hayase, MD[b], Noel G. Boyle, MD, PhD[b]

KEYWORDS

- Epicardial • Hybrid surgical approach • Ventricular tachycardia • Ablation

KEY POINTS

- A hybrid surgical approach to epicardial ablation of ventricular tachycardia (VT) should be considered in patients who have had prior cardiac surgery or failed percutaneous epicardial access attempts.
- Comprehensive preprocedure multidisciplinary work-up should be done with particular emphasis on the likely site of origin of the clinical arrhythmia.
- Surgical approaches do not provide complete access to the epicardial surface, and the site of surgical access should be tailored to reach the relevant substrate location.
- Three-dimensional anatomic mapping should be performed using conventional ablation and mapping catheters, but surgical ablation tools can be used where larger lesion sets are needed.
- The hybrid surgical approach for VT ablation can be performed with acceptable safety and efficacy.

INTRODUCTION

Epicardial mapping and ablation is an established option for the treatment of ventricular and, more recently, atrial arrhythmias.[1,2] The method of percutaneous epicardial access for electrophysiology (EP) procedures was first described by Sosa and colleagues[3] in 1996 for the treatment of ventricular tachycardia (VT) in the setting of chagasic cardiomyopathy. With growing experience in epicardial interventions for ventricular arrhythmias, it is now well recognized that the main limitation of the approach is the presence of pericardial adhesions. Adhesions are usually seen in the context of prior cardiac surgery but can also occur in patients with pericardial disease without prior surgery.[4]

Open surgical access has been used to successfully circumvent limitations with epicardial access and has been shown to allow safe and efficacious epicardial ablation in the treatment of VT.[5] This review describes the hybrid surgical approach—its indications, risks, and outcomes.

INDICATIONS FOR EPICARDIAL AND HYBRID ACCESS

The indications for epicardial interventions for ventricular arrhythmia are based on the electrocardiographic (ECG) morphology of the ventricular arrhythmia,[6–8] prior unsuccessful endocardial ablation, prior mapping indicating an epicardial focus, epicardial scar on cardiac contrast magnetic resonance imaging, or substrates known to be associated with epicardial circuits (such as Chagas cardiomyopathy or arrhythmogenic right ventricular cardiomyopathy). A suggested schema is shown in **Fig. 1**.

In a multicenter study of predominantly percutaneous epicardial ablation from 3 tertiary centers, 86% had prior failed endocardial ablations. The

[a] Cardiology Academic Group, St. George's University of London, Cranmer Terrace, London SW17 0QT, UK;
[b] UCLA Cardiac Arrhythmia Center, UCLA Health System, David Geffen School of Medicine at UCLA, Los Angeles, CA, USA
* Corresponding author.
E-mail address: ali@sgul.ac.uk

Card Electrophysiol Clin 12 (2020) 383–390
https://doi.org/10.1016/j.ccep.2020.05.002

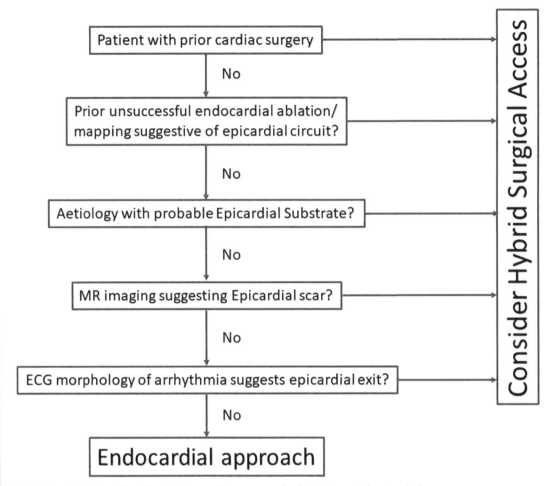

Fig. 1. Flowchart depicting the decision-making process for hybrid surgical epicardial access.

most common indications for epicardial ablation as a percentage of all patients undergoing epicardial VT ablation were arrhythmogenic right ventricular cardiomyopathy 41%, dilated cardiomyopathy 35%, other nonischemic cardiomyopathies 18%, ischemic cardiomyopathy 16%, and normal heart 6%.[9] The population where hybrid surgical access is an option, however, is skewed predominantly toward to patients who have had prior cardiac surgery.

In the largest series of hybrid surgical epicardial access from UCLA Medical Center, the commonest indications were prior coronary artery bypass grafting (45%), valve surgery (22%), and the presence of a left ventricular assist device (LVAD) (10%).[10] In that series, 95% had undergone prior attempt at endocardial ablation, 34% of whom had multiple ablations. Therefore, the substrate compared with percutaneous epicardial cohorts is naturally driven by patients with ischemic cardiomyopathy and with valvular nonischemic cardiomyopathyes who have had prior cardiac surgery.

Although conventional cardiac surgical patients comprise a majority of hybrid surgical patients, niche indications also have arisen with expanding experience. Left ventricle (LV) summit arrhythmias are known to be challenging, particularly when arising from the inaccessible area, basal to the epicardial course of the anterior interventricular vein, where close proximity to the left coronary system and sometimes deep intramural origin provide substantial obstacles to successful ablation.[11] Although several alternative percutaneous strategies have been developed to circumvent this problem, such as bipolar ablation, half normal saline catheter irrigation, and ablation delivery through angioplasty wires, a hybrid surgical approach also may be considered. A hybrid approach is advantageous, where direct visualization and dissection of the left main coronary artery is required to deliver ablation directly beneath the artery.

A hybrid surgical approach also should be considered for the no-entry LV. This situation can arise in the presence of double mechanical valves limiting both retrograde aortic and transmitral approaches.[12] Furthermore, surgical exposure also can circumvent problems, where LV endocardial access to the critical substrate is limited by percutaneous devices for structural heart disease, such as LVADs.[13]

PREPROCEDURE PLANNING

When considering hybrid surgical epicardial access, it is essential to weigh the benefits and risks and tailor the approach to each individual patient. Comprehensive preprocedure evaluation with imaging, including review of prior procedural mapping, and a multidisciplinary team approach are required in every case. Preprocedure imaging ideally should comprise scar localization by late gadolinium contrast magnetic resonance imaging and three-dimensional (3-D) computed tomography (CT) reconstruction, particularly in patients with coronary artery bypass grafts.

It is essential to gather as much data as possible on the probable site of origin of clinically recorded tachycardias and the likelihood of an epicardial origin. These can be derived from evaluation of the clinical tachycardia from 12-lead ECG morphology.[6–8] Attention should be given to the frontal plane axis because this enables a patient-tailored approach to the surgical access site, as discussed later. Preprocedure noninvasive programmed stimulation through an implantable cardioverter defibrillator also can be considered to supplement this process if no 12-lead ECG of the tachycardia morphology has been recorded.

Detailed review of mapping data from any prior ablation procedures should be undertaken. Data from substrate mapping with unipolar voltage settings may reveal the extent of epicardial substrate in nonischemic cardiomyopathy.[14] Specifically, lack of good pace map match, response to entrainment, or a broad endocardial breakout during activation mapping may suggest an epicardial site of origin. In cases of LV summit arrhythmias, preprocedure detailed activation and/or pace mapping of the anterior interventricular vein and its septal branches or the left anterior descending artery and septal perforators should be performed to identify the site of origin.[15]

PROCEDURAL CONSIDERATIONS
Facilities

When considering hybrid surgical access, due consideration must be given to the location of the procedure. The ability to rapidly convert patients to cardiopulmonary bypass must be available.

Procedures can be routinely undertaken in the EP laboratory with cardiac bypass facilities on standby. This is necessary because fluoroscopy is still needed to perform intraprocedural coronary angiography to ensure safe delivery of ablation energy because often only a small region of myocardium can be visualized directly. Furthermore, coronary arteries often are covered by epicardial fat and can be difficult to discern. In 1 study, procedure times were on average 7 hours in total; therefore, case mix in the laboratory should be scheduled to account for the significant investment of time that is needed for these procedures.[10]

Access Site

Two principal surgical approaches can be used to gain access: the subxiphoid approach and the limited thoracotomy approach. Key considerations for both approaches are summarized in **Table 1**. The subxiphoid approach is performed through an incision over the midline of the epigastrium at the level of the subxiphoid process. Individual patient anatomy may require extension to a partial sternotomy or removal of the xiphoid process in order to achieve adequate exposure. Dissection through the subcutaneous tissue, the linea alba, and the diaphragmatic pericardial surface is undertaken. Access through the pericardium is undertaken by sharp dissection. Adhesion lysis under direct vision is performed to gain access to the inferior and posterior LV epicardial surface. Once the epicardium is accessed, a sheath then can be placed to continue mapping and ablation as with a percutaneous approach.

The limited thoracotomy approach differs from the subxiphoid approach in several aspects. First, double lung ventilation may be required in order to enable left lung deflation to aid pericardial exposure. Access usually is undertaken through the third to fifth intercostal space and is determined by patient-specific position of the heart, as seen on preprocedure fluoroscopy. An incision over the chosen intercostal space is performed and extended through the subcutaneous tissue and fascia in order to reach the pericardium. In contrast to the subxiphoid approach, significant adhesions are encountered more often, where the parietal pericardium is strongly adhered to the epicardial surface, requiring careful dissection. A modification to the thoracotomy approach has been reported using video-assisted thoracoscopy.[16,17] This approach was described using a non–rib-displacing limited thoracotomy through the third intercostal space and allows direct visualization of the epicardial surface through a smaller incision.

Table 1
Comparison of subxiphoid and limited thoracotomy surgical access.

	Subxiphoid	Limited Thoracotomy
Ventilation	Double lung	Single lung may be required
ECG	Usual placement of electrodes	Displaced ECG electrodes
LV segments accessed	Inferior/inferolateral segments	Anterior/anterolateral and apical segments—tailor intercostal space to location of substrate.
Adhesions	Mild	May need extensive dissection with need for oversewing
3-D mapping	Impedance or magnetic can be used	Impedance based system may give distorted geometry if large retractors required.
Ablation	Conventional EP catheters for mapping and ablation	Conventional EP catheters for mapping and ablation but may experience frequent steam pops. Surgical tools under direct vision can be used after mapping with EP catheters.

Each of the 2 principal surgical access routes enables only a small region of the epicardial surface to be viewed directly (**Fig. 2**). The key difference between the 2 approaches is their ability to favor access to certain myocardial segments. In the largest series on hybrid surgical ablation, comparison of the mapped surface area during hybrid surgical access compared with percutaneous epicardial access demonstrated that only 36% of the total epicardial surface of the heart could be mapped through surgical access, highlighting the importance of careful preprocedure planning.[10] When comparing a subxiphoid with a thoracotomy approach, the subxiphoid approach favored access to the inferior and inferolateral LV segments but rarely the anterior and anterolateral LV segments. In contrast, the thoracotomy approach more frequently provided access to the anterior and anterolateral segments as well as the apex. More widespread access overall could be achieved, most likely as a result of tailoring the intercostal space to the myocardial segments likely to encompass the tachycardia substrate.

Mapping and Ablation

The choice of mapping system for hybrid procedures is based on operator preference and some procedural considerations. For the 12-lead ECG placement, a subxiphoid approach does not alter the placement of the electrodes. A thoracotomy approach, however, may necessitate displacing or losing some ECG electrodes with the resultant change in morphology of any induced arrhythmia; therefore, comparison to preexisting VT morphologies and pace mapping may be limited. Once surgical access is obtained and hemostasis has been achieved satisfactorily, full heparinization to attain an activated clotting time of greater than 300 s can be undertaken to facilitate endocardial LV mapping if required.

The options for mapping as for a percutaneous approach are between conventional mapping under fluoroscopy, impedance (Navx/EnSite Mapping, Abbott Medical, St. Paul, Minnesota) and/or magnetic (Carto, Biosense Webster, Diamond Bar, California) 3-D–based mapping systems. Magnetic-based and impedance-based systems have been used for hybrid surgical procedures with both approaches. An impedance-based system, however, may produce more distorted geometry when dealing with open chest/thoracotomy procedures due to changes in thoracic impedance when the chest cavity is opened and displacement of reference patches. On the other hand, the use of surgical equipment, such as large retractors may interfere with a magnetic-based system and, therefore, might be more suited to a surgical subxiphoid or thoracoscopic approach.

During VT induction, it is important to be aware that failure of external defibrillation may occur during hybrid surgical procedures due to the introduction of air within the pericardial space, which can occur with both subxiphoid and thoracotomy approaches. In 1 series, this was noted to occur in 2 of 10 cases, requiring internal defibrillation through the implantable cardioverter defibrillator.[5]

Although substrate, activation, and pace mapping require the use of conventional ablation or dedicated multipolar mapping catheters, more options exist for delivering ablation energy. These

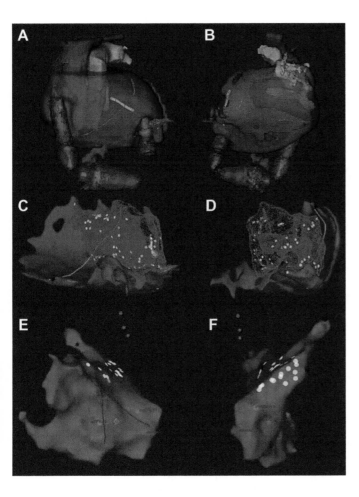

Fig. 2. Representative geometry from the same patient in which subxiphoid access and then at a later date, anterior thoracotomy was used. CT merged models in anteroposterior (*A*) and posteroanterior (*B*) views of the LV epicardium (*orange*), LVAD (*blue*), SVC (*purple*), and aorta (*yellow*) are shown with the overlying geometry of the LV epicardium (*green*). Subxiphoid access with CT model removed. Right anterior oblique (*C*) and left anterior oblique (*D*) views of the endocardial LV geometry (*gray* wire mesh) and epicardial geometry (*green*). Red dots indicate path of epicardial access through subxiphoid approach. Anterior thoracotomy approach in the same patient at a later date. Right anterior oblique (*E*) and left anterior oblique (*F*) views of the epicardial geometry. Brown line represents the course of the LAD artery and its diagonal branch. White dots indicate ablation lesions. (*From* Li A, Hayase J, Do D, et al. Hybrid surgical vs percutaneous access epicardial ventricular tachycardia ablation. *Heart Rhythm.* 2018;15(4):512-519; with permission.)

range from open irrigated radiofrequency (RF) ablation catheters used for percutaneous mapping and ablation to surgical ablation tools. Ablation also can be performed using RF or cryothermal energy (**Fig. 3**). Options for surgical tools include the Isolator Coolrail bipolar surgical linear ablation pen (AtriCure, West Chester, Ohio).[18] This device is an internally irrigated catheter with 30-mm parallel electrodes through which bipolar energy is delivered. Ablation lesions have a large surface area with a depth of approximately 4 mm to 5 mm.[19] The use of surgical cryoablation also has been reported using the Surgifrost Surgical Cryoablation System (Medtronic CryoCath LP).[20] This system comprises a malleable metal probe with an adjustable insulation sleeve that can vary the length of the ablation zone. Cooling is achieved by Argon gas to attain temperatures down to −150°, resulting in deep lesion formation. A similar cryoprobe, CryoICE (Atricure, Mason, Ohio), also has been described.[13,21] The advantage of a malleable probe is the option to create linear lesion formation or to mold the probe into a loop for lesions with a larger surface

area. Furthermore, cryoablation may provide better catheter stability during ablation.

Ablation through standard irrigated RF ablation catheters can also be performed for example, FlexAbility catheter (Abbott Medical, Santa Clara, California); Thermcool SF (Biosense Webster). During subxiphoid surgical approach, the ablation catheter is maneuvered through a sheath placed in the pericardium as in the percutaneous approach and ablation usually is performed in a similar fashion. During thoracotomy access/during ablation under direct vision, however, high impedance and frequent steam pops can occur, likely due to insufficient surrounding irrigation because standard catheters are designed primarily for the blood pool but have been successfully used in the epicardial space where irrigation fluid can surround and cool the catheter tip adequately.[5] The RF generator cutoff, therefore, may need to be adjusted to allow for high impedance during energy delivery for thoracotomy procedures.

The choice between conventional and surgical ablation catheters is dependent on the extent of

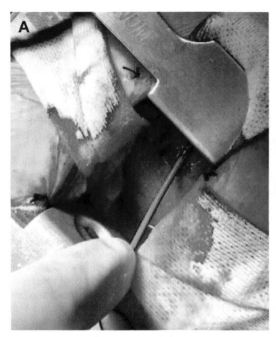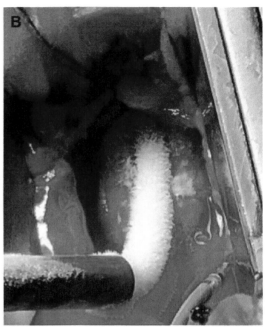

Fig. 3. Examples of ablation tools for hybrid procedures. (*A*) Open-irrigated ablation used during anterior thoracotomy (*B*) Cryoprobe ablation catheter used during anterior thoracotomy. Ice crystals can be visualized on the probe and epicardial surface during freezing. A multipolar mapping catheter also can be seen in the bottom right corner of the photo.

substrate and the level of precision required. Surgical ablation tools generally require ablation to be performed under direct vision through a thoracotomy approach, which requires sufficient surgical exposure that may expand to full median sternotomy. Surgical tools are unable to record electrograms, pace, or be visualized in a 3-D mapping system. They can ablate large areas of substrate, however, and achieve deep lesions in a shorter time period. Conventional ablation catheters can be utilized with both surgical access approaches with little modification needed for subxiphoid approach and can deliver RF in a targeted manner, which may be advantageous when dealing with arrhythmias close to critical structures, as in cases of LV summit arrhythmias.

COMPLICATIONS

Even when planned carefully, hybrid surgical access for VT ablation, although safe, may have significant associated risks. Postcardiotomy pleuritic pain is almost universal in this group of patients, and surgical access requires a longer postprocedure recovery period with a risk of wound infection and, therefore, longer length of stay in hospital. In the largest series of surgical access cases, 20% of cases experienced complications.[10] The most frequent complication was bleeding due to

ventricular wall damage during blunt dissection of adhesions where the pericardium was intensely adhered to the epicardial surface and occurred exclusively during an anterior thoracotomy approach, which required simple oversewing. When compared with a propensity-matched cohort undergoing percutaneous epicardial ablation, there was no statistical difference in complication rates seen, although numbers may be too small to draw firm conclusions.[10]

ALTERNATIVE STRATEGIES TO SURGICAL ACCESS

In patients with prior cardiac surgery, some centers have shown that a percutaneous epicardial access approach is feasible. Extreme caution should be exercised, however, when utilizing this approach and the authors do not advocate this approach outside of experienced centers without immediate surgical support and cardiopulmonary bypass on standby. The main concern of this approach is the presence of intense adhesions postcardiotomy that limit access to the epicardial surface and require adhesion lysis with the mapping/ablation catheter. Adhesion lysis should be performed with extreme caution due to the risk of bleeding and disruption of coronary artery bypass grafts, potentially leading to catastrophic complications.[22]

Several case series have been published on percutaneous epicardial access post–coronary surgery and post–noncoronary cardiac surgery.[23–26] Although feasible, the rate of access failure and complications are higher (up to 22%).[24,26] The authors, therefore, do not use this approach routinely.

OUTCOMES

Acute procedural success in the small number of hybrid surgical ablation case series has been reported as 50% to 60%.[10,20] In a series of 40 patients, 50% achieved complete success, 30% partial success and 5% (2 patients) with failure to eliminate the clinical arrhythmia due to proximity to the left coronary artery.[10] Furthermore, there did not appear to be differences in outcome between subxiphoid or thoracotomy approaches. When compared with a propensity-matched group of percutaneous epicardial ablation procedures, 1-year ablation outcomes were similar between percutaneous and surgical groups, with 37% versus 43% reaching the primary endpoint of VT recurrence; 50% reached a combined endpoint of VT recurrence, death, or cardiac transplantation/ventricular assist device implantation, with no difference between groups.[10]

SUMMARY

Patients under consideration for hybrid surgical access ablation represent the most challenging end of the spectrum of patients undergoing VT ablation, because they usually have failed 1 or more attempts at endocardial ablation and/or also have failed percutaneous epicardial access. Preprocedure work-up in these patients must be comprehensive and multidisciplinary. Prior identification of the likely site of origin of VT is paramount to the success of the procedure and determines the method of surgical access. Current surgical approaches provide incomplete access to localized areas of the epicardial surface. Despite this, in carefully selected patients, surgical hybrid ablation is efficacious and has an acceptable safety profile with similar acute and long-term outcomes to that of percutaneous epicardial access patients.

DISCLOSURE

The authors have no conflicts of interest to disclose.

REFERENCES

1. Boyle NG, Shivkumar K. Epicardial interventions in electrophysiology. Circulation 2012;126(14):1752–69.
2. Jiang R, Buch E, Gima J, et al. Feasibility of percutaneous epicardial mapping and ablation for refractory atrial fibrillation: insights into substrate and lesion transmurality. Heart Rhythm 2019;16(8):1151–9.
3. Sosa E, Scanavacca M, d'Avila A, et al. A new technique to perform epicardial mapping in the electrophysiology laboratory. J Cardiovasc Electrophysiol 1996;7(6):531–6.
4. Li A, Buch E, Boyle NG, et al. Incidence and significance of adhesions encountered during epicardial mapping and ablation of ventricular tachycardia in patients with no history of prior cardiac surgery or pericarditis. Heart Rhythm 2018;15(1):65–74.
5. Michowitz Y, Mathuria N, Tung R, et al. Hybrid procedures for epicardial catheter ablation of ventricular tachycardia: value of surgical access. Heart Rhythm 2010;7(11):1635–43.
6. Berruezo A, Mont L, Nava S, et al. Electrocardiographic recognition of the epicardial origin of ventricular tachycardias. Circulation 2004;109(15):1842–7.
7. Bazan V, Bala R, Garcia FC, et al. Twelve-lead ECG features to identify ventricular tachycardia arising from the epicardial right ventricle. Heart Rhythm 2006;3(10):1132–9.
8. Bazan V, Gerstenfeld EP, Garcia FC, et al. Site-specific twelve-lead ECG features to identify an epicardial origin for left ventricular tachycardia in the absence of myocardial infarction. Heart Rhythm 2007;4(11):1403–10.
9. Sacher F, Roberts-Thomson K, Maury P, et al. Epicardial ventricular tachycardia ablation: a multicenter safety study. J Am Coll Cardiol 2010;55(21):2366–72.
10. Li A, Hayase J, Do D, et al. Hybrid surgical vs percutaneous access epicardial ventricular tachycardia ablation. Heart Rhythm 2018;15(4):512–9.
11. Yamada T, Doppalapudi H, Litovsky SH, et al. Challenging radiofrequency catheter ablation of idiopathic ventricular arrhythmias originating from the left ventricular summit near the left main coronary artery. Circ Arrhythm Electrophysiol 2016;9(10). https://doi.org/10.1161/CIRCEP.116.004202.
12. Soejima K, Nogami A, Sekiguchi Y, et al. Epicardial catheter ablation of ventricular tachycardia in no entry left ventricle. Circ Arrhythm Electrophysiol 2015;8(2):381–9.
13. Diamantakos E, Harvey R, Shivkumar K, et al. Structural interventions and potential unforeseen limits on access to ventricular tachycardia substrates. JACC Clin Electrophysiol 2019;5(8):996–7.

14. Hutchinson MD, Gerstenfeld EP, Desjardins B, et al. Endocardial unipolar voltage mapping to detect epicardial ventricular tachycardia substrate in patients with nonischemic left ventricular cardiomyopathy. Circ Arrhythm Electrophysiol 2011;4(1):49–55.

15. Cheung JW, Anderson RH, Markowitz SM, et al. Catheter ablation of arrhythmias originating from the left ventricular outflow tract. JACC Clin Electrophysiol 2019;5(1):1–12.

16. Aksu T, Erdem Guler T, Yalin K. Successful ablation of an epicardial ventricular tachycardia by video-assisted thoracoscopy. Europace 2015;17(7):1116.

17. Vroomen M, Maesen B, La Meir M, et al. Hybrid ablation of ventricular tachycardia: a single-centre experience. J Atr Fibrillation 2019;11(5):2118.

18. Mathuria NS, Vaseghi M, Buch E, et al. Successful ablation of an epicardial ventricular tachycardia using a surgical ablation tool. Circ Arrhythm Electrophysiol 2011;4(6):e84–6.

19. Wood MA, Ellenbogen AL, Pathak V, et al. Efficacy of a cooled bipolar epicardial radiofrequency ablation probe for creating transmural myocardial lesions. J Thorac Cardiovasc Surg 2010;139(2):453–8.

20. Anter E, Hutchinson MD, Deo R, et al. Surgical ablation of refractory ventricular tachycardia in patients with nonischemic cardiomyopathy. Circ Arrhythm Electrophysiol 2011;4(4):494–500.

21. Mulloy DP, Bhamidipati CM, Stone ML, et al. Cryoablation during left ventricular assist device implantation reduces postoperative ventricular tachyarrhythmias. J Thorac Cardiovasc Surg 2013; 145(5):1207–13.

22. Jincun G, Faguang Z, Weibin H, et al. Outside-in subepicardial dissection during percutaneous epicardial ventricular tachycardia ablation. Circ Arrhythm Electrophysiol 2016;9(10):e004499.

23. Sosa E, Scanavacca M, D'Avila A, et al. Nonsurgical transthoracic epicardial approach in patients with ventricular tachycardia and previous cardiac surgery. J Interv Card Electrophysiol 2004;10(3):281–8.

24. Roberts-Thomson KC, Seiler J, Steven D, et al. Percutaneous access of the epicardial space for mapping ventricular and supraventricular arrhythmias in patients with and without prior cardiac surgery. J Cardiovasc Electrophysiol 2010;21(4): 406–11.

25. Tschabrunn CM, Haqqani HM, Cooper JM, et al. Percutaneous epicardial ventricular tachycardia ablation after noncoronary cardiac surgery or pericarditis. Heart Rhythm 2013;10(2):165–9.

26. Killu AM, Ebrille E, Asirvatham SJ, et al. Percutaneous epicardial access for mapping and ablation is feasible in patients with prior cardiac surgery, including coronary bypass surgery. Circ Arrhythm Electrophysiol 2015;8(1):94–101.

Epicardial Ablation via Arterial and Venous Systems

Venkatakrishna N. Tholakanahalli, MD, FHRS

KEYWORDS

• Ventricular arrhythmias • Intracoronary • Arterial • Venous • Ablation

KEY POINTS

- Intracoronary artery and venous mapping helps identify the area of interest for ventricular arrhythmias or atrial arrhythmias.
- Successful mapping through these routes enhances precision for intervention and may decrease the need to access the epicardial space in general and in post–cardiac surgery patients when access is limited.
- Ethanol injection, coil embolization, and radiofrequency ablation can be used as potential options with this approach.
- Mapping with these techniques enhances precision to intervene regardless of whether the mapped site is the ultimate ablation site.

INTRODUCTION

Ventricular arrhythmias (VA) increase morbidity and mortality in structural heart disease and can cause morbidity in structurally normal hearts. Catheter ablation of VAs can be effective endocardially given the accessibility via transaortic and transseptal approaches into the left ventricle (LV) and directly through the venous system to the right ventricle (RV). VAs inaccessible from an endocardial approach often arise or have critical components on the epicardium or in the midmyocardium. Vallés and colleagues[1] described criteria to identify epicardial origin or exit of VAs based on several criteria with a common theme of delayed intrinsicoid deflection, prolonged QRS duration, and presence or absence of Q waves with variable sensitivity and specificity. The yield of these criteria is better for VAs in patients with idiopathic and nonischemic cardiomyopathy and less predictable with ischemic scar-mediated VAs.

Presumed epicardial arrhythmias typically require thorough mapping epicardially and endocardially in order to execute appropriate therapeutic strategies. The approach to percutaneous epicardial ablation is well known (and covered in detail elsewhere in this issue) and requires careful consideration based on morphology of VAs, and often is done after failure to approach through the endocardial route. In some cases, intra–coronary arterial (CA) and coronary sinus venous (CSV) mapping/intervention may be highly valuable for intramyocardial sites of origin or epicardial sites of origin without having to access epicardial space. Even when interventions within CA or CSV routes are not possible, mapping may guide intervention endocardially. In one series, Baman and colleagues[2] reported that idiopathic VAs arising from an epicardial site of origin were identified in 15% of the patients through the CSV system. Another observation from the cohort of Mountantonakis and colleagues[3] showed that

Advanced Interventional Cardiac Electrophysiology, LAA Closure program and EP Laboratory, Minneapolis VA Health Care System, University of Minnesota, 111C, One Veterans Dr. Minneapolis MN 55417, USA
E-mail address: thola001@umn.edu

Card Electrophysiol Clin 12 (2020) 391–399
https://doi.org/10.1016/j.ccep.2020.06.006
1877-9182/20/Published by Elsevier Inc.

9% of idiopathic VAs are linked to CSV (53% great cardiac vein [GCV], 40% anterior interventricular vein [AIV], 7% middle cardiac vein [MCV]). The true incidence of arterial proximity to the arrhythmia site of origin is unclear, but ongoing studies continue to provide insight.

ANATOMY

CA and CSV anatomy closely follow each other, providing a global epicardial accessibility to potentially map many VAs, which (especially in idiopathic cases) seem to have predilections to specific sites. The sites are shown in **Fig. 1**.[4] Percutaneous epicardial mapping, although it has advantages, sometimes is limited by epicardial fat (**Fig. 2**A).

Mapping of VAs via CSV tributaries and CAs also narrows down the locations where these arrhythmias arise or exit, which enables clinicians to precisely identify sites where potential interventional therapies can be accomplished. The structures adjacent to sites where VAs can potentially be mapped through veins and arteries are discussed later in this article in relation to site-specific mapping.

MAPPING TOOLS

Previously, the pathfinder Cardima catheter (Fremont, CA) was used in many of the original studies, but it is no longer available. Instead, CA or CSV mapping can be performed using any angioplasty wire (0.356 mm [0.014 in]), covered with uninflated angioplasty balloon over the wire with ~5 mm of the wire tip exposed and the other end connected to alligator clip. This method allows unipolar signals to be recorded against an indifferent electrode within the inferior vena cava[5] (**Fig. 3**A**).

Intracoronary wire mapping using 0.356-mm (0.014-in) VisionWire (Biotronik SE & CO KG, Berlin, Germany) was originally performed by Tholakanahalli and colleagues[6] in a septal perforator branch. The advantage of this wire is that the tip is exposed (15 mm) but the body of the wire is insulated and therefore does not require an angioplasty balloon. Similar to an angioplasty wire, the proximal end can be connected to an alligator clip to record unipolar signals with indifferent electrode in the inferior vena cava. Alternatively, a second VisionWire can be placed in the coronary artery or vein closer to the first one to make a bipolar electrode pair for bipolar signals, although the distance between bipolar electrodes is greater than 15 mm[6] (see **Fig. 3**A**).

Other tools that can be used to map include Map-iT 4/3.3 Fr. Decapolar 2 mm, 2-5-2 mm, or 2-8-2 mm diagnostic catheter (Access point technologies, Rogers, MN) and any diagnostic catheter can potentially be used in venous territory if feasible by caliber.

A 7-Fr mapping catheter, Decanav 2-8-2 mm, 10-pole catheter (Biosense-Webster, Irvine, CA),

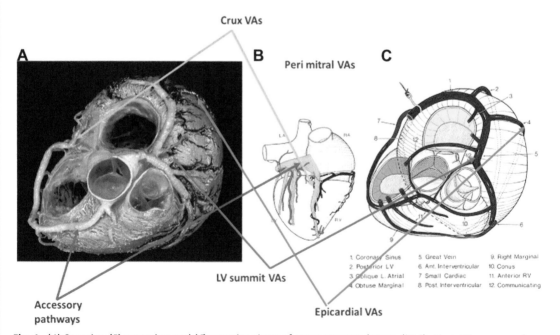

Fig. 1. (*A*) Superior, (*B*) posterior, and (*C*) superior views of coronary vasculature distribution. VAs commonly approached through arterial or venous system and accessory pathways are shown. (*Adapted from* McAlpine WA. Heart and coronary arteries. In: New York: Springer-Verlag; 1975; with permission.)

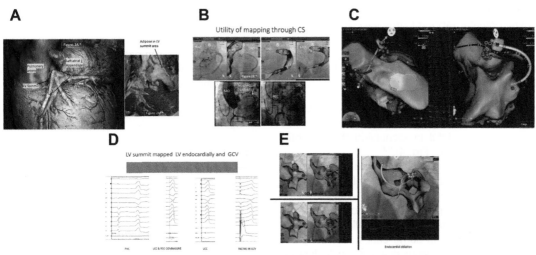

Fig. 2. Mapping of LV summit region. (*A**) LV summit region. (*A***) Adipose deposition in the LV summit region. (*B*) Mapping of LV summit. (*B**) CSV angiogram in relation to right ventricular outflow tract (RVOT) and overlapping coronary sinus (CS) geometry created with ablation catheter. (*B***) shows a multipolar catheter in CS with distal tip in GCV-AIV region, aortic root angiogram, and ablation catheter in right coronary cusp (RCC). (*C*) A Map-iT multipolar catheter in CSV-AIV and ablation catheter in GCV mapping. (*D*) Premature ventricular complex (PVC), which is mapped through GCV by pacing, left coronary cusp (LCC), and LCC and RCC commissure. (*E*) The mapped PVC being ablated endocardially. LAO, left anterior oblique; RAO, right anterior oblique. ([*2A*] *Illustration courtesy* UCLA Cardiac Arrhythmia Center, Wallace A. McAlpine MD collection)

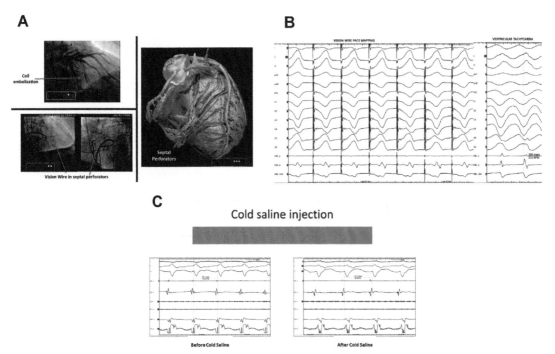

Fig. 3. Mapping of septal VA through septal perforators of CA. (*A**) Coil embolization. (*A***) VisionWire mapping through septal perforators. (*A****) Cardiac anatomy of left anterior descending coronary artery with septal perforators. (*B*) Pace mapping through a septal VisionWire compared with spontaneous VA. (*C*) Slowing of ventricular tachycardia with cold saline injection. ([*3A****] *Illustration courtesy* UCLA Cardiac Arrhythmia Center, Wallace A. McAlpine MD collection).

or Inquiry decapolar 2-5-2 mm spacing 4-Fr diagnostic catheter (Abbott Cardiovascular, Plymouth MN) can also be used.

CONFIRMING OPTIMAL LOCATION FOR INTERVENTION

As with other VA, entrainment, pace mapping, mid-diastolic potentials, and late potential mapping can be helpful in identifying the potential target sites (**Fig. 3**B; **Fig. 4**).[5,6]

Additional techniques can be used when assessing the optimal site of ablation through intracoronary arterial or venous vessels. One such method is repeated termination of VAs with cold saline injection through balloon-occluded arterial branches.[5] In some cases, VAs may not terminate, but may slow down in cycle length[6] (**Fig. 3**C).

INTERVENTIONAL TECHNIQUES
Unipolar Ablation Through Coronary Veins

Ablation of VAs through coronary veins is a well-known concept with direct current (DC) ablation[7] or radiofrequency energy[8] for accessory pathways.

Radiofrequency energy in the current practice is delivered mainly using an irrigated-tip catheter at a power of 15 to 25 W. Other catheters used are 5, 6, or 7 Fr. Non–irrigated-tip catheters (Blazer, Boston Scientific, Natick, MA; Mariner, Medtronic Inc, Minneapolis, MN) or a standard 8.5-Fr. irrigated-tip catheter cannot be advanced in a coronary venous tributary. The main issue with ablation in these structures is sudden increase in impedance caused by slow flow, which in some cases can be overcome by increasing the limits of impedance on the radiofrequency generator.

Chemical Ablation

Injection of ethanol 96% to 98% in 1-mL increments up to 4 mL if permissible based on vein sizes (and slightly less in arterial approach) is an important modality for treating these arrhythmias. Typically, an angioplasty balloon is used to occlude the targeted vessel to prevent backflow and alcohol is injected (American Regent Inc, Shirley, NY; or Akorn Inc, Lake Forest, IL). This process may take up to 30 minutes to have a permanent effect. Brugada and colleagues[9] first described use of intracoronary arterial ethanol injection to

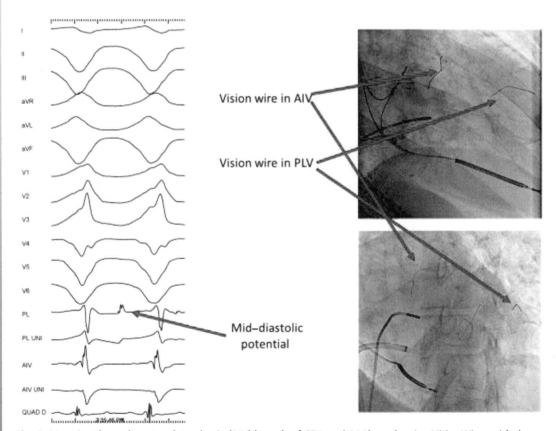

Fig. 4. Mapping through posterolateral vein (PLV) branch of CSV, and AIV branch using VisionWires with demonstration of mid-diastolic potential recorded from posterolateral branch as shown.

permanently stop VAs. The concept can be used through arterial or venous routes.

Coil Embolization

Coil embolization is a technique described originally by Tholakanahalli and colleagues,[6] mainly for intraseptal VAs. The technique is useful for CA intervention therapies. CV coil embolization has not been described, but theoretically may not be helpful. Once the specific target vessel is identified, balloon occlusion of the targeted vessel followed by contrast injection (1:10 dilution; 1–2 mL) assessed by transesophageal echocardiogram helps assess the distribution of the vessel targeted.[6] The balloon catheter can be exchanged with courier microcatheter (Codman Neurovascular, Codman and Shurtleff, Inc, Raynham, MA). Coils typically used are Mircuspere, Deltapush (Codman Neurovascular). Once deployed, contrast injection helps determine whether there is occlusion of the vessel. Testing for VAs from 30 minutes to 1 hour may provide the acute success assessment.[6] If the watershed area of the vessel encompasses the critical isthmus site or the focus of interest, coil embolization should be beneficial.

Simultaneous Unipolar Versus Bipolar Ablation

CSV mapping is extremely helpful when dealing with midmyocardial substrates, but delivery of energy through the veins may not be sufficient to reach the critical site. Simultaneous unipolar ablation[10] and bipolar ablation[11] have been described as useful options in these challenging patients.

For simultaneous unipolar ablation, irrigated-tip ablation catheters can be positioned in the GCV with a second ablation catheter in aortomitral continuity for VAs involving the LV summit. This technique has been described as beneficial when activation maps are equal in both situations with an associated wall thickness greater than 8 mm.[10]

Futyma and colleagues[11] described bipolar ablation involving placement of catheters in the GCV and LV endocardium for LV summit VAs. A 3.5-mm ablation catheter is placed in GCV at the earliest site of activation and a 4-mm ablation catheter in the endocardium of the LV at the earliest activation site of endocardial aspect. Careful assessment of the proximity of coronary arteries is performed with right anterior oblique (RAO) (42°) caudal (20°) views, and left anterior oblique (32°) projection helps to assess catheter position and relationship to the coronary arteries. If there is more than 5 mm distance from the arteries, bipolar ablation can be safely performed, starting with 10 W to a maximum of 27 W with

impedance decrease from 190 to 220 Ω to 140 to 180 Ω for successful elimination of VAs. This technique has not been described in other epicardial locations but it could be considered in difficult situations.

Other Techniques

Recently a technique has been described using radiofrequency energy delivered through a coronary reentry system developed to treat coronary artery chronic total occlusions by perforating an arterial branch into an intramyocardial location.[12] This technique involves positioning of an intracoronary guidewire into a septal perforator and a stingray LP device (Boston Scientific, Marlborough, MA) is positioned at the proximal portion of the perforator branch. The balloon used provides support to drive the guidewire directly into the myocardium of interest and deliver radiofrequency energy.

SITE-SPECIFIC MAPPING AND ABLATION
Left Ventricular Summit

CSV mapping is extremely valuable to identify the best site for ablation in patients with VAs arising from the LV summit area. The LV summit, as best described by McAlpine,[4] involves the area bound by the bifurcation of the left main coronary artery to form the left anterior descending coronary artery and left circumflex artery, with the base of the triangle demarcated by the transecting AIV, which drains into GCV. This is a complex area for ablation epicardially because it is an inaccessible area because of coronary artery proximity (see **Fig. 2**A*),[4] and epicardial fat (see **Fig. 2**A**) limits the biophysics of ablation. The accessible zones of the LV summit are beyond this region more laterally and apically. Epicardial ablation can be attempted in the accessible zone, but most cases are best approached through the GCV/AIV, left coronary cusp (LCC), anterior LV beneath the LCC, or anterior right ventricular outflow tract (RVOT).[13] The definition of the best activation site can be crystallized with mapping through CSV anatomy involving GCV and AIV to bracket the activation timing as well as anterior communicating branch between GCV and lesser cardiac vein, which traverses behind the RVOT (**Fig. 2**B–D).

Mapping in this area can be attempted using a multipolar catheter, as described earlier, or wire mapping if venous tributaries are small. The precision of mapping increases the success rate for ablation. If coronary arteries are not in close relationship (at least 5 mm), radiofrequency ablation using an open-irrigated ablation catheter from the GCV can be attempted (see **Fig. 2**C). If electrogram (EGM) characteristics are suggestive of midmyocardial arrhythmia origin, bipolar ablation between the GCV and LV endocardium has been described as well.[11] LV endocardial unipolar ablation with high-power energy delivered continuously for more than 3 minutes may be effective, as may simultaneous unipolar ablation (**Fig. 2**E). Alcohol injection into the anterior communicating branch if the location shows early activation can be effective in some patients.[11]

Left Ventricular Crux

The VAs arising from LV crux area are unique idiopathic VAs, nicely described by Kawamura and colleagues.[14] The locations of these VAs are best mapped through the MCV if feasible. There are 2 described subtypes of crux VAs. Basal crux VAs present with left bundle branch block (LBBB) or right bundle branch block (RBBB) morphology in V1 but have unique signature V2 with R greater than S wave and the rest of the precordial leads having a predominant R or Rs morphology with negative inferior leads. Apical crux VA presents with LBBB or RBBB pattern in V1 with V2 R greater than S and rS pattern in V4 to V6 or QS pattern in the apical leads[4] (**Fig. 5**). These VAs may have epicardial electrocardiogram features. Mapping can be performed for both subtypes via the MCV. The apical version may be successfully ablated with an epicardial approach; however, the basal version often must be targeted via the venous system.

Ventricular Septal Ventricular Arrhythmias

Although the current article involves epicardial mapping via veins and arteries, epicardial vessels and their branches provide excellent access to intramural substrates. Septal perforators are hence extremely valuable routes through which septal VAs can be mapped. Further, the critical site of an arrhythmia may be distant from its exit and therefore an epicardial VA may exit the epicardium but have a critical septal component.

Mapping can be performed as originally described by Segal and colleagues[5] using angioplasty wires with a noninflated balloon used to cover its body with ~5-mm tip of wire exposed, which provides the electrode tip for mapping septal perforators. Alternatively, a VisionWire (Biotronik SE & CO KG, Berlin, Germany) can be used to collect unipolar or bipolar EGMs, and pacing techniques/entrainment mapping can also be performed. Similarly, venous routes can potentially be used to map these areas.[15] Interventions of septal VAs can be achieved with alcohol injection or coil embolization (see **Fig. 3**A).[4,6] Tavares and Valderrábano[15] showed retrograde ethanol infusion for VAs arising from the LV summit region and septal region with successful outcomes. As described by McAlpine,[4] communicating venous branches between the GCV and lesser cardiac vein take a course behind the pulmonary artery through the septum and provide a valuable site for mapping septal VAs.[16]

Use of Arterial/Venous Mapping to Facilitate Mapping of Epicardial and Endocardial Ventricular Arrhythmias

Mapping of VAs associated with structural heart disease may be facilitated by placing a multipolar catheter in the coronary sinus tributaries[17] or arteries.[5] Placing a mapping catheter in a surrogate for the epicardial space (artery or vein) helps

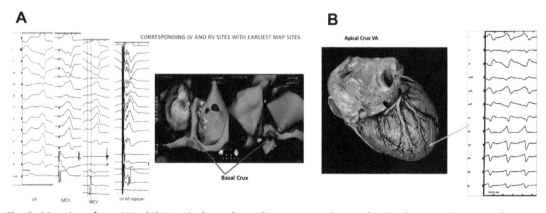

Fig. 5. Mapping of crux VAs. (*A*) Ventricular tachycardia, pace mapping, and activation mapping, as well as pace mapping endocardially adjacent to the site on LV septal side. (*Right*) 3D electroanatomic mapping with MCV, RV, and LV geometry and location of VA from basal crux. (*B*) Apical crux anatomic location and morphology of associated VA. inf, inferior. ([*B*] *Illustration courtesy* UCLA Cardiac Arrhythmia Center, Wallace A. McAlpine MD collection.)

identify and map epicardial VAs and to determine whether epicardial access is necessary. The same is true more broadly for endocardial activation as well (see **Figs.** 3B and 4; **Figs.** 6A and 7).

Perimitral Ablation: Mitral Flutter, Vein of Marshall Trigger, or Tachycardia

There are some atrial arrhythmias (AAs) that need mapping/intervention through the CSV. One important example is perimitral atrial flutter involving mitral isthmus. Ablation success for this AA depends on completion of an ablation line from the left inferior pulmonary vein to the mitral annulus. It is often incomplete because of suboptimal ablation of the isthmus closest to the coronary sinus caused by the cooling effect of atrial tissue from blood flow within the CSV. Successful ablation is often achieved by ablating within the CSV at the site corresponding with atrial ablation in the mitral isthmus region and, if needed, performing balloon occlusion of the coronary sinus to impede cooling and allow completion of the ablation line.[18] The second approach, as described by Lee and colleagues,[19] is ablation of the ostium of the vein of Marshall (VOM) and additional endocardial ablation at the site mapped from the coronary sinus. The third approach involves cannulating the VOM and balloon occlusion and subsequent alcohol injection[15] (**Fig.** 6B). Targeting the VOM may be helpful for mitral isthmus flutters as well as VOM triggers for atrial fibrillation.

Right Coronary Artery and Coronary Sinus Mapping of Accessory Pathways

In a series described by Dhala and colleagues,[20] in 50 consecutive patients with posteroseptal accessory pathways, mapping/ablation was approached through the coronary venous system and the pathways mapped in proximity to the coronary sinus ostia and further into the body of the coronary sinus. The posteroseptal accessory pathways not amenable for ablation within the venous system were successfully ablated with epicardial access in a series described by Scanavacca and colleagues.[21,22]

Right-sided accessory pathways are traditionally difficult for catheter ablation mainly because of difficulty in precise mapping caused by anatomic restraints. A technique to overcome this challenge was elegantly described by Shah and colleagues,[23] using a microcatheter in the right coronary artery in a pediatric population and

A

Coronary sinus mapping alcohol injection

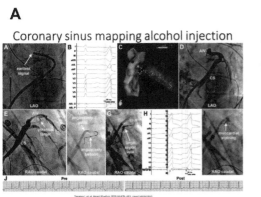

B

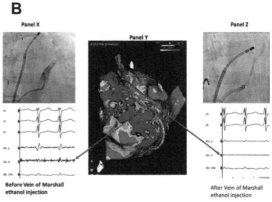

Fig. 6. (A) Successful venous ethanol ablation of a left ventricular summit VT using a septal branch of the AIV. The earliest endocardial activation time (30 ms) was recorded in the AIV. A: Fluoroscopic view showing the position of the multipolar catheter in this location. B: Recorded earliest endocardial signal. C: Three dimensional activation maps showing the earliest activation time in the AIV. D, E: Coronary venograms were performed to delineate the CS, GCV, and AIV, similar to **Fig. 1**. A potential target venule is identified arising from the AIV (septal branch). F–H: Signals from this potential target venule are recorded using a Balanced Middleweight wire (see text for description). The signal obtained from the wire preceded the QRS by 40 ms. In this case, the septal vein was too large, and contrast injection did not lead to myocardial staining. I: After the wire was removed, the balloon was gently pushed to create a small intramural venule perforation that would allow for contrast extravasation and myocardial staining. Ethanol was then delivered. J: Rhythm strips before (left) and after (right) ethanol injection show elimination of PVCs. (B) Panel X showing VOM with injection of contrast in CSV with fractionated electrograms demonstrated endocardially on the ridge using ablation catheter where VOM epicardially traversing. Panel Y shows 3D electroanatomic mapping with bipolar voltage demonstrating ablation catheter location in relation to coronary sinus and VOM. Panel Z showing balloon inflation and injection of ethanol into VOM with demonstration of loss of electrograms on ablation catheter positioned endocardially on the ridge adjacent to VOM. ([A] Reproduced with permission Tavares L et al. Heart Rhythm. 2019;16:478-483)

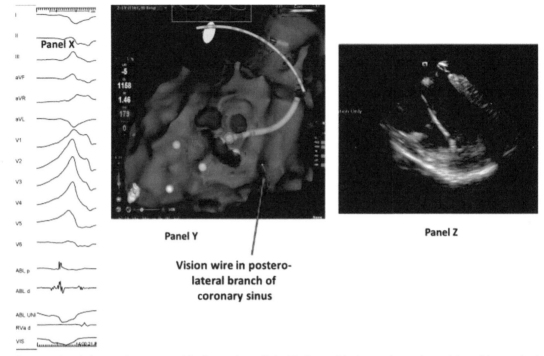

Fig. 7. Epicardial mapping as a guide for endocardial ablation. Ablation catheter is positioned beneath the lateral edge of posteromedial papillary muscle in the intracardiac echo on panel Z, electroanatomic mapping in panel Y with demonstration of vision wire epicardially. Unipolar electrograms demonstrated by vision wire in postero lateral CSV tributary and electrograms on ablation catheter.

using supporting sheaths to reach the successful endocardial ablation site. Similarly, Olgun and colleagues[24] described the use of an octapolar microcatheter in the right coronary artery in children. The risk of coronary artery injury for ablations, particularly if performed in the coronary sinus (CS) for accessory pathways, is inversely proportional to the distance between the coronary artery and the ablation site, as expected.[25]

COMPLICATIONS

Although venous or arterial intracoronary mapping has been shown to be safe in many small studies,[5,6,17] caution is required. Like any intravascular procedure, there is potential dissection and perforation risk while injecting contrast, advancing wires, or accessing the vessel using guide sheaths. Alcohol injection may cause acute complications related to backflow into larger vascular territories.

SUMMARY

Epicardial ablation via the arterial and venous systems provides an excellent opportunity to map and intervene on complex arrhythmias involving epicardial origin, areas inaccessible by a standard epicardial approach, and arrhythmias of intramural origin.

DISCLOSURE

The author has nothing to disclose.

REFERENCES

1. Vallès E, Bazan V, Marchlinski FE. ECG criteria to identify epicardial ventricular tachycardia in nonischemic cardiomyopathy. Circ Arrhythm Electrophysiol 2010;3:63–71.
2. Baman TS, Ilg KJ, Gupta SK, et al. Mapping and ablation of epicardial idiopathic ventricular arrhythmias from within the coronary venous system. Circ Arrhythm Electrophysiol 2010;3:274–9.
3. Mountantonakis SE, Frankel DS, Tschabrunn CM, et al. Ventricular arrhythmias from the coronary venous system: prevalence, mapping and ablation. Heart Rhythm 2015;12:1145–53.
4. McAlpine WA. Heart and coronary arteries. New York: Springer-Verlag; 1975.
5. Segal OR, Wong T, Chow AWC, et al. Intra-coronary guidewire mapping – a novel technique to guide ablation of human ventricular tachycardia. J Interv Card Electrophysiol 2007;18:143–54.

6. Tholakanahalli VN, Bertog S, Roukoz H, et al. Catheter ablation of ventricular tachycardia using intracoronary wire mapping and coil embolization: Description of a new technique. Heart Rhythm 2013;10:291–5.

7. Fisher JD, Brodman R, Kim SG, et al. Attempted nonsurgical electrical ablation of accessory pathways via the coronary sinus in the Wolff-Parkinson-White syndrome. J Am Coll Cardiol 1984;4:685–94.

8. Huang SK, Graham AR, Bharati S, et al. Short and long-term effects of trans-catheter ablation of the coronary sinus by radiofrequency energy. Circulation 1988;78:416–27.

9. Brugada P, de Swart H, Smeets JL, et al. Transcoronary chemical ablation of ventricular tachycardia. Circulation 1989;79:475–82.

10. Yamada T, Maddoxx WR, McElderry T, et al. Radiofrequency catheter ablation of idiopathic ventricular arrhythmias originating from intramural foci in the left ventricular outflow tract. Circ Arrhythm Electrophysiol 2015;8:344–52.

11. Futyma P, Sander J, Ciapala K, et al. Bipolar radiofrequency ablation delivered from coronary veins and adjacent endocardium for treatment of refractory left ventricular summit arrhythmias. J Interv Card Electrophysiol 2019. https://doi.org/10.1007/s10840-019-00609-9.

12. Romero J, Carlos Diaz J, Hayase J, et al. Intramyocardial radiofrequency ablation of ventricular arrhythmias using intracoronary wire mapping and a coronary reentry system: Description of a novel technique. Heart Rhythm Case Rep 2018;4:285–92.

13. Enriquez A, Malavassi F, Supple G, et al. How to map and ablate left ventricular summit arrhythmias. Heart Rhythm 2017;14-1:141–8.

14. Kawamura M, Gerstenfeld EP, Vedantham V, et al. Idiopathic ventricular arrhythmia originating from the cardiac crux or inferior septum epicardial idiopathic ventricular arrhythmia. Circ Arrhythm Electrophysiol 2014;7:1152–8.

15. Tavares L, Valderrábano M. Retrograde ethanol ablation for ventricular tachycardia. Heart Rhythm 2019;16:4780483.

16. Komatsu Y, Nogami A, Shinoda Y, et al. Idiopathic ventricular arrhythmias originating from the vicinity of the communicating vein of cardiac venous systems at the left ventricular summit. Circ Arrhythm Electrophysiol 2018;11:e005386.

17. De Paola AAV, Melo WDS, Tavora MZP, et al. Angiographic and electrophysiologic substrates for ventricular tachycardia mapping through the coronary veins. Heart 1998;79:59–63.

18. Wong KCK, Jones M, Qureshi N, et al. Balloon occlusion of the distal coronary sinus facilitates mitral isthmus ablation. Heart Rhythm 2011;8:833–9.

19. Lee JH, Nam GB, Kim M, et al. Radiofrequency catheter ablation targeting the vein of Marshall in difficult mitral isthmus ablation or pulmonary vein isolation. J Cardiovasc Electrophysiol 2017;28:386–93.

20. Dhala AA, Deshpande SS, Bremner S, et al. Transcatheter ablation of posteroseptal accessory pathways using a venous approach and radiofrequency energy. Circulation 1994;90:1799–810.

21. Scanavacca MI, Sternick EB, Pisani C, et al. Accessory atrioventricular pathways refractory to catheter ablation: Role of percutaneous epicardial approach. Circ Arrhythm Electrophysiol 2015;8:128–36.

22. Mao J, Moriarty JM, Mandapati R, et al. Catheter ablation of accessory pathways near the coronary sinus: Value of defining coronary arterial anatomy. Heart Rhythm 2015;12(3):508–14.

23. Shah MJ, Jones TK, Cecchin F. Improved localization of right-sided accessory pathways with microcatheter-assisted right coronary artery mapping in children. J Cardiovasc Electrophysiol 2004;15:1238–43.

24. Olgun H, Karagoz T, Celiker A. Coronary microcatheter mapping of coronary arteries during radiofrequency ablation in children. J Interv Card Electrophysiol 2010;27:75–9.

25. Stavrakis S, Jackman WM, Nakagawa H, et al. Risk of coronary artery injury with radiofrequency ablation and cryoablation of epicardial posteroseptal accessory pathways within the coronary venous system. Circ Arrhythm Electrophysiol 2014;7:113–9.

Epicardial Ablation Biophysics and Novel Radiofrequency Energy Delivery Techniques

Rachel Debenham, MD[a], Wendy S. Tzou, MD, FHRS[b],*

KEYWORDS

- Catheter ablation • Epicardial ablation • Ventricular arrhythmia • Ablation biophysics
- Radiofrequency ablation • Cryoablation

KEY POINTS

- Important differences exist between endocardial and epicardial environments that lead to differences in ablation biophysics, whether using radiofrequency or cryothermal energy.
- Absence of convective thermal conduction properties associated with circulating blood is a major difference in epicardial ablation compared with endocardial ablation.
- Various techniques exist to manipulate relative impedances of myocardium, ambient fluid, and the radiofrequency ablation circuit itself, in order to enhance lesion formation during epicardial ablation.

INTRODUCTION

Both radiofrequency (RF) and cryothermal energy have been used in catheter ablations to treat atrial and ventricular arrhythmias, from both the endocardium and the epicardium.[1,2] The underlying mechanisms leading to focused myocyte death and ablation efficacy differ between the 2 energy sources, with the most obvious and simplest difference being that RF ablation works through tissue heating, whereas cryothermal ablation is carried out by tissue freezing. However, key differences also exist in the ambient environments and structures of the endocardial and pericardial spaces. These differences affect the approach to epicardial catheter ablation using either energy source. Understanding these differences as well as a basic understanding of endocardial ablation biophysics is critical to understanding how ablation approaches differ on the epicardium. In this article, these concepts are reviewed in the context of ventricular arrhythmia ablation.

UNDERSTANDING DIFFERENCES: EPICARDIUM VERSUS ENDOCARDIUM

Anatomic features of the epicardium have been highlighted in a prior article and will not be covered in detail here except to emphasize features that have impact on ablation biophysics and efficacy. First, the ventricular epicardium tends to be smoother, without the same degree of ridges, pouches, trabeculations, or other intracavitary structures that may confound catheter movement or stability during endocardial ablation, especially endocardial ventricular ablation. Second, the epicardium is covered with fat in varying distribution and thickness, but primarily near the atrioventricular and interventricular grooves, following the distribution of the coronary arteries. Last, but not

[a] Internal Medicine, University of Colorado School of Medicine, 12401 East 17th Avenue, MS B-136, Aurora, CO 80045, USA; [b] Cardiac Electrophysiology, University of Colorado School of Medicine, 12401 East 17th Avenue, MS B-136, Aurora, CO 80045, USA
* Corresponding author.
E-mail address: wendy.tzou@cuanschutz.edu
Twitter: @Zo_EP2 (W.S.T.)

Card Electrophysiol Clin 12 (2020) 401–408
https://doi.org/10.1016/j.ccep.2020.05.006
1877-9182/20/© 2020 Elsevier Inc. All rights reserved.

least, the pericardial space is absent of circulating blood.

The cumulative impact of these characteristic differences is that (1) passive convective effects of ablation encountered when ablating on the endocardium are reduced substantially, (2) standard use of active convective cooling (ie, open-irrigated ablation) during RF ablation may lead to smaller ablation lesions, and (3) impedance differences can be manipulated to potentially augment epicardial RF ablation size, even when ablating within regions of epicardial fat.[3]

ENDOCARDIAL RADIOFREQUENCY ABLATION BIOPHYSICS: BACK TO THE BASICS

Since its introduction as a means to perform nonsurgical and directed arrhythmia therapy in the 1980s, RF ablation has become the primary source used in catheter ablations. RF ablation involves the transfer of electrical current into tissue, which produces a small rim of resistive heating at the electrode-tissue interface. Thermal heat conduction from this point source then proceeds in radial distribution, with rates of temperature increase dictated by proximity to the source; tissue closer to the heating source will experience more rapid increase, whereas the rate of heating of tissues farther away is slower. Importantly, a durable RF lesion, that is, one in which irreversible myocardial nonviability is achieved, occurs when the tissue temperature reaches $\geq 50^\circ$C. The radius of thermal conduction from the RF source at which a tissue temperature of 50°C is reached, otherwise known as the 50° isotherm, determines the size/depth of a durable RF lesion.[4,5] Factors that promote extension of this 50° isotherm radius, and therefore increased RF ablation lesion size, include increased size of the RF electrode or catheter tip, and higher power, contact force, and duration with which RF energy is continuously applied through the electrode.[6–8]

In the setting of circulating blood, additional factors may limit RF ablation efficacy or safety (**Fig. 1**). First, circulating blood, which is composed mostly of water, produces a convective cooling effect, which draws heat away from the RF source and away from targeted tissue, thus limiting RF lesion size; in regions of higher blood flow or relative catheter instability, this inefficiency in heat transfer is magnified substantially.[9,10]

Second, high temperatures can be produced at the electrode tip-tissue interface during RF ablation; when temperatures exceed 100°C, the water contained in surrounding blood can boil, and red blood cells can degrade, resulting in coagulum and char formation at the electrode-tissue interface. The denatured protein adheres to the catheter-tip surface and electrically insulates it, increases the impedance to current flow, and reduces the effective surface area for RF current conduction; smaller RF lesions result, as does increased risk of systemic embolism of the unintended ablation byproducts.[4,11]

The high-temperature phenomenon at the electrode and tissue interface also can occur when ablating in regions with low blood flow (eg, pouches or within coronary veins), leading to increases in impedance and limited power delivery. Finally, excessive heating can produce temperatures greater than 100°C below the surface of targeted tissue, water within which also can boil and erupt, disrupting surrounding tissue planes and producing an often audible sound. These so-called steam pops are often accompanied by an acute increase in impedance, likely attributable to a sudden introduction of vaporized water into the active RF circuit, and can result in cardiac perforation and tamponade, as well increased risk for acute thrombus formation and thromboembolism.[11]

A critical advance in RF ablation catheter design to overcome the issue of coagulum and char formation is active cooling of the electrode tip during RF application. Although this approach could potentially augment unwanted convective cooling effects at the tip-tissue interface, such localized cooling also increases the ability to deliver higher power for longer durations, promoting higher temperature formation deeper within tissue, thus allowing for a larger 50° isotherm radius (see **Fig. 1**). In preclinical models, cooled- or irrigated-tip RF ablation increased lesion sizes by up to 50% compared with non-cooled-tip ablation using a standard 3.5- or 4-mm tip electrode.[8,12] Initially available catheter designs included a closed-loop system, in which the electrode cooling occurred internally with a recirculating solution of dextrose 5% in water (D5W) within the catheter, and an open-irrigation system, in which heparinized normal saline (NS) is irrigated outwardly, through six 0.4-mm irrigation pores positioned around the electrode tip.[13,14] Preclinical studies have suggested a higher rate of steam pops and char formation because of higher electrode-tissue interface temperatures with the closed-tip cooled ablation catheters, especially when ablating with higher power.[13,15] Currently, open-irrigated ablation catheters are more widely clinically available and more widely used. Given the high volumes of fluid that may be introduced during open-irrigated ablation, especially during prolonged ablation cases, low-flow open-irrigated catheters have been introduced in which smaller

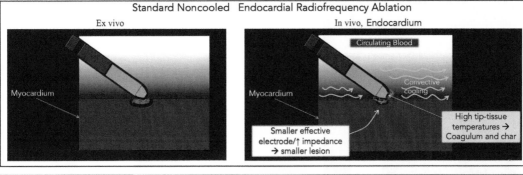

Fig. 1. Impact of active cooling of the RF ablation catheter tip during ablation. In idealized settings (*upper left*), RF current delivered to myocardium results in a rim of resistive heating, and the radial, thermal conduction of this heat then is responsible for most of the lesion that forms; the size of the 50° isotherm is impacted largely by the temperature achieved at the heating energy source. In endocardial ablation (*upper right*), circulating blood can limit RF lesion size because of effects of passive convective cooling and red blood cell degradation because of high temperatures at the RF electrode-tissue interface, leading to coagulum and char on the RF electrode. Cumulative effects produce a smaller lesion. When the RF electrode is actively cooled (*lower*), tip-tissue temperatures during RF delivery are lower; char and coagulum are less likely to form, and higher power and current can be delivered, allowing for larger 50° isotherm radius and larger lesions compared with noncooled RF ablation.

volumes of NS are irrigated through more porous electrode tips, which allows for more comprehensive electrode-tip cooling but with less fluid required to achieve it.

ADDITIONAL BIOPHYSICAL CONSIDERATIONS DURING RADIOFREQUENCY ABLATION

Solutions containing charged ions, including NS, possess a small ionic charge and can conduct electrical current. When open-irrigated RF ablation is performed using NS as the irrigant, some of the RF current is conducted away from myocardium and into the ambient NS cloud that surrounds the ablation electrode.[16–18] Along those lines, the impedance in solutions containing a higher concentration of charged particles (ie, NS) is lower compared with those with lower concentrations of charged ions. Half-normal saline (HNS) as well as D5W have relatively higher impedances compared with NS and, importantly, have higher impedances relative to myocardium (**Fig. 2**).[17,18] Consequently, more RF current in the context of open irrigation using HNS or D5W is directed toward myocardium compared with NS, because less RF current is

conducted away by surrounding medium; preclinical studies have demonstrated that larger lesions are comparatively formed (see **Fig. 2**).[16–18] In clinical use, HNS irrigation has also been demonstrated to have improved acute as well as longer-term efficacy in achieving ablation success, particularly when NS open irrigation is unsuccessful, and very commonly when critical arrhythmia elements are suspected to be midmyocardial.[19]

Baseline impedance within an RF circuit, which is inversely related to the potential size of RF lesions that can be created, can also be decreased simply by repositioning or adding grounding patches closer to the site of ablation.[20,21] In other words, placement of impedance patches closer to the heart, or in a position that promotes RF current vector toward the cardiac region of interest, is a simple method for augmenting RF ablation size and potentially improving outcomes, especially among cases in which deep, intramural substrate must be targeted.[21,22]

EPICARDIAL RADIOFREQUENCY ABLATION

In the pericardial space, absence of circulating blood effectively eliminates passive convective

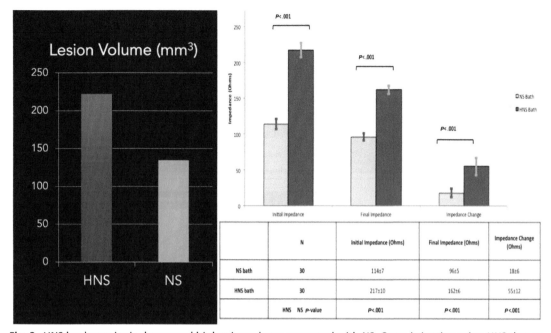

Fig. 2. HNS has lower ionic charge and higher impedance compared with NS. Open irrigation using HNS thus results in greater current delivery to the myocardium and larger lesions compared with NS. (*Adapted from* Nguyen DT, Nguyen K, Zheng L, Schuller JL, Zipse MM, Tzou WS and Sauer WH. Effect of Environmental Impedance Surrounding a Radiofrequency Ablation Catheter Electrode on Lesion Characteristics. *J Cardiovasc Electrophysiol.* 2017;28:564-569; with permission.)

cooling when RF energy is delivered. Epicardial RF ablation without active cooling of the electrode increases the propensity for high tip-tissue interface temperatures to be reached, thus limiting overall power delivery in temperature-controlled systems; although the potential for coagulum and char formation owing to red-blood cell degradation is less than with endocardial ablation, increases in impedance as well as steam pops can still occur and limit ablation lesion size.[23]

Preclinical studies have demonstrated that significantly larger epicardial lesions can be formed with active, closed-loop cooling of the RF electrode during ablation, in areas both with and without epicardial fat, compared with noncooled RF ablation, although with potentially higher risk of steam pops.[23] However, the same may not apply when using open-irrigation cooling; in a porcine in vivo study examining ablation lesions created by ThermoCool SmartTouch, ThermoCool SmartTouch-SF (Biosense Webster, Diamond Bar, CA, USA), or FlexAbility (Abbott, Minneapolis, MN, USA) open-irrigated RF catheters, the size of epicardial lesions did not differ significantly when using low irrigation flow rates (5 mL/min) versus high flow rates (15 mL/min); however, the larger the volume of intrapericardial fluid retained during RF ablation, the smaller the lesions were (**Fig. 3**).[24]

This seeming paradox makes sense when considering the differences in environmental impedance inherent to the irrigation fluid used within the respective electrode-cooling systems (D5W in closed-loop cooled RF systems and NS in standard, open-irrigated RF ablation), as well as the volume of irrigated fluid within the pericardial space during RF delivery (**Fig. 4**A, B).[16–18,24] In the case of standard open-irrigated RF epicardial ablation using NS, higher volumes of intrapericardial NS during ablation produces significantly smaller RF lesions and actually neutralizes the effect of higher power on creating larger lesions.[24]

Interestingly, when lower ionic concentration irrigant is used and the pericardial space is filled with this fluid (HNS or D5W), not only are larger and deeper lesions created in the myocardium in comparison to those created using NS irrigation, but there is a theoretically decreased risk of pericarditis and even lung injury because of the preferential conduction of RF current toward myocardium and away from these adjacent structures (**Fig. 4**).[3] In other words, the higher impedance environment created by the layer of HNS or D5W may produce a layer of insulation between the RF catheter and adjacent, cardiac, and noncardiac structures, by both increasing the relative distance between the RF energy source and

No Intrapericardial Fluid   Intrapericardial Fluid Present

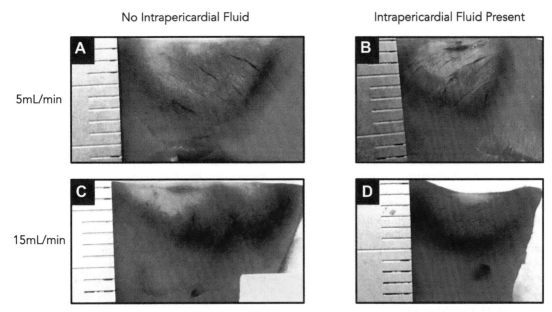

Fig. 3. In vivo porcine epicardial RF ablation experiment demonstrating that RF lesions were significantly larger when ablating in the absence (*panels A and C*) compared with presence (*panels B and D*) of intrapericardial fluid. RF lesion sizes did not differ significantly between flow rates of 5 (*panels A and B*) and 15 (*panels C and D*) mL/ min. (*Adapted from* Aryana A, O'Neill PG, Pujara DK, Singh SK, Bowers MR, Allen SL and d'Avila A. Impact of irrigation flow rate and intrapericardial fluid on cooled-tip epicardial radiofrequency ablation. *Heart Rhythm.* 2016;13:1602-11; with permission.)

surrounding structures and preferentially directing flow away from them and toward the lower-impedance myocardium. Maintenance of fluid within the pericardial space also can reduce risk of injury to the left phrenic nerve,[25] the location of which should be identified to avoid injury before ablation. Use of HNS in open-irrigated RF epicardial ablation also can produce significantly deeper

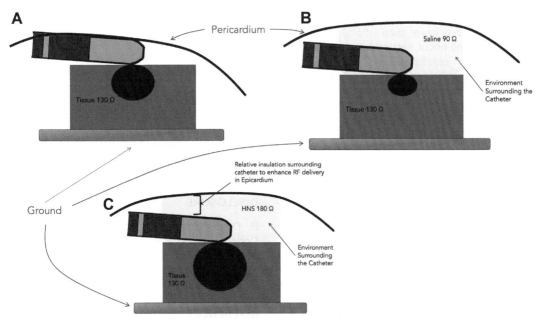

Fig. 4. Impact of intrapericardial fluid content (*A* = absence; *B* NS irrigant; *C* = HNS irrigant) and associated impedance and RF ablation lesion size given relative impedance differences promoting current flow in the direction of lower resistance. HNS irrigant (*C*) may also confer a relative shielding effect to collateral structures, including the lung, phrenic nerve, and pericardium itself. (*Courtesy of* Dr. William H. Sauer.)

lesions compared with NS-irrigated ablation in areas with epicardial fat thickness of up to 3 mm, which is comparable to depths achieved even with bipolar ablation.[3] Depth of ablation lesions achieved using any of the commercially available RF catheters becomes more dramatically limited in areas with epicardial fat thickness of greater than 3 mm.[3] However, ablation of such regions spanning the left ventricle might theoretically be avoided given frequent proximity of major coronary arteries within regions of thick epicardial adipose; epicardial ablation within 5 mm of a coronary artery is not recommended given the potential for significant arterial injury as well as ineffective ablation.[2] Caution should always be exercised when applying techniques to augment RF lesion size, because they also are associated with a higher rate of steam pops and potential for associated complications.[16–19]

EPICARDIAL CRYOABLATION

Another clinically used energy source for ablation is cryothermal energy. Several complex mechanisms are involved in the ability of cryothermal energy to induce focal myocyte death.[26,27] A stepwise process occurs, which initially leads to slowing in metabolism, disrupted ion-pump function, and increased intracellular acidity. These processes can be reversible, especially if cooling occurs briefly and to a temperature of no more than -30°C, which allows cryoablation in "mapping mode" to assess relative safety or efficacy of ablation at a given site.[28]

At temperatures lower than -55°C, more irreversible changes occur, related to ice crystal formation, which results in a combination of distortion of membranes, nuclei, and organelles, and eventually to dysfunction, with the mitochondria being the most sensitive. Freeze-thaw cycles perpetuate additional permanent damage, because thawing of the ice leads to increased volume and hyperosmolality, which disrupt membrane integrity and promote further cellular destruction.[26,27] Over a period of hours to weeks, processes of hemorrhage and inflammation, and then replacement fibrosis occur; resulting lesions usually are more sharply demarcated and homogeneous with respect to replacement fibrosis, and they tend to be less disruptive to adjacent architecture, compared with RF.[26,27,29] The final size and permanence of cryoablation lesions directly correlate with size of the cryoprobe, tissue temperature achieved, rate of freezing, the duration with which it is sustained, and the use of multiple freeze-thaw cycles.[27,29,30] The intensity of cooling (lowest temperature and fastest rate) is greatest at the site at which the catheter and tissue are in contact; freezing spreads radially from this site forming a temperature gradient, with progressively slower and less cooling at more distant sites, which, by extension, are more prone to reversible rather than irreversible effects.[27] Contemporary systems now cool more quickly and efficiently to -80°C, but the presence of any proximate heat source, which is most impactful when performing endocardial cryoablation within warm blood, can limit its efficacy in comparison to RF ablation, especially when the desired target is deep within thicker myocardium.[27,30,31]

With respect to epicardial cryoablation, cryoenergy applied near a heat source (eg, coronary artery) has been shown to produce more shallow lesions.[30] However, more remote warming can also occur from endocardium to epicardium and may account for less marked effect than anticipated with focal epicardial cryoablation when ablating with a percutaneously inserted standard cryocatheter over the epicardial left ventricle[29] or even with open surgical epicardial ablation using a linear probe; for truly intramural sources, this phenomenon can be problematic. Cardioplegia in selected cases of open-surgical ablation with cryothermal energy has been used to maximize the potential transmurality and durability of epicardial cryoablation.[32]

SUMMARY

Beyond greater complexity and anatomic differences involved in epicardial compared with endocardial access and ablation, key differences exist in environments of the intracardiac and pericardial spaces that affect the biophysics of ablation. These differences must be considered when determining the best approach/techniques for epicardial ablation. RF energy delivery to the epicardium can be enhanced with the use of actively cooled ablation catheters; this effect can be augmented further with use of fluids with lower ionic concentration and higher impedance, including HNS and D5W.

DISCLOSURE

R. Debenham: Nothing to disclose. W.S. Tzou: Consultant or speaker honoraria from Abbott, Biosense Webster, Boston Scientific, Medtronic; Research funding from Boston Scientific, Biosense Webster, Abbott.

REFERENCES

1. Calkins H, Hindricks G, Cappato R, et al. 2017 HRS/EHRA/ECAS/APHRS/SOLAECE expert consensus

statement on catheter and surgical ablation of atrial fibrillation. Heart Rhythm 2017;14:e275–444.

2. Cronin EM, Bogun FM, Maury P, et al. 2019 HRS/EHRA/APHRS/LAHRS expert consensus statement on catheter ablation of ventricular arrhythmias. Heart Rhythm 2019;21(8):1143–4.

3. Zipse MM, Edward JA, Zheng L, et al. Impact of epicardial adipose tissue and catheter ablation strategy on biophysical parameters and ablation lesion characteristics. J Cardiovasc Electrophysiol 2020;31(5):1114–24.

4. Haines DE, Watson DD, Verow AF. Electrode radius predicts lesion radius during radiofrequency energy heating. Validation of a proposed thermodynamic model. Circ Res 1990;67:124–9.

5. Whayne JG, Nath S, Haines DE. Microwave catheter ablation of myocardium in vitro. Assessment of the characteristics of tissue heating and injury. Circulation 1994;89:2390–5.

6. Haines DE. Determinants of lesion size during radiofrequency catheter ablation: the role of electrode-tissue contact pressure and duration of energy delivery. J Cardiovasc Electrophysiol 1991;2:509–15.

7. Yokoyama K, Nakagawa H, Shah DC, et al. Novel contact force sensor incorporated in irrigated radiofrequency ablation catheter predicts lesion size and incidence of steam pop and thrombus. Circ Arrhythm Electrophysiol 2008;1:354–62.

8. Nakagawa H, Yamanashi WS, Pitha JV, et al. Comparison of in vivo tissue temperature profile and lesion geometry for radiofrequency ablation with a saline-irrigated electrode versus temperature control in a canine thigh muscle preparation. Circulation 1995;91:2264–73.

9. Strickberger SA, Hummel J, Gallagher M, et al. Effect of accessory pathway location on the efficiency of heating during radiofrequency catheter ablation. Am Heart J 1995;129:54–8.

10. Jain MK, Wolf PD. A three-dimensional finite element model of radiofrequency ablation with blood flow and its experimental validation. Ann Biomed Eng 2000;28:1075–84.

11. Haines DE, Verow AF. Observations on electrode-tissue interface temperature and effect on electrical impedance during radiofrequency ablation of ventricular myocardium. Circulation 1990;82:1034–8.

12. Ruffy R, Imran MA, Santel DJ, et al. Radiofrequency delivery through a cooled catheter tip allows the creation of larger endomyocardial lesions in the ovine heart. J Cardiovasc Electrophysiol 1995;6:1089–96.

13. Yokoyama K, Nakagawa H, Wittkampf FH, et al. Comparison of electrode cooling between internal and open irrigation in radiofrequency ablation lesion depth and incidence of thrombus and steam pop. Circulation 2006;113:11–9.

14. Calkins H, Epstein A, Packer D, et al. Catheter ablation of ventricular tachycardia in patients with structural heart disease using cooled radiofrequency energy. J Am Coll Cardiol 2000;35:1905–14.

15. Cooper JM, Sapp JL, Tedrow U, et al. Ablation with an internally irrigated radiofrequency catheter: learning how to avoid steam pops. Heart Rhythm 2004;1:329–33.

16. Nguyen DT, Olson M, Zheng L, et al. Effect of irrigant characteristics on lesion formation after radiofrequency energy delivery using ablation catheters with actively cooled tips. J Cardiovasc Electrophysiol 2015;26:792–8.

17. Nguyen DT, Nguyen K, Zheng L, et al. Effect of environmental impedance surrounding a radiofrequency ablation catheter electrode on lesion characteristics. J Cardiovasc Electrophysiol 2017;28:564–9.

18. Nguyen DT, Gerstenfeld EP, Tzou WS, et al. Radiofrequency ablation using an open irrigated electrode cooled with half-normal saline. J Am Coll Cardiol 2017;3:1103–10.

19. Nguyen DT, Tzou WS, Sandhu A, et al. Prospective multicenter experience with cooled radiofrequency ablation using high impedance irrigant to target deep myocardial substrate refractory to standard ablation. J Am Coll Cardiol 2018;4:1176–85.

20. Barkagan M, Rottmann M, Leshem E, et al. Effect of baseline impedance on ablation lesion dimensions. Circ Arrhythm Electrophysiol 2018;11:e006690.

21. Shapira-Daniels A, Barkagan M, Rottmann M, et al. Modulating the baseline impedance: an adjunctive technique for maximizing radiofrequency lesion dimensions in deep and intramural ventricular substrate: an adjunctive technique for maximizing radiofrequency lesion dimensions in deep and intramural ventricular substrate. Circ Arrhythm Electrophysiol 2019;12:e007336.

22. Futyma P, Kulakowski P. Frontal placement of dispersive patch for effective ablation of arrhythmia originating from the anterior right ventricular outflow tract. J Interv Card Electrophysiol 2017;49:327.

23. D'Avila A, Houghtaling C, Gutierrez P, et al. Catheter ablation of ventricular epicardial tissue: a comparison of standard and cooled-tip radiofrequency energy. Circulation 2004;109:2363–9.

24. Aryana A, O'Neill PG, Pujara DK, et al. Impact of irrigation flow rate and intrapericardial fluid on cooled-tip epicardial radiofrequency ablation. Heart Rhythm 2016;13:1602–11.

25. Di Biase L, Burkhardt JD, Pelargonio G, et al. Prevention of phrenic nerve injury during epicardial ablation: comparison of methods for separating the phrenic nerve from the epicardial surface. Heart Rhythm 2009;6:957–61.

26. Lustgarten DL, Keane D, Ruskin J. Cryothermal ablation: mechanism of tissue injury and current

experience in the treatment of tachyarrhythmias. Prog Cardiovasc Dis 1999;41:481–98.

27. Khairy P, Dubuc M. Transcatheter cryoablation part I: preclinical experience. Pacing Clin Electrophysiol 2008;31:112–20.

28. Friedman PL. Catheter cryoablation of cardiac arrhythmias. Curr Opin Cardiol 2005;20:48–54.

29. D'Avila A, Aryana A, Thiagalingam A, et al. Focal and linear endocardial and epicardial catheter-based cryoablation of normal and infarcted ventricular tissue. Pacing Clin Electrophysiol 2008;31:1322–31.

30. Lustgarten DL, Bell S, Hardin N, et al. Safety and efficacy of epicardial cryoablation in a canine model. Heart Rhythm 2005;2:82–90.

31. Di Biase L, Al-Ahamad A, Santangeli P, et al. Safety and outcomes of cryoablation for ventricular tachyarrhythmias: results from a multicenter experience. Heart Rhythm 2011;8:968–74.

32. Anter E, Hutchinson MD, Deo R, et al. Surgical ablation of refractory ventricular tachycardia in patients with non-ischemic cardiomyopathy. Circ Arrhythm Electrophysiol 2011;4:494–500.

Epicardial Ablation Complications

Nicola Tarantino, MD[a], Domenico G. Della Rocca, MD[b,*], Michela Faggioni, MD[c,d],
Xiao-Dong Zhang, MD, PhD[a], Sanghamitra Mohanty, MD[b], Alisara Anannab, MD[b,e],
Ugur Canpolat, MD[b,f], Huseyin Ayhan, MD[b,g], Mohamed Bassiouny, MD[b], Anu Sahore, MD[b],
Kudret Aytemir, MD[f], Annahita Sarcon, MD[h], Giovanni B. Forleo, MD, PhD[i], Carlo Lavalle, MD[j],
Rodney P. Horton, MD[b], Chintan Trivedi, MD, MPH[b], Amin Al-Ahmad, MD[b],
Jorge Romero, MD[a], David J. Burkhardt, MD[b], Joseph G. Gallinghouse, MD[b],
Luigi Di Biase, MD, PhD[a,b,k], Andrea Natale, MD[b,l,m,n]

KEYWORDS

- Percutaneous • Epicardial approach • Complications • Cardiac arrhythmia

KEY POINTS

- Percutaneous epicardial approach has become an adjunctive tool for electrophysiologists to treat disparate cardiac arrhythmias.
- It is essential to know the prevalence, risk factors, and prevention strategies of potential undesired events occurring during the epicardial puncture, catheter manipulation, and in the postprocedure period.
- The reported complication rate ranges from less than 1% to 17.5%, and can occur at any stage of the epicardial intervention.

INTRODUCTION

Since its first description by Sosa and colleagues,[1] the percutaneous epicardial approach has become an adjunctive tool for electrophysiologists to treat disparate cardiac arrhythmias, including accessory pathways, atrial tachycardia, and particularly ventricular tachycardia (VT).[2-5] This novel technique prompted a strong impulse to perform epicardial access as an alternative strategy for pacing and defibrillation, left atrial appendage exclusion, heart failure with preserved ejection fraction, and genetically engineered tissue delivery.[6-10] However, because of the incremental risk of major complications compared with standalone endocardial ablation, it is still practiced in a limited number of highly experienced centers across the world.[11,12]

The authors N. Tarantino and D.G. Della Rocca contributed equally to this work.

Funding: None declared.

[a] Arrhythmia Services, Department of Medicine, Montefiore Medical Center, Albert Einstein College of Medicine, 110 East 210th Street, Bronx, NY 10467, USA; [b] Texas Cardiac Arrhythmia Institute, St. David's Medical Center, 919 East 32nd Street, Austin, TX 78705, USA; [c] Icahn School of Medicine at Mount Sinai, New York, NY, USA; [d] James J Peters Veterans Affairs Medical Center, Bronx, NY, USA; [e] Department of Cardiovascular Intervention, Central Chest Institute of Thailand, Nonthaburi, Thailand; [f] Department of Cardiology, Hacettepe University Faculty of Medicine, Sıhhiye, Ankara 06100, Turkey; [g] Department of Cardiology, Faculty of Medicine, Yıldırım Beyazıt University, Ankara, Turkey; [h] Division of Electrophysiology, University of California San Francisco, San Francisco, CA, USA; [i] Department of Cardiology, Azienda Ospedaliera-Universitaria "Luigi Sacco", Milano, Italy; [j] Department of Cardiology, Policlinico Universitario Umberto I, Policlinico Street, Roma 155-00161, Italy; [k] Department of Clinical and Experimental Medicine, University of Foggia, Foggia, Italy; [l] Interventional Electrophysiology, Scripps Clinic, La Jolla, CA, USA; [m] Department of Cardiology, MetroHealth Medical Center, Case Western Reserve University School of Medicine, Cleveland, OH, USA; [n] Division of Cardiology, Stanford University, Stanford, CA, USA.

* Corresponding author. 3000 N Interstate Highway 35 Suite 700, Austin, TX 78705.

E-mail address: domenicodellarocca@hotmail.it

Card Electrophysiol Clin 12 (2020) 409–418
https://doi.org/10.1016/j.ccep.2020.06.004

Given the risk, it is essential to know the prevalence, risk factors, and prevention strategies of potential undesired events occurring during the epicardial puncture, catheter manipulation, and in the postprocedure period. Classification criteria of the complications adopted by various investigators are based on the severity (major vs minor, depending on the extent or irreversibility of the damage), anatomy (intrapericardial, extrapericardial, and extrathoracic), or on the temporal relationship (acute vs delayed when occurring 48 hours after the procedure).

This article focuses on studies concerning epicardial ablation of VT, and a brief anatomic description of the mediastinal structures encountered during epicardial access and ablation is offered and followed, when possible, by an explanation of pathophysiologic mechanisms for each type of complication. Adverse events associated with, but not directly caused by, epicardial access (eg, groin site complications, atrioventricular blocks caused by combined endocardial maneuvers) are considered unrelated to the epicardial procedure and are not discussed.

EPIDEMIOLOGY AND OVERVIEW

The reported complication rate ranges from less than 1% to 17.5%, (**Table 1**) and can occur at any stage of the epicardial intervention (eg, pericardial access, catheter manipulation, ablation).[13,14] The wide variability is attributable to heterogeneous technical approaches (inferior vs anterior access), different center experience, the definition of complication (ie, minor vs major [ie, effusion volume in cubic centimeters]), and nature of the analyzed studies, most of which are retrospective and single centered. Nevertheless, periprocedural fatal events are uncommon overall (0%–3%). For instance, in a retrospective single-center study enrolling 54 patients, 6 patients (9%) experienced major pericardial effusion, but the only periprocedural fatal event was ascribed to prolonged anesthesia in a patient with preexisting renal failure, and therefore was not related to the epicardial intervention.[15] In another, larger tertiary single-center series, the rate of severe effusion (200–1300 cm^3) was slightly lower (<7%), but all the subjects were treated with pericardial drain, and no death was recorded.[16] Upadhyay and colleagues[17] found equally reassuring results even in their pediatric population, noting only 1 accidental uncomplicated pleural puncture among 10 epicardial procedures.

From the analysis of multicenter cohorts, the incidence of major complications is lower, probably as a result of larger cohorts or greater extent of recall bias. A European multicenter study by Della Bella and colleagues[18] observed a prevalence of major and minor periprocedural complications in 9 (4.1%) and 17 (7.8%) patients, respectively. Cardiac tamponade caused by accidental right ventricle (RV) tear during the epicardial sheath exchange occurred in 8 out of 218 (3.7%) patients undergoing a hybrid endocardial-epicardial approach; however, only 2 of them required surgical repair. In the same cohort, only 1 patient experienced subdiaphragmatic hematoma necessitating surgical intervention. In contrast, uneventful RV needle puncture occurred in 5% and, more importantly, there were no procedure-related deaths.

Another multicenter retrospective study, by Sacher and colleagues,[19] recognized epicardial bleeding secondary to RV puncture in 7 (4.5%) of 136 patients. As minor complications, 23 (17%) patients experienced RV puncture without sequelae, and 2 patients reported accidental pleural catheterization. No constrictive pericarditis, phrenic nerve injury, or deaths were reported.

A unique spectrum of anecdotal complications may occur from epicardial access/mapping/ablation, such as pleuropericardial/peritoneal-pericardial fistula, pneumopericardium, intrapericardial wire fracture, coronary perforation, and hepatic hematoma. However, because these complications are rare, a precise estimate of their frequency is not available.[20–23]

ACCESS-RELATED COMPLICATIONS

Epicardial access can be performed by an inferior or anterior approach, the former less frequently performed because of presumed additional risk to injury infradiaphragmatic organs and vessels; however, limited data are available. A retrospective series showed that, overall, complications tended to occur more frequently with an inferior approach compared with the anterior access (9% vs 5%, P = .55).[22] Furthermore, Keramati and colleagues found that the anterior approach causes less pericardial bleeding than the initial inferior Sosa technique[1] (P = .002). However, the mortalities were comparable (0% vs 1%, P = .31),[13] and the anterior approach can be associated with abdominal and mediastinal organs damage as well (see **Table 1**).

Abdominal Organ Injury

Characteristically caused by the inferior approach, abdominal complications are as rare as they are under-recognized. Using this technique, the needle is directed dorsally, crossing in sequence the skin, subxiphoid space, the Larrey foramina of the diaphragm, and ultimately the inferior aspect of the pericardium. As such, if initial access is shallow and through the Larrey foramina, the diaphragm does not need to be perforated. The needle can be directed more posteriorly thereafter, in order to gain inferior access to the pericardium. The close relationship between the diaphragm and abdominal organs accounts for the accidental hepatic or gastric perforation, hemoperitoneum, peritoneum-pericardium fistula, and RV-to-abdomen fistula.[22,23] Gastric perforation in the setting of epicardial ablation has never been reported; however, it has been described in a case of explorative pericardiocentesis.[24] Hepatic perforation or hematoma might be asymptomatic, given the parenchymal elasticity, and can be managed conservatively; however, serious bleeding should be always sought in case of hemodynamic instability. Likewise, pericardial-peritoneum fistula should be suspected in a case of abdominal pain and distension.[20,22] In the case of hemodynamic instability without signs of tamponade, intracardiac echocardiography (ICE) can be maneuvered by pulling back the probe in the inferior vena cava to assess for hemoperitoneum or liver hematoma,[23] whereas fluoroscopic assessment can be of help to identify air in the pericardium or peritoneum.

Vascular Injury

Several vessels can be encountered during the epicardial access, and even the anterior approach is not risk free. By pointing the needle toward the left shoulder but with a less acute angle (with respect to the chest wall), the puncture spares the infradiaphragmatic structures; however, other more superficial supradiaphragmatic vascular branches can be harmed, such as the superior epigastric vessel (terminal branch of the left internal mammary artery [LIMA]), which usually runs beneath and slightly lateral to the ensiform process in front of the transversus abdominis muscle,[25] the xiphoid artery, or the musculophrenic artery, the musculophrenic artery being more lateral and therefore less prone to be in the trajectory of the needle.[26,27] The LIMA usually lies medially at the level of the sixth costosternal articulation or lower, featuring a superficial course in a craniocaudal direction, so much so it could be reached once the needle crosses the sternal insertion of the diaphragm and lands in the retrosternal space.[28] To avoid damage to the LIMA, the needle should be directed deeper and more laterally once it is under the costochondral margin.[26] The pericardiophrenic artery, a branch of the LIMA, travels along the lateral pericardial silhouette along with

the phrenic nerve and vein, and is unlikely to be injured unless the needle is advanced more medially and cranially at the base of the heart.[29] Moreover, along with arteries, associated veins running parallel to the LIMA can be damaged, even though the clinical consequences of selective vein injury are unknown.[26]

As the needle passes the fibrous pericardium, an epicardial vessel can be injured, causing acute myocardial ischemia and dramatic tamponade.[23] Electrocardiogram (ECG) and ICE monitoring are of utmost importance during this step. In addition, coronary graft lesion is a theoretic risk during epicardial access in patients with previous coronary-aortic bypass graft.[30] However, percutaneous epicardial access is rarely performed in the postsurgical population.

Right Ventricle Injury, Acute Pericardial Effusion and Tamponade

Inadvertent RV puncture is common, occurring in as many as 17% of the patients reported by Sacher and colleagues.[19] However, consequent significant bleedings (>80 cm³) were limited to 4 procedures (n = 136 patients).[19] In contrast, in the study by Tung and colleagues,[16] 6.7% had significant periprocedural bleeding, but only 1 was associate with known RV puncture, and no patient required surgical intervention. Della Bella and colleagues[18] counted the same condition in 5% of the cases, although none of them developed hemopericardium, whereas Schmidt and colleagues[31] reported 1 fatal event related to RV puncture.

Risk can be limited by injecting a small amount of contrast along the track of the needle tip, showing indentation of the external pericardium followed by outlining of the cardiac borders once the needle advances into the cavity. Wire insertion in the pericardial space should follow the left cardiac borders in left oblique fluoroscopic view, thus confirming the extracardiac position of the needle and preventing further accidental dilation and cannulation of RV free wall. In rare instances, repetitive unsuccessful epicardial punctures can generate a reversible RV pseudoaneursym,[23] which can be suspected in cases of chronic chest pain after an epicardial procedure. According to a nonrandomized analysis, the incidence of inadvertent RV puncture seems to diminish in parallel with the experience of the operator (from 24% to 10%; P = .07).[19]

Rare Mediastinal Complications

Incidence of pleural catheterization is estimated as 1.5% of cases, usually not complicated by pneumothorax.[19] One case of pleural inflammatory-hemorrhagic effusion associated with hemopericardium in the setting of a pericardial reactive autoimmune syndrome has been reported,[22] whereas pleuropericardial fistula was described in 3 isolated cases.[16,32,33]

In addition, intrapericardial guidewire fracture with rescue retrieve was a novel complication reported by Killu and colleagues.[22]

CATHETER MANIPULATION AND ABLATION-RELATED COMPLICATIONS
Vascular Injury

Epicardial coronary vessels can be damaged not only during energy delivery (thermal injury) but also during catheter manipulation (mechanical injury) (see **Table 1**). All the thermal sources used in electrophysiology may denature the protein content of the adventitia, impair the local innervation and muscular tone, or activate coagulation.[34] Some patients may be susceptible to coronary vasospasm caused by mapping catheter mechanical trauma with dramatic consequences.[23] Major branches are less likely to be compromised by temperature variations, because of the convective cooling effect of blood flow,[32] but coronary angiography is still mandatory before ablation, and a distance less than 12 mm from the ventricular target to the arterial course should be avoided.[18,35] In 1 series by Sacher and colleagues,[19] 1 case (0.6%) of asymptomatic subcritical coronary stenosis of an anomalous branch of the right coronary artery was attributed to thermal injury by cryoablation; however, no primary revascularization was needed. Sosa and Scanavacca[36] described 1 episode (1 out of 215 patients) of an acute coronary syndrome (non–Q wave infarct) following radiofrequency (RF) application in proximity with a marginal branch.

Accidental coronary vein laceration during sheath manipulation is an uncommon event, and it has been reported in 2 series, with 1 patient requiring surgical intervention.[19,23] Characteristically, the effusion of venous origin features slow accumulation of blood, thus leading to delayed diagnosis and intervention. This bleeding mechanism may be under-reported because mild venous injury may be self-limited, and the cause of self-limited bleeding is often not determined.

Phrenic Nerve Palsy

The right phrenic nerve (PN) runs close to the superior vena cava and the right superior pulmonary vein, then descends along the right atrium and the lateral wall of the RV until reaching the right hemidiaphragm.[37] The left PN generally passes laterally to the left atrial appendage (LAA), and then deviates either anteriorly or anterolaterally over the left ventricle (LV) to insert into the homolateral diaphragmatic dome behind the cardiac apex. A posterior trajectory has also been described, passing behind the LAA neck and directing toward the inferior wall of the LV.[38] In addition, despite being an extrapericardial structure, the PN is, on average, less than 5 mm distant from the epicardial aspect of the LV (3.4 mm from the middle cardiac vein, 6.3 mm from the anterior intraventricular vein).[36,39] As a result of its anatomic relationship, and the marginal incidence of VT arising from the margin of the RV, the left PN is more likely to be injured during epicardial ablations (see **Table 1**).

The PN is enveloped by myelin sheath showing heat sink–like properties, to the extent that it can absorb and subsequently dissipate heat even when the RF delivery is terminated. An elegant experiment in a canine model showed that transient injury could occur at low temperatures within a distance of about 10 mm, whereas the likelihood of permanent damage was proportional to the duration of the lesion (38 $\pm$ 32 vs 92 $\pm$ 83 seconds).[40] Direct PN contact with an irrigated catheter could acutely damage the PN, but permanent lesions were principally observed at a higher temperature (47 C$\pm$ 3°C vs 51 C$\pm$ 6°C; $P = .002$).

In our opinion, the time and temperature relationship of the permanent injury accounts for the rarity and generally favorable prognosis of this complication in the setting of cardiac ablation,[41] in particular with an epicardial approach, in which the continuous contraction and "swinging" of the heart and the presence of catheter irrigation fluid in the pericardial cavity can disperse the thermal energy. PN palsy was found in only 1 patient out of 50 in the cohort analyzed by Tung and colleagues,[16] and as an isolated case in another retrospective study with 116 procedures.[16,22] In contrast, failures of substrate-based ablation because of the vicinity to the PN are more common. According to Della Bella and colleagues,[18] the presence of the PN course identified with pace mapping prevented energy delivery at the selected site in 1% to 7% of the cases.[42] Furthermore, the same group showed that nerve-sparing ablation (of lesions in sites adjacent to the PN capture course) is inferior to PN balloon displacement in terms of procedural success and, additionally, is associated with a higher chance of PN compromise (3 out of 12 vs 0 out of 13 patients treated with the alternative strategy; P = nonsignificant). In contrast, a case of PN injury despite the pericardial instillation of saline was reported by Killu and colleagues,[22] who pointed out possible damage of the pericardiophrenic artery as an ischemic mechanism of the complication.

Cardiac Tamponade

Acute cardiac tamponade is the most life-threatening complications, ranging from less than 1% to 3.7% of the procedures,[15,16,18,19] although the highest percentages are associated with a combined endoepicardial approach. Immediate pericardial drainage is indicated, and periodic monitoring of the pericardial space with ICE is essential to prevent any abrupt hemodynamic decline secondary to tamponade.

POSTPROCEDURAL AND FOLLOW-UP COMPLICATIONS
Pericardial Syndromes and Miscellaneous

Precordial pain is the most frequent postprocedure symptom, being observed between 21% and 29% of cases.[18,34] Sacher and colleagues[19] observed 1 case of delayed tamponade 10 days after the procedure in a patient with an International Normalized Ratio (INR) of 11. Constrictive pericarditis, major pericardial reaction, and chronic pericarditis up to 9 months after the procedure have been also documented, and pericardiectomy was often required.[19,22,43,44] It is worth emphasizing that some of these late presentations developed despite systematic antiinflammatory prophylaxis (with steroid and nonsteroid agents, including colchicine) during the postoperative period and at discharge, and immunoglobulins were successfully used in 1 patient, advocating an autoimmune cause (post–cardiac injury syndrome).

Rarely, accidental air entrapment during catheter exchange may produce pneumopericardium and increase the defibrillation thresholds in patients with a preexisting device.[45] A chest radiograph may be of greater value than routine cardiac ultrasonography for this purpose. Negative pressure should be applied to evacuate all the air and the device should be interrogated.

RISK FACTORS AND PREVENTIVE STRATEGIES

Contrary to what might be expected, obesity does not represent a risk factor for complications in epicardial access, as indicated in an elegant original investigation by the Mayo clinic group. Wan and colleagues[46] retrospectively reviewed 152 electrophysiologic epicardial procedures and subdivided the population according to the body mass index (BMI). Although cardiovascular risk factors (hypertension, diabetes mellitus, sleep apnea, elderly age) were considerably more prevalent in obese patients, no difference in complications was noted (9.8% vs 8.7% vs 12.3%, in the normal, overweight, and obese groups, respectively;

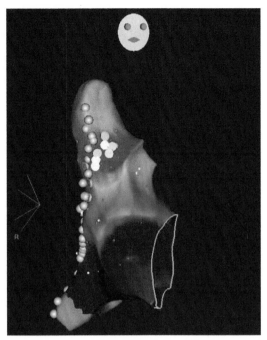

Fig. 1. Locations of PN capture using high-output bipolar pacing can be marked on the electroanatomic map and used as a reference throughout the procedure. Pacing is usually performed at 20 mA and with a pulse width of 10 milliseconds.

$P = .83$). However, the study revealed that high BMI might technically compromise the epicardial puncture, as shown by a non–statistically significant trend toward an inferior rather than anterior epicardial approach in moderately to severely obese patients (49% vs 61%; $P = .12$). Likewise,

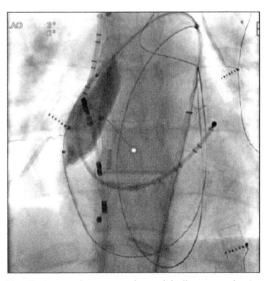

Fig. 2. A vascular or esophageal balloon can be inflated in the pericardial space until PN capture is lost.

Table 1
Prevalence of Epicardial Ablation-Related Complications

Complication	Frequency (%)	Reference	Preventive Strategy
RV puncture	5 17 4.5	Della Bella et al,[18] 2011 Sacher et al,[19] 2010 Castaño et al,[34] 2011	• Controlled apnea • Pressure-sensitive needle • Contrast injection • Real-time transthoracic ultrasonography or ICE • Continuous ECG monitoring
Acute hemopericardium	4.5[a] 6.7 11.1 10 21 7.1	Sacher et al,[19] 2010 Tung et al,[16] 2013 Pandian et al,[15] 2017 Sosa et al,[59] 1998 Sosa et al,[60] 2000 Sarkozy et al,[61] 2013	• Continuous ICE • Anticoagulation management as per guidelines (see text)
Acute tamponade	5.5 3.7[b] 5.3	Pandian et al,[15] 2017 Della Bella et al,[18] 2011 Sarkozy et al,[61] 2013	• Continuous ICE • Anticoagulation management as per guidelines (see text)
Delayed tamponade	0.6 0.9	Sacher et al.[19] 2010 Killu et al,[22] 2013	• Close follow-up
Coronary artery perforation	Case report	Koruth et al,[23] 2011	• Continuous ECG monitoring
Coronary artery spasm and occlusion	0.6 0.3 0.4	Sacher et al.[19] 2010 Koruth et al,[23] 2011 Castaño et al,[34] 2011	• Continuous ECG monitoring
Coronary Vein Laceration	0.3 0.7	Sacher et al.[19] 2010 Koruth et al,[23] 2011	• Continuous ICE
Pleural catheterization	10 1.5	Upadhyay et al,[17] 2017 Sacher et al.[19] 2010	• Contrast injection • Fluoroscopy-guided wire advancement
PN palsy	0.5 0.9 5.8[d] 25[c]	Tung et al,[16] 2013 Killu et al,[22] 2013 Spencer et al.[39] 2015 Bunch et al,[40] 2005	• Epicardial balloon inflation • Partially insulated ablation catheter • Continuous saline irrigation • PN pacing • Nerve-sparing ablation
Pleuropericardial fistula	0.5 case report Case report	Tung et al,[16] 2013 Killu et al,[30] 2015 Schmidt et al,[31] 2010	—
Abdominopericardial fistula	0.9	Killu et al,[22] 2013	• Anterior access
RV abdominal fistula	0.3	Koruth et al,[23] 2011	• Anterior access • ICE monitoring of abdominal cavity in absence of other causes of hemodynamic instability
RV pseudoaneurysm	0.3	Koruth et al,[23] 2011	• Clinical and imaging follow-up
Subxiphoid hematoma	0.5 0.5 0.4	Tung et al,[16] 2013 Della Bella et al,[18] 2011 Castaño et al,[34] 2011	• Anterior access
Hepatic hematoma	0.9 0.6 3	Killu et al,[22] 2013 Mathuria et al,[33] 2010 Killu et al,[30] 2015	• Anterior access • Preoperative chest and abdomen CT scan

(continued on next page)

Table 1
(continued)

Complication	Frequency (%)	Reference	Preventive Strategy
Esophagopleural fistula	Case report	Adam et al,[44] 2016	• Esophageal temperature monitoring • Gastric protection (PPI?)
Defibrillation threshold increase	Case report	Javaheri et al,[43] 2012	• Fluoroscopy • Pericardiocentesis and air evacuation • Device interrogation and reprogramming
Precordial pain	21 29 >50	Della Bella et al,[18] 2011 Castaño et al,[34] 2011 Sacher et al.[19] 2010	• NSAIDs, steroids, colchicine
Intrapericardial wire fracture	0.9	Killu et al,[22] 2013	• Wire size >0.635 mm (0.025 in)
Death	1.8[e] 3[f]	Pandian et al,[15] 2017 Killu et al,[30] 2015	—

Abbreviations: CT, computed tomography; NSAIDs, nonsteroidal antiinflammatory drugs; PPI, proton pump inhibitor.
[a] Two cases caused by RV puncture.
[b] In patients with combined endoepicardial approach.
[c] Three patients out of 12, with 2 transient and 1 permanent palsy.
[d] All transient.
[e] Not attributable to the procedure itself.
[f] One secondary to RV puncture, the other caused by electromechanical dissociation.

performing the procedure under general anesthesia does not diminish the complication rate compared with conscious sedation only, as shown in 170 patients undergoing VT ($P = 1$) or premature ventricular complex ablation ($P = .12$),[47] although the retrospective analysis failed to record the frequency of accidental RV puncture. The risk of the latter might be decreased with controlled apnea or by the use of novel technology such as the pressure-sensor needle (EpiAccess System by EpiEP, Inc, New Haven, CT), as shown by our group.[48]

Some investigators have hypothesized that pericardial adhesions secondary to previous pericardiectomy or pericarditis may facilitate fistulization to another cavity, as in the case of pericardial-peritoneal fistula.[22] In this regard, the limited experience of patients with prior cardiac surgery or pericardial syndrome suggests that epicardial access is feasible in a variable percentage, between 33% and 98% of cases.[15,29,46] Nevertheless, catheter manipulation is constrained and electroanatomic mapping is often inadequate (3% of patients without adhesions vs 85% of patients with adhesions; $P<.001$). Accordingly, procedural failure is more likely (68% vs 48%; $P = .02$), although no difference was observed in terms of complications rate.[49] In this challenging setting, epicardial access can still be achieved by limited surgical subxiphoid pericardial window access, with direct exposure

of diaphragmatic pericardium.[15,19,50] Percutaneous left parasternal approach has been anecdotally reported and can represent a valid alternative in expert hands.[51]

PN protection strategies (**Fig. 1**) have been described by various investigators, adopting mechanical or thermodynamic solutions, such as PN displacement by epicardial balloon inflation (**Fig. 2**), ablation with a partially insulated catheter, or continuous saline irrigation, or simply by monitoring the PN capture while pacing from the left subclavian vein.[52–55] Despite the efforts, the aforementioned techniques are not always feasible, and also the safety has not been successfully compared with controls.[40,49]

Interestingly, uninterrupted anticoagulation does not seem to be an absolute contraindication to epicardial VT ablation, as shown in 2 recent retrospective series that reported similar complication rates and periprocedural bleeding in subjects with warfarin and unfractionated heparin.[56,57] Nonetheless, international guidelines recommend to maintain INR less than 1.5 for warfarin and discontinue direct anticoagulation at least 48 hours before the procedure.[58]

SUMMARY

Percutaneous epicardial ablation offers a groundbreaking therapeutic resource for interventional electrophysiologists; however, awareness of all the potential complications along with developing adequate skillset, technologies for prevention, and management of any adverse events is paramount (**Table 1**).

CONFLICTS OF INTEREST

Dr J.D. Burkhardt is a consultant for Biosense Webster and Stereotaxis. Dr A. Natale has received speaker honoraria from Boston Scientific, Biosense Webster, St. Jude Medical, Biotronik, and Medtronic; and is a consultant for Biosense Webster, St. Jude Medical, and Janssen. All other authors have reported that they have no relationships relevant to the contents of this article to disclose.

REFERENCES

1. Sosa E, Scanavacca M, d'Avila A, et al. A new technique to perform epicardial mapping in the electrophysiology laboratory. J Cardiovasc Electrophysiol 1996;7(6):531–6.
2. Scanavacca MI, Sternick EB, Pisani C, et al. Accessory atrioventricular pathways refractory to catheter ablation: role of percutaneous epicardial approach. Circ Arrhythm Electrophysiol 2015;8(1):128–36.
3. Ban JE, Park TY, Park SW. Percutaneous epicardial ablation of incessant atrial tachycardia originating from the left atrial appendage. J Thorac Dis 2016; 8(11):E1551–4.
4. Schweikert RA. Epicardial ablation of supraventricular tachycardia. Card Electrophysiol Clin 2010;2(1): 105–11.
5. Cardoso R, Aryana A, Singh SM, et al. Epicardial ablation of ventricular tachycardia: a review. Korean Circ J 2018;48(9):778–91.
6. Syed FF, DeSimone CV, Ebrille E, et al. Percutaneous epicardial pacing using a novel insulated multielectrode lead. JACC Clin Electrophysiol 2015; 1(4):273–83.
7. Clark BC, Opfermann JD, Davis TD, et al. Single-incision percutaneous pericardial ICD lead placement in a piglet model. J Cardiovasc Electrophysiol 2017;28(9):1098–104.
8. Litwinowicz R, Bartus M, Burysz M, et al. Long term outcomes after left atrial appendage closure with the LARIAT device-Stroke risk reduction over five years follow-up. PLoS One 2018;13(12): e0208710.
9. Borlaug BA, Carter RE, Melenovsky V, et al. Percutaneous pericardial resection: a novel potential treatment for heart failure with preserved ejection fraction. Circ Heart Fail 2017;10(4):e003612.
10. Garcia JR, Campbell PF, Kumar G. A minimally invasive, translational method to deliver hydrogels to the

heart through the pericardial space. JACC Basic Transl Sci 2017;2:601–9.
11. Roten L, Sacher F, Daly M, et al. Epicardial ventricular tachycardia ablation for which patients? Arrhythm Electrophysiol Rev 2012;1(1):39–45.
12. Romero J, Cerrud-Rodriguez RC, Di Biase L, et al. Combined endocardial-epicardial versus endocardial catheter ablation alone for ventricular tachycardia in structural heart disease: a systematic review and meta-analysis. JACC Clin Electrophysiol 2019;5(1):13–24.
13. Keramati AR, DeMazumder D, Misra S, et al. Anterior pericardial access to facilitate electrophysiology study and catheter ablation of ventricular arrhythmias: a single tertiary center experience. J Cardiovasc Electrophysiol 2017;28(10): 1189–95.
14. Lin CY, Chung FP, Lin YJ, et al. Safety and efficacy of epicardial ablation of ventricular tachyarrhythmias: experience from a Tertiary Referral Center in Taiwan. Acta Cardiol Sin 2018;34(1):49–58.
15. Pandian J, Kaur D, Yalagudri S, et al. Safety and efficacy of epicardial approach to catheter ablation of ventricular tachycardia - an institutional experience. Indian Heart J 2017;69(2):170–5.
16. Tung R, Michowitz Y, Yu R, et al. Epicardial ablation of ventricular tachycardia: an institutional experience of safety and efficacy. Heart Rhythm 2013; 10(4):490–8.
17. Upadhyay S, Walsh EP, Cecchin F, et al. Epicardial ablation of tachyarrhythmia in children: experience at two academic centers. Pacing Clin Electrophysiol 2017;40(9):1017–26.
18. Della Bella P, Brugada J, Zeppenfeld K, et al. Epicardial ablation for ventricular tachycardia: a European multicenter study. Circ Arrhythm Electrophysiol 2011;4(5):653–9.
19. Sacher F, Roberts-Thomson K, Maury P, et al. Epicardial ventricular tachycardia ablation a multicenter safety study. J Am Coll Cardiol 2010;55(21): 2366–72.
20. Natanzon SS, Beinart R, Nof E. Peritoneal pericardial fistula post epicardial ventricular tachycardia ablation. Europace 2019. https://doi.org/10.1093/europace/euz164 [pii:euz164].
21. Hsieh CH, Ross DL. Case of coronary perforation with epicardial access for ablation of ventricular tachycardia. Heart Rhythm 2011;8(2):318–21.
22. Killu AM, Friedman PA, Mulpuru SK, et al. Atypical complications encountered with epicardial electrophysiological procedures. Heart Rhythm 2013; 10(11):1613–21.
23. Koruth JS, Aryana A, Dukkipati SR, et al. Unusual complications of percutaneous epicardial access and epicardial mapping and ablation of cardiac arrhythmias. Circ Arrhythm Electrophysiol 2011;4(6): 882–8.

24. Alpat S, Sahinoglu T, Uysal S, et al. Long and wrong way: unintended pericardial catheter insertion through stomach. J Cardiol Cases 2014; 10(2):66–8.

25. Baudoin YP, Hoch M, Protin XM, et al. The superior epigastric artery does not pass through Larrey's space (trigonum sternocostale). Surg Radiol Anat 2003;25(3–4):259–62.

26. Nagamatsu Y, Mori S, Fukuzawa K, et al. Anatomical characteristics of the superior epigastric artery for epicardial ablation using the anterior approach. J Cardiovasc Electrophysiol 2019; 30(8):1339–40.

27. Vaidya VR, Asirvatham SJ. Epicardial access: adjusting the approach as we discover complications. J Cardiovasc Electrophysiol 2019;30(8):1341–4.

28. Henriquez-Pino JA, Gomes WJ, Prates JC, et al. Surgical anatomy of the internal thoracic artery. Ann Thorac Surg 1997;64(4):1041–5.

29. Picichè M. Noncoronary collateral myocardial blood flow: the human heart's forgotten blood supply. Open Cardiovasc Med J 2015;9:105–13.

30. Killu AM, Ebrille E, Asirvatham SJ, et al. Percutaneous epicardial access for mapping and ablation is feasible in patients with prior cardiac surgery, including coronary bypass surgery. Circ Arrhythm Electrophysiol 2015;8(1):94–101.

31. Schmidt B, Chun KR, Baensch D, et al. Catheter ablation for ventricular tachycardia after failed endocardial ablation: epicardial substrate or inappropriate endocardial ablation? Heart Rhythm 2010; 7(12):1746–52.

32. Bisbal F, Villuendas R, de Diego O, et al. Iatrogenic pleuropericardial communication: a rare complication of percutaneous epicardial mapping. HeartRhythm Case Rep 2017;3(4):196–8.

33. Mathuria N, Buch E, Shivkumar K. Pleuropericardial fistula formation after prior epicardial catheter ablation for ventricular tachycardia. Circ Arrhythm Electrophysiol 2012;5(1):e18–9.

34. Castaño A, Crawford T, Yamazaki M, et al. Coronary artery pathophysiology after radiofrequency catheter ablation: review and perspectives. Heart Rhythm 2011;8(12):1975–80.

35. Yamada T. Catheter ablation of epicardial ventricular tachycardia. J Arrhythm 2014;30:262–71.

36. Sosa E, Scanavacca M. Epicardial mapping and ablation techniques to control ventricular tachycardia. J Cardiovasc Electrophysiol 2005;16(4): 449–52.

37. Mears JA, Lachman N, Christensen K, et al. The phrenic nerve and atrial fibrillation ablation procedures. J Atr Fibrillation 2009;2:176.

38. Ernst S, Sanchez-Quintana D, Ho SY. Anatomy of the pericardial space and mediastinum: relevance to epicardial mapping and ablation. Card Electrophysiol Clin 2010;2(1):1–8.

39. Spencer JH, Goff RP, Iaizzo PA. Left phrenic nerve anatomy relative to the coronary venous system: implications for phrenic nerve stimulation during cardiac resynchronization therapy. Clin Anat 2015; 28(5):621–6.

40. Bunch TJ, Bruce GK, Mahapatra S, et al. Mechanisms of phrenic nerve injury during radiofrequency ablation at the pulmonary vein orifice. J Cardiovasc Electrophysiol 2005;16(12):1318–25.

41. Bai R, Patel D, Di Biase L, et al. Phrenic nerve injury after catheter ablation: should we worry about this complication? J Cardiovasc Electrophysiol 2006; 17(9):944–8.

42. Okubo K, Trevisi N, Foppoli L, et al. Phrenic nerve limitation during epicardial catheter ablation of ventricular tachycardia. JACC Clin Electrophysiol 2019; 5(1):81–90.

43. Javaheri A, Glassberg HL, Acker MA, et al. Constrictive pericarditis presenting as a late complication of epicardial ventricular tachycardia ablation. Circ Heart Fail 2012;5:e22–3.

44. Adam O, Singh A, Balkhy H, et al. Late presentation of constrictive pericarditis after limited epicardial ablation for inappropriate sinus tachycardia. HeartRhythm Case Rep 2016;2(5):441–5.

45. Yamada T, McElderry HT, Platonov M, et al. Aspirated air in the pericardial space during epicardial catheterization may elevate the defibrillation threshold. Int J Cardiol 2009;135(1):e34–5.

46. Wan SH, Killu AM, Hodge DO, et al. Obesity does not increase complication rate of percutaneous epicardial access. J Cardiovasc Electrophysiol 2014;25(11):1174–9.

47. Killu AM, Sugrue A, Munger TM, et al. Impact of sedation vs. general anaesthesia on percutaneous epicardial access safety and procedural outcomes. Europace 2018;20(2):329–36.

48. Di Biase L, Burkhardt JD, Reddy V, et al. Initial international multicenter human experience with a novel epicardial access needle embedded with a real-time pressure/frequency monitoring to facilitate epicardial access: feasibility and safety. Heart Rhythm 2017;14(7):981–8.

49. Li A, Buch E, Boyle NG, et al. Incidence and significance of adhesions encountered during epicardial mapping and ablation of ventricular tachycardia in patients with no history of prior cardiac surgery or pericarditis. Heart Rhythm 2018;15(1):65–74.

50. Soejima K, Couper G, Cooper JM, et al. Subxiphoid surgical approach for epicardial catheter-based mapping and ablation in patients with prior cardiac surgery or difficult epicardial access. Circulation 2004;110(10):1197–201.

51. Miyamoto K, Noda T, Aiba T, et al. Parasternal intercostal approach as an alternative to subxiphoid approach for epicardial catheter ablation: a case report. HeartRhythm Case Rep 2015;1(3):150–5.

52. Kumar S, Barbhaiya CR, Baldinger SH, et al. Epicardial phrenic nerve displacement during catheter ablation of atrial and ventricular arrhythmias: procedural experience and outcomes. Circ Arrhythm Electrophysiol 2015;8(4):896–904.

53. Killu AM, Naksuk N, Syed FF, et al. Feasibility of directional percutaneous epicardial ablation with a partially insulated catheter. J Interv Card Electrophysiol 2018;53(1):105–13.

54. Neven K, Fernandez-Armenta J, Andreu D, et al. Epicardial ablation: prevention of phrenic nerve damage by pericardial injection of saline and the use of a steerable sheath. Indian Pacing Electrophysiol J 2014;14(2):87–93.

55. Santangeli P, Marchlinski FE. Left phrenic nerve pacing from the left subclavian vein: novel method to monitor for left phrenic nerve injury during catheter ablation. Circ Arrhythm Electrophysiol 2015;8(1):241–2.

56. Sawhney V, Breitenstein A, Ullah W, et al. Epicardial catheter ablation for ventricular tachycardia on uninterrupted warfarin: a safe approach for those with a strong indication for peri-procedural anticoagulation? Int J Cardiol 2016;222:57–61.

57. Nakamura T, Davogustto GE, Schaeffer B, et al. Complications and anticoagulation strategies for percutaneous epicardial ablation procedures. Circ Arrhythm Electrophysiol 2018;11(11):e006714.

58. Sticherling C, Marin F, Birnie D, et al. Antithrombotic management in patients undergoing electrophysiological procedures: a European Heart Rhythm Association (EHRA) position document endorsed by the ESC Working Group Thrombosis, Heart Rhythm Society (HRS), and Asia Pacific Heart Rhythm Society (APHRS). Europace 2015;17(8):1197–214.

59. Sosa E, Scanavacca M, D'Avila A, et al. Endocardial and epicardial ablation guided by nonsurgical transthoracic epicardial mapping to treat recurrent ventricular tachycardia. J Cardiovasc Electrophysiol 1998;9(3):229–39.

60. Sosa E, Scanavacca M, d'Avila A, et al. Nonsurgical transthoracic epicardial catheter ablation to treat recurrent ventricular tachycardia occurring late after myocardial infarction. J Am Coll Cardiol 2000;35(6):1442–9.

61. Sarkozy A, Tokuda M, Tedrow UB, et al. Epicardial ablation of ventricular tachycardia in ischemic heart disease. Circ Arrhythm Electrophysiol 2013;6(6):1115–22.

The Future of Percutaneous Epicardial Interventions

Roshan Karki, MBBS, Paul A. Friedman, MD, Ammar M. Killu, MBBS*

KEYWORDS

• Percutaneous • Epicardial • Pericardial • Innovation

KEY POINTS

- The pericardial space provides a unique vantage point to various cardiac structures.
- The use of percutaneous pericardial interventions is likely to increase with improvement of safety and efficacy profile.
- There is ongoing innovation of percutaneous pericardial techniques in left atrial appendage closure, hybrid ablation of atrial and ventricular arrhythmias, device therapies, and treatment of heart failure.
- A systematic surveillance of the percutaneous pericardial tools and techniques and their outcomes is important to guide further development of this field.

 Video content accompanies this article at http://www.cardiacep.theclinics.com.

INTRODUCTION

Since it was first described by Sosa and colleagues[1] in 1996, the percutaneous access of the "dry" pericardial space has been increasingly used in interventional electrophysiologic procedures. Given its unique anatomic position, the pericardial space allows access to almost every region of the epicardium and offers opportunities for the development of novel ablative and device therapies among other interventional techniques.[2,3] Because the pericardial space does not directly communicate with the central circulation, catheter-based left atrial or left ventricular procedures can be performed without anticoagulation, and it also serves as an alternative route for delivery of drugs.[4] Furthermore, the pericardial space can serve as a buffer whereby a balloon is percutaneously placed to protect injury of extracardiac structures during endocardial ablation.[5]

The use of percutaneous pericardial interventions, although increasing, remains limited to major medical centers because of the associated procedural risks. Although operator experience is paramount, there have been efforts to develop tools and techniques to mitigate such risks. Electroanatomic mapping and fusion with computed tomography imaging has been demonstrated to be feasible as an adjunct to fluoroscopy to reduce right ventricular puncture.[6] The Food and Drug Administration has approved EpiAccess needle (EpiEP, New Haven, CT), which has distal sensors for real-time monitoring of pressure and frequency for safer access into the pericardial space.[7] The use of a long micropuncture needle (needle-in-needle technique)[8] instead of Tuohy needle (Havel's Inc, Cincinnati, OH) has been associated with lower risk of large pericardial effusions. Pericardial carbon dioxide insufflation through a coronary vein or the right atrium has

Division of Cardiovascular Diseases and Internal Medicine, Mayo Clinic, 200 1st Street, Rochester, MN 55905, USA
* Corresponding author.
E-mail address: Killu.Ammar@mayo.edu
Twitter: @roshankarkimd (R.K.); @drpaulfriedman (P.A.F.); @akillumd (A.M.K.)

Card Electrophysiol Clin 12 (2020) 419–430
https://doi.org/10.1016/j.ccep.2020.04.007

also been described as another strategy to enlarge the virtual space for safe pericardial entry.[9] As the ease of access and safety profile of percutaneous pericardial interventions improve, so too will adoption of the procedures by electrophysiologists.

Since we last reviewed this subject a decade ago,[2] there has been a significant advance in percutaneous pericardial interventions. We hereby discuss a few of these important works that will likely shape this arena for years to come.

PERCUTANEOUS PERICARDIAL ACCESS

The subxiphoid puncture (**Fig. 1**) remains the standard approach for percutaneous pericardial access and has been extensive described. One of the advantages of this approach is avoidance of lung tissue, thus substantially reducing the risk of pneumothorax. A new technique[10] requiring a lateral puncture has been described and involves the use of a balloon device to displace the underlying lung (**Fig. 2**). The balloon sheath is introduced into the pericardial space by standard subxiphoid approach, and the balloon is inflated with contrast. Under fluoroscopic guidance, a needle is inserted into the left intercostal space and maneuvered until there is indentation on the balloon, which is then punctured. A guidewire is then passed through the needle and used to advance a sheath. Although there is need for subxiphoid access to perform the lateral access, it is used as a bail-out strategy when access to the transverse sinus or left atrial

appendage (LAA) is difficult with traditional approach.

EPICARDIAL ECHOCARDIOGRAPHY GUIDANCE

Epicardial mapping and ablation are often performed for treatment of complex ventricular arrhythmias and accessory pathways. Intracardiac echocardiography (ICE) has revolutionized the ability for real-time monitoring during electrophysiologic procedures thereby improving safety and efficacy. However, visualization of intrapericardial tools by ICE is limited in the absence of pericardial fluid, and eliminated in the presence of air. Epicardial coronary arteries are subject to damage during pericardial procedures, and often require coronary angiography to assess their proximity to the ablation catheter. At some centers, this requires the complexity of coordination with interventional colleagues, and it subjects the patient to risks of contrast exposure, increased radiation, and angiography-associated complications. Furthermore, reliance on distance from the vessel using two-dimensional views is imperfect, and angiography provides limited tissue characterization (eg, presence of epicardial fat). We developed a prototype multipurpose pericardial sheath that is used to advance an ICE probe for high-resolution visualization of coronary arteries and myocardial substrate so ablation is safely and effectively performed (Video 1).[11] This 12F

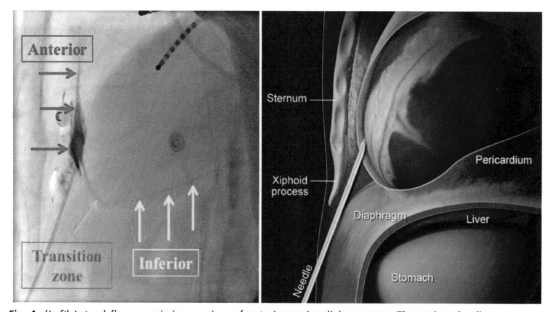

Fig. 1. (*Left*) Lateral fluoroscopic image view of anterior pericardial puncture. The various landing zones are highlighted. (*Right*) Cartoon demonstration of left panel.

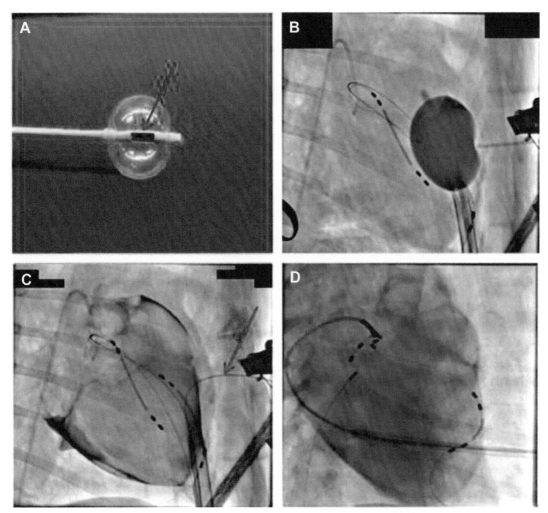

Fig. 2. Percutaneous lateral pericardial access. (*A*) Inflated ballon device with red arrow showing the window to pass a guidewire. (*B*) Balloon device in pericardial space, inflated with contrast, and with indentation by a lateral access needle. (*C*) Guidewire (orange arrow) retrieved through the anterior pericardial access. (*D*) Sheath (with ablation catheter) in pericardial space through the lateral access. (*From* Isath A, Abudan Al-Masry A, Sugrue A, et al. Lateral Percutaneous Epicardial Access With a Novel Technique. *JACC Clinical electrophysiology.* 2018;4(8):1115-1116; with permission.)

catheter sheath, an iteration of a previously described sheath,[12] has three windows at the distal end to allow epicardial echocardiography (**Fig. 3**). Each window is surrounded by a partially insulated electrode that is used to record local electrograms and deliver energy for radiofrequency ablation or electroporation. It also has a stabilizing balloon and a flange on either side of balloon, to minimize any collateral damage. We were able to successfully perform epicardial echocardiography via this sheath, and perform ablation without acute coronary arterial damage in canine models. It needs further modifications for reliable delivery of ablative energy and demonstration of safety and efficacy in chronic animal models.

PERICARDIAL APPROACHES TO TREATMENT OF ATRIAL FIBRILLATION
Epicardial Cooling for Painless Atrial Defibrillation

Although external cardioversion has been the standard of care for termination of uncontrolled or symptomatic atrial fibrillation (AF), it is not feasible when episodes are frequent, and may require frequent health care use. The efficacy of antiarrhythmic drugs for AF termination and maintenance of sinus rhythm has been modest at best. Although there is great enthusiasm for ablative therapy for AF, it has been predominantly used in younger cohorts,[13] compared with the age distribution of AF in most Western societies, and it is

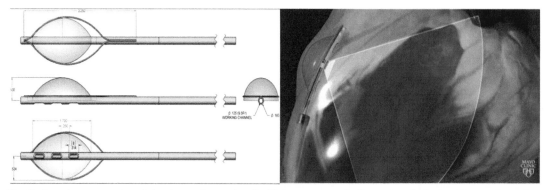

Fig. 3. Percutaneous epicardial echocardiography. (*Left*) A prototype balloon sheath device. The undersurface has three windows bordered by electrodes for mapping and ablation. The outer surface has stabilizing balloon and flanges. (*Right*) The balloon sheath device in the pericardial space with echocardiography probe in position. (*From* Sugrue A, Vaidya VR, Padmanabhan D, et al. A novel percutaneous stabilizing sheath for minimal invasive epicardial echocardiography and ablation. *J Interv Card Electrophysiol.* 2019; with permission.)

associated with frequent recurrences. Early termination of AF prevents adverse remodeling, and may foster maintenance of sinus rhythm. Therefore, device therapy with low-energy internal atrial defibrillation emerged as an option. Although effective, atrial defibrillation has not been well tolerated because of shock-related chest discomfort. Myocardial cooling offers an attractive alternative for potentially painless atrial defibrillation through its effect on temperature-sensitive channels[14] and prolongation of atrial ERP.[15] Yambe and colleagues[16] demonstrated that a device using Peltier elements (dissimilar semiconductors that are electrified to create a thermal gradient) with transcutaneous energy transmission system is used to terminate AF. We made a similar observation in open-chest canine models that it is feasible to achieve rapid myocardial cooling using double-stack Peltier elements and avoid extreme heating using a heat-sink (**Fig. 4**).[17] We also determined that the oblique sinus is the preferred location because of its proximity to the left atrium, pulmonary veins, and ganglionic plexi (GP). We then performed a prospective study[18] in which

we induced AF in open-chest canine models and attempted termination of AF with a device placed in the oblique sinus that would decrease the temperature to 5C versus a control device that would maintain normal temperature. We found that rapid myocardial cooling by the pericardial device in oblique sinus was more effective in terminating AF compared with control subjects. Given that Peltier elements are made smaller than 1.0 mm^3, are configured into different shapes, have good longevity, and do not require circulating refrigerants, they hold great promise for incorporation into a battery-powered device that is delivered percutaneously into the oblique sinus. The development of such a device would signal a significant advance in the management of AF.

Epicardial Mapping and Ablation of Atrial Fibrillation

Catheter ablation is the standard of care in patients with drug-refractory symptomatic AF, but has a significant recurrence rate. The recurrence is attributed to reconnection of pulmonary vein–

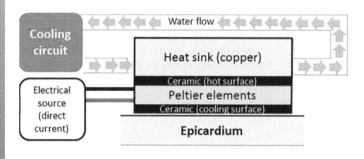

Fig. 4. The Peltier effect occurs when electric current is passed through a circuit of thermocouple (semiconductors or Peltier elements sandwiched between two ceramic plates) to cool the epicardial side. It does produce heat toward parietal pericardium, which is neutralized by a copper heat sink. (*From* Naksuk N, Killu AM, Gaba P, et al. Effect of epicardial cooling Peltier elements on atrial conduction: A proof-of-concept study for a potentially painless method of atrial defibrillation. *Heart rhythm.* 2016;13(11):2253-2258; with permission.)

left atrial conduction and non–pulmonary vein isolation (PVI) triggers. Jiang and colleagues[19] studied feasibility of percutaneous epicardial mapping and ablation of the left atrium during endocardial ablation. In their case series, epicardial mapping of posterior left atrium and inferior pulmonary veins within the oblique sinus demonstrated nontransmurality with an endocardial ablation alone. Epicardial ablation to create box lesions in the posterior wall and to terminate mitral isthmus dependent flutter was successfully demonstrated. In addition, there has been rising interest in hybrid procedures[20] where epicardial ablation is performed by surgeons using minimally invasive techniques, and followed by endocardial catheter ablation to identify any potential gaps. Future innovations and advancements in energy delivery are likely to make such techniques entirely percutaneous. Such percutaneous hybrid approaches have a potential role for treatment of refractory or recurrent AF despite prior ablation, and need larger prospective clinical studies.

Autonomic Neuromodulation of Atrial Fibrillation

Stimulation of GP, located in the epicardial fat pad, has been shown to cause firing in the pulmonary veins and induce AF by causing dispersion, and shortening, of the atrial effective refractory period.[21] Adjunctive anatomy-guided endocardial radiofrequency ablation of GP combined with PVI has been shown to have incremental benefit over PVI alone in paroxysmal and persistent/longstanding persistent AF.[22,23] However, the need for higher power to endocardially ablate GP can potentially result in incomplete autonomic blockade that can be proarrhythmic, and collateral damage of extracardiac structures. Therefore, the epicardial ablation of GP seems to be an effective atrial myocardial sparing option. The epicardial delivery of direct current for irreversible

electroporation of GP has been shown to be highly effective to acutely achieve complete denervation in preclinical studies.[24,25] Then, a medium-term study was performed whereby the pulsed field ablation of GP was performed in dog models with follow-up of 120 days.[26] Using a steerable sheath through the pericardial access, specially designed 8F nitinol finger and glove catheters (**Fig. 5**) were advanced to deliver electroporation (NanoKnife system, AngioDynamics, Latham, NY). The GP were identified in specific anatomic locations, such as transverse sinus (great artery GP), oblique sinus (retroaortic GP), vein of Marshall GP, and right periaortic space (right superior and inferior GP). Direct current energy (1000 V, 100 microsecond pulse width, 10 pulses) was delivered to GP resulting in increased atrial effective refractory period. At the end of the study period, 95.2% of the GP were noted to have pathologically confirmed durable lesions with minimal atrial myocardial injury. The effectiveness and safety of percutaneous epicardial autonomic neuromodulation with pulsed field ablation need further studies.

Percutaneous Left Atrial Appendage Ligation

In patients who are unable to take long-term oral anticoagulants, LAA occlusion has emerged as an alternative strategy for prevention of AF-related stroke.[27] Driven by the greater morbidity and higher Rankin score associated hemorrhagic as opposed to ischemic strokes, and the dramatic reduction in hemorrhagic stroke with LAA closure, there was a drop in cardiovascular risk, and in the 4-year extended follow-up of the PROTECT AF trial, reduction in mortality.[28] The Achilles heel of endocardial LAA occlusion is development of device-related thrombus that, although uncommon (3.7%), is associated with a higher risk of stroke and systemic embolism, and requires treatment with anticoagulation.[29] Whether endocardial

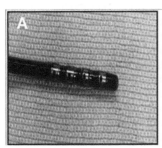 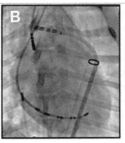 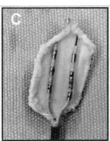 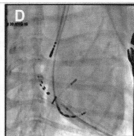

Fig. 5. Catheters for epicardial ablation of ganglionic plexus. (*A*) 8F finger catheter. (*B*) Fluoroscopy of finger catheter in the transverse sinus. (*C*) 8F glove catheter. (*D*) Fluoroscopy of glove catheter in the oblique sinus. (*From* Padmabhan et al. Electroporation of epicardial autonomic ganglia: Safety and efficacy in medium-term canine models. *J Cardiovasc Electrophysiol.* 2019;30(4):607-615; with permission.)

LAA occlusion with an alternative device, such as the Amplatzer Amulet (Abbott, Chicago, IL), will have better efficacy and safety compared with the Watchman device will be answered by Amulate IDE Trial (NCT02879448).[30] Entirely percutaneous pericardial LAA closure is an attractive alternative because it leaves no endocardial foreign body that will be a nidus for device-related thrombus or infection, and mitigates catheter-related air or thromboembolism.

The Lariat device (SentreHEART, Redwood, CA) was originally approved by the Food and Drug Administration for suture-based soft tissue approximation and has been used for percutaneous LAA closure in humans under investigational device exemption.[31] The deployment of the Lariat device requires a combined epicardial and endocardial approach. A balloon is placed in the LAA over a magnet-tipped guidewire placed via trans-septal access. Subxiphoid access is obtained using the anterior approach and another magnet-tipped pericardial guidewire is introduced via pericardial sheath and approximated with the tip of the endocardial guidewire. Using the pericardial guidewire as monorail, the Lariat snare is advanced over the LAA. The suture is released and cinched after confirming optimal position by transesophageal echocardiography. In a large multicenter registry of 712 patients, Lakkireddy and colleagues[32] demonstrated the Lariat device to be successfully deployed in 95.5% of patients, of whom 98% had successful LAA exclusion. However, there were 24 cardiac perforations (10 patients required open heart surgery) and one device-related death. The LAA closure by Lariat device has also been shown to have other salutary physiologic effects, such as reverse left atrial remodeling,[33] reduction of AF burden, and reduction of blood pressure. Given that many patients with AF have hypertension, and that hypertension is a stroke risk factor, blood pressure reduction as a side effect of LAA closure might enhance therapeutic effectiveness, although at present this is speculative. We previously demonstrated complete disappearance of LAA electrograms after LAA exclusion.[34,35] Han and colleagues[36] showed a significant acute reduction of bipolar and unipolar LAA voltages after LAA exclusion by Lariat device. Therefore, LAA ligation by Lariat device could have incremental value over PVI for management of AF as suggested by LAA-AF Registry. An ongoing multicenter randomized trial, the aMAZE study (NCT02513797), is designed to answer this question and will provide important guidance in this direction.

The Sierra ligation system (Aegis Medical Innovations Inc, Vancouver, Canada) is an entirely percutaneous LAA ligation system and should not require anticoagulation. We initially described this electrical navigation system–guided technique in canine models.[2,34,35] The LAA closure system used in this technique has two components: a grasper with articulating jaw to record atrial electrograms and a ligator that is loaded with a support wire. After subxiphoid puncture via anterior approach, the device is advanced to the LAA, the location of which is confirmed by atrial electrogram recording, which is then grasped with the articulating jaw. Once the LAA is controlled by the grasper, a hollow loop suture containing the support wire is advanced over and up to the base of LAA. The loop is then cinched down, the wire is removed, and the suture is secured by suture clip after a complete LAA ligation is confirmed by transesophageal echocardiography and disappearance of left atrial electrograms. The Sierra ligation system was approved for human studies under investigational device exemption and underwent initial enrollments in LASSO-AF Trial (NCT02583178).

PERCUTANEOUS PERICARDIAL PACEMAKERS AND DEFIBRILLATORS

Cardiac implantable electronic devices are routinely implanted to primarily treat bradycardia, optimize heart failure management, and prevent arrhythmic deaths. Although transvenous systems remain the dominant modality supported by many years of experience, they may not be technically possible in patients with venous stenosis/occlusion, tricuspid valve prosthesis, or complex congenital heart disease, and may not be preferred in those with a history of endovascular infection or severe tricuspid valve regurgitation. Moreover, the anatomic limitation to implant the left ventricular lead in the optimal coronary sinus branch remains one of most vexing problems causing failure of cardiac resynchronization therapy in heart failure patients. Although conduction system pacing has recently emerged as a possible alternative, whether the efficacy and long-term performance of traditional biventricular pacing can be replicated is yet to be seen. Leadless pacemakers and subcutaneous implantable cardioverters defibrillator have provided limited solutions because most current devices have limited dual functionality for pacing and shocking function. Today, many patients undergo surgical implantation of an epicardial lead, which is associated with a significant rate of lead failure and morbidity associated with surgery.

There have been preclinical and clinical studies to develop minimally invasive techniques for epicardial lead implantation.[37,38] A percutaneous pericardial approach can provide a minimally invasive vantage point for implantation of such devices at a desired location. There have been some reports of percutaneous epicardial implantation of defibrillator leads.[39] An ideal percutaneously delivered pericardial pacing and defibrillation system should (1) be easy to deliver to a desired site; (2) be reliably stable to avoid dislodgement; (3) deliver energy in a directional manner to avoid painful extracardiac stimulation; (4) avoid compression of the cardiac chambers, vessels, or extracardiac structures; (5) be less irritable so there is no significant pericarditis or pericardial adhesions; (6) have reliable long-term performance without need for frequent replacement; and (7) be easy to extract if needed. We briefly discuss various tools and techniques that have been studied in the last decade

and will pave the way for future development of percutaneous epicardial pacemakers and defibrillators.

Partially Insulated Multielectrode Lead for Directional Pacing

Pacing with a percutaneously delivered epicardial lead can cause extracardiac stimulation leading to inadvertent diaphragmatic contraction and discomfort. We designed a fork-shaped multielectrode lead (**Fig. 6**A, B) that is partially insulated to direct the electric field toward the myocardium.[40] The lead has supportive nitinol loops to provide stability and is contoured to the natural cardiac surface. A steerable sheath, placed through subxiphoid access via anterior approach, was used to deploy the lead in various positions in animal models. We showed that pacing from the

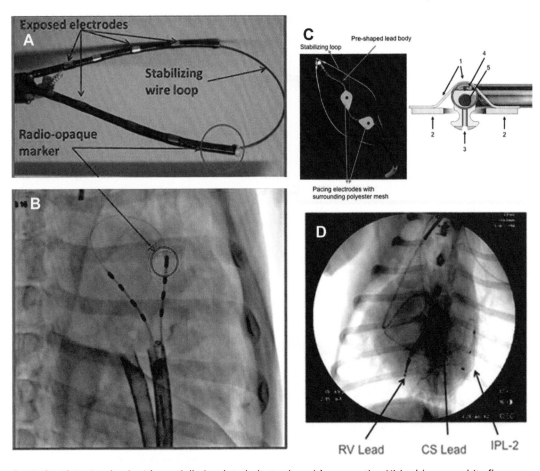

Fig. 6. (*A, B*) Pacing lead with partially insulated electrodes with supportive Nitinol loops and its fluoroscopy. (From Syed FF et al. Percutaneous Epicardial Pacing using a Novel Insulated Multi-electrode Lead. JACC Clinical electrophysiology. 2015; 1(4): 273-283; with permission) (*C,D*) Partially insulated passive fixation epicardial lead and its fluoroscopy. (*From* John et al. Acute and chronic performance evaluation of a novel epicardial pacing lead placed by percutaneous subxiphoid approach in a canine model. *Circulation Arrhythmia and electrophysiology.* 2015;8(3):659-666; with permission.)

electrodes directed onto the myocardium had better sensing amplitude and capture threshold but did not cause significant extracardiac stimulation. John and colleagues[41] also tested intrapericardial passive-fixation leads for pacing in canine models and demonstrated electrical performance similar to that of transvenous leads. The leads were partially insulated to prevent phrenic stimulation. However, the initial design had issues with stability, which was addressed in the second iteration (**Fig. 6**C, D).

Partially Insulated Epicardial Defibrillation Systems

For the same reason described previously, we also developed two prototypes of partially insulated defibrillation leads and tested them in preclinical animal models.[42] The first prototype included a forked lead with defibrillation coil and partially insulated with a cover of polyether block amide

insulation (Pebax, Arkema, King of Prussia, PA) (**Fig. 7**A, B). A fixation screw was used for active fixation. The second prototype was a defibrillation mesh (**Fig. 7**C, D) made of nitinol wire. It was partially insulated with a urethane balloon attached to the frame and mesh. Of the 130 shocks delivered, 84 were successful with mean energy for 75% chance of defibrillation of 13.7 ± 6.6 J for the forked lead and 7.7 ± 7.3 J for the mesh lead. This proof-of-concept study demonstrated the feasibility of a percutaneously placed epicardial system with directional epicardial delivery of energy for defibrillation.

Transverse Sinus Lead for Pacing

An important challenge with percutaneous epicardial pacing lead implantation is lead dislodgement. Similar to transvenous system, screw-in active fixation has been explored but could cause ventricular arrhythmias and has theoretic risk of injury to

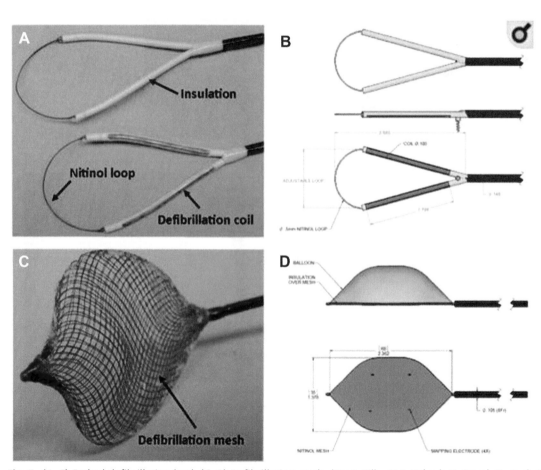

Fig. 7. (*A, B*) Forked defibrillation lead. (*C, D*) Defibrillation mesh. (*From* Killu AM, Naksuk N, Starek Z, et al. A Novel Defibrillation Tool: Percutaneously Delivered, Partially Insulated Epicardial Defibrillation. *JACC Clinical electrophysiology*. 2017;3(7):747-755; with permission.)

coronary arteries. A self-expanding system can potentially cause cardiac/coronary compression and phrenic nerve impingement. The pericardial reflections provide a vantage point to supplant some of these limitations. In particular, the transverse sinus open at medial and lateral borders is used to secure the lead. We designed a polyethylene terephthalate multielectrode lead (**Fig. 8**) with a suture-like configuration.[43] In the most recent iteration, we used leads with eight electrodes to avoid far-field phrenic capture. We used two pericardial sheaths: one commercially available steerable sheath for introduction of lead, and the other prototype sheath for capture and externalization of the lead. The prototype lead was advanced over the transverse sinus from the left to right and captured on the right,

secured, and externalized. An important advantage of this approach is the opportunity for four-chamber cardiac pacing, with no foreign material in the central circulation, minimizing thromboembolic risk.

LIMITED ANTERIOR PERICARDIAL RESECTION FOR HEART FAILURE WITH PRESERVED EJECTION FRACTION

Heart failure with preserved ejection fraction (HFpEF), which accounts for about 50% of patients with heart failure, is characterized by elevated left ventricular end-diastolic pressure at rest or during exercise. Numerous clinical trials have failed to identify an effective drug treatment for HFpEF. In animal models, removal of

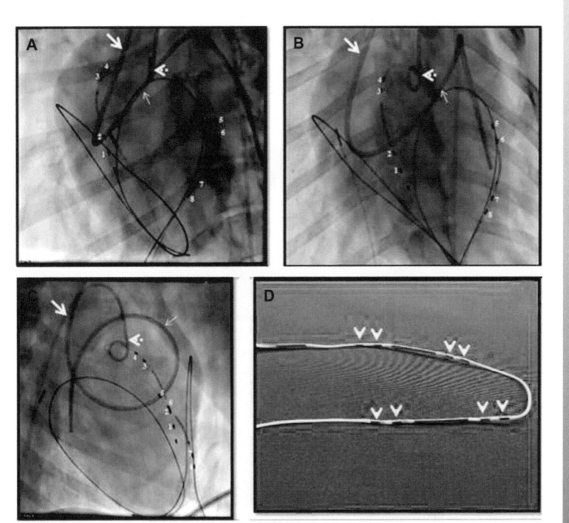

Fig. 8. (*A–C*) The fluoroscopy of the pacing lead across transverse sinus (*arrows*). (*D*) Prototype multipolar pacing lead. (*From* Vaidya VR, Sugrue A, Padmanabhan D, et al. Percutaneous epicardial pacing using a novel transverse sinus device. *J Cardiovasc Electrophysiol.* 2018;29(9):1308-1316.; with permission.)

pericardial constraints by pericardiectomy has been shown to improve the left ventricular compliance, although myocardial properties remain unchanged. Our institution has developed and tested a minimally invasive approach to pericardial resection.[44,45] Using the subxiphoid approach, percutaneous pericardial access was obtained in normal dogs and porcine models of HFpEF. Then, a device with a scissor-like cutting tool and capability of pacing phrenic nerve was deployed in the pericardial space, and a limited anterior pericardial resection was performed (**Fig. 9**). In both closed-chest models, limited anterior pericardiectomy was shown to significantly attenuate the elevation of left ventricular end-diastolic pressure following a saline load. This novel therapeutic strategy shows promise, but it is not clear if the improvement of left ventricular diastolic reserve will sustain long term. However, more preclinical studies are warranted to demonstrate salutary effects, acute and chronic, on exercise hemodynamics, and before it is translated for human use. The procedure is currently undergoing early human evaluation.

FUTURE DIRECTIONS

The experience in percutaneous access of pericardial space for ablation of ventricular arrhythmias and accessory pathways, and ongoing advance in minimally invasive surgical pericardial procedures, have led to better understanding of this unique anatomic space and growth of interventional pericardiology. There are several novel tools and techniques in development for ablation and device treatment of arrhythmias, LAA ligation, heart failure treatment, intrapericardial drug delivery, and epicardial biopsy. Prior cardiac surgery may limit the use of this technique.[46] Future development of techniques to prevent adhesions during surgery and tools to access and remove adhesions may help this important cohort. With increasing use and complexity of procedures, systematic assessment of these techniques and their outcomes is warranted. To this effect, we have established a percutaneous pericardial registry, which is one way to critically analyze and accurately determine outcomes.

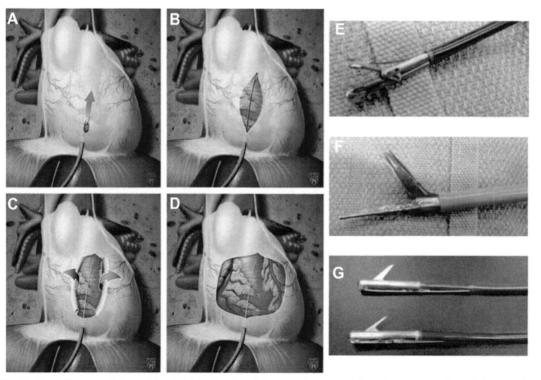

Fig. 9. (*A–D*) Passage of the cutting tool in the sheath by anterior approach and reverse cutting of the anterior parietal pericardium. (*E–G*) Scissor-like cutting tool. (*From* Borlaug BA, Carter RE, Melenovsky V, et al. Percutaneous Pericardial Resection: A Novel Potential Treatment for Heart Failure With Preserved Ejection Fraction. *Circulation Heart failure*. 2017;10(4); with permission.)

DISCLOSURE

Drs R. Karki and A.M. Killu do not have financial disclosures relevant to this article. Dr P.A. Friedman is a coinventor of epicardial cooling technology licensed to MediCool, and epicardial leads.

SUPPLEMENTARY DATA

Supplementary data related to this article can be found online at https://doi.org/10.1016/j.ccep.2020.04.007.

REFERENCES

1. Sosa E, Scanavacca M, d'Avila A, et al. A new technique to perform epicardial mapping in the electrophysiology laboratory. J Cardiovasc Electrophysiol 1996;7(6):531–6.

2. Stanton CM, Asirvatham SJ, Bruce CJ, et al. Future developments in nonsurgical epicardial therapies. Card Electrophysiol Clin 2010;2(1):135–46.

3. Hirano M, Yamamoto H, Hasebe Y, et al. Development of a novel shock wave catheter ablation system: a validation study in pigs in vivo. Europace 2018;20(11):1856–65.

4. Garcia JR, Campbell PF, Kumar G, et al. Minimally invasive delivery of hydrogel-encapsulated amiodarone to the epicardium reduces atrial fibrillation. Circ Arrhythmia Electrophysiol 2018;11(5):e006408.

5. Nakahara S, Ramirez RJ, Buch E, et al. Intrapericardial balloon placement for prevention of collateral injury during catheter ablation of the left atrium in a porcine model. Heart Rhythm 2010;7(1):81–7.

6. Bradfield JS, Tung R, Boyle NG, et al. Our approach to minimize risk of epicardial access: standard techniques with the addition of electroanatomic mapping guidance. J Cardiovasc Electrophysiol 2013;24(6):723–7.

7. Di Biase L, Burkhardt JD, Reddy V, et al. Initial international multicenter human experience with a novel epicardial access needle embedded with a real-time pressure/frequency monitoring to facilitate epicardial access: feasibility and safety. Heart Rhythm 2017;14(7):981–8.

8. Gunda S, Reddy M, Pillarisetti J, et al. Differences in complication rates between large bore needle and a long micropuncture needle during epicardial access: time to change clinical practice? Circ Arrhythmia Electrophysiol 2015;8(4):890–5.

9. Silberbauer J, Gomes J, O'Nunain S, et al. Coronary vein exit and carbon dioxide insufflation to facilitate subxiphoid epicardial access for ventricular mapping and ablation: first experience. JACC Clin Electrophysiol 2017;3(5):514–21.

10. Isath A, Abudan Al-Masry A, Sugrue A, et al. Lateral percutaneous epicardial access with a novel technique. JACC Clin Electrophysiol 2018;4(8):1115–6.

11. Sugrue A, Vaidya VR, Padmanabhan D, et al. A novel percutaneous stabilizing sheath for minimal invasive epicardial echocardiography and ablation. J Interv Card Electrophysiol 2020;57(3):453–64.

12. Killu AM, Naksuk N, Syed FF, et al. Feasibility of directional percutaneous epicardial ablation with a partially insulated catheter. J Interv Card Electrophysiol 2018;53(1):105–13.

13. Packer DL, Mark DB, Robb RA, et al. Effect of catheter ablation vs antiarrhythmic drug therapy on mortality, stroke, bleeding, and cardiac arrest among patients with atrial fibrillation: the CABANA randomized clinical trial. JAMA 2019;321(13):1261–74.

14. Holland WC, Klein RL. Effects of temperature, Na and K concentration and quinidine on transmembrane flux of K42 and incidence of atrial fibrillation. Circ Res 1958;6(4):516–21.

15. Smeets JL, Allessie MA, Lammers WJ, et al. The wavelength of the cardiac impulse and reentrant arrhythmias in isolated rabbit atrium. The role of heart rate, autonomic transmitters, temperature, and potassium. Circ Res 1986;58(1):96–108.

16. Yambe T, Sumiyoshi T, Koga C, et al. New implantable therapeutic device for the control of an atrial fibrillation attack using the Peltier element. Conf Proc IEEE Eng Med Biol Soc 2012;2012:5741–4.

17. Naksuk N, Killu AM, Gaba P, et al. Effect of epicardial cooling Peltier elements on atrial conduction: a proof-of-concept study for a potentially painless method of atrial defibrillation. Heart Rhythm 2016;13(11):2253–8.

18. Witt CM, Dalton S, O'Neil S, et al. Termination of atrial fibrillation with epicardial cooling in the oblique sinus. JACC Clin Electrophysiol 2018;4(10):1362–8.

19. Jiang R, Buch E, Gima J, et al. Feasibility of percutaneous epicardial mapping and ablation for refractory atrial fibrillation: insights into substrate and lesion transmurality. Heart rhythm 2019;16(8):1151–9.

20. Kiser AC, Landers MD, Boyce K, et al. Simultaneous catheter and epicardial ablations enable a comprehensive atrial fibrillation procedure. Innovations (Phila) 2011;6(4):243–7.

21. Scherlag BJ, Yamanashi W, Patel U, et al. Autonomically induced conversion of pulmonary vein focal firing into atrial fibrillation. J Am Coll Cardiol 2005;45(11):1878–86.

22. Katritsis DG, Pokushalov E, Romanov A, et al. Autonomic denervation added to pulmonary vein isolation for paroxysmal atrial fibrillation: a randomized clinical trial. J Am Coll Cardiol 2013;62(24):2318–25.

23. Pokushalov E, Romanov A, Katritsis DG, et al. Ganglionated plexus ablation vs linear ablation in patients undergoing pulmonary vein isolation for persistent/long-standing persistent atrial fibrillation: a randomized comparison. Heart Rhythm 2013;10(9):1280–6.

24. DeSimone CV, Madhavan M, Venkatachalam KL, et al. Percutaneous autonomic neural modulation: a novel technique to treat cardiac arrhythmia. Cardiovasc Revasc Med 2013;14(3):144–8.

25. Madhavan M, Venkatachalam KL, Swale MJ, et al. Novel percutaneous epicardial autonomic modulation in the canine for atrial fibrillation: results of an efficacy and safety study. Pacing Clin Electrophysiol 2016;39(5):407–17.

26. Padmanabhan D, Naksuk N, Killu AK, et al. Electroporation of epicardial autonomic ganglia: safety and efficacy in medium-term canine models. J Cardiovasc Electrophysiol 2019;30(4):607–15.

27. January CT, Wann LS, Calkins H, et al. 2019 AHA/ACC/HRS focused update of the 2014 AHA/ACC/HRS guideline for the management of patients with atrial fibrillation: a report of the American College of Cardiology/American Heart Association task force on clinical practice guidelines and the Heart Rhythm Society. J Am Coll Cardiol 2019;74(1):104–32.

28. Reddy VY, Sievert H, Halperin J, et al. Percutaneous left atrial appendage closure vs warfarin for atrial fibrillation: a randomized clinical trial. JAMA 2014;312(19):1988–98.

29. Dukkipati SR, Kar S, Holmes DR, et al. Device-related thrombus after left atrial appendage closure. Circulation 2018;138(9):874–85.

30. Lakkireddy D, Windecker S, Thaler D, et al. Rationale and design for AMPLATZER amulet left atrial appendage occluder IDE randomized controlled trial (Amulet IDE Trial). Am Heart J 2019;211:45–53.

31. Bartus K, Bednarek J, Myc J, et al. Feasibility of closed-chest ligation of the left atrial appendage in humans. Heart Rhythm 2011;8(2):188–93.

32. Lakkireddy D, Afzal MR, Lee RJ, et al. Short and long-term outcomes of percutaneous left atrial appendage suture ligation: Results from a US multicenter evaluation. Heart Rhythm 2016;13(5):1030–6.

33. Dar T, Afzal MR, Yarlagadda B, et al. Mechanical function of the left atrium is improved with epicardial ligation of the left atrial appendage: insights from the LAFIT-LARIAT Registry. Heart Rhythm 2018;15(7):955–9.

34. Friedman PA, Asirvatham SJ, Dalegrave C, et al. Percutaneous epicardial left atrial appendage closure: preliminary results of an electrogram guided approach. J Cardiovasc Electrophysiol 2009;20(8):908–15.

35. Bruce CJ, Stanton CM, Asirvatham SJ, et al. Percutaneous epicardial left atrial appendage closure: intermediate-term results. J Cardiovasc Electrophysiol 2011;22(1):64–70.

36. Han FT, Bartus K, Lakkireddy D, et al. The effects of LAA ligation on LAA electrical activity. Heart Rhythm 2014;11(5):864–70.

37. Kumthekar RN, Opfermann JD, Mass P, et al. Percutaneous epicardial placement of a prototype miniature pacemaker under direct visualization: an infant porcine chronic survival study. Pacing Clin Electrophysiol 2020;43(1):93–9.

38. Haydin S, Saygi M, Ergul Y, et al. Subxiphoid approach to epicardial implantation of implantable cardioverter defibrillators in children. Pacing Clin Electrophysiol 2013;36(8):926–30.

39. Jacob S, Lieberman RA. Percutaneous epicardial defibrillation coil implantation: a viable technique to manage refractory defibrillation threshold. Circ Arrhythmia Electrophysiol 2010;3(2):214–7.

40. Syed FF, DeSimone CV, Ebrille E, et al. Percutaneous epicardial pacing using a novel insulated multielectrode lead. JACC Clin Electrophysiol 2015;1(4):273–83.

41. John RM, Morgan K, Brennecke LH, et al. Acute and chronic performance evaluation of a novel epicardial pacing lead placed by percutaneous subxiphoid approach in a canine model. Circ Arrhythmia Electrophysiol 2015;8(3):659–66.

42. Killu AM, Naksuk N, Starek Z, et al. A novel defibrillation tool: percutaneously delivered, partially insulated epicardial defibrillation. JACC Clin Electrophysiol 2017;3(7):747–55.

43. Vaidya VR, Sugrue A, Padmanabhan D, et al. Percutaneous epicardial pacing using a novel transverse sinus device. J Cardiovasc Electrophysiol 2018;29(9):1308–16.

44. Borlaug BA, Carter RE, Melenovsky V, et al. Percutaneous pericardial resection: a novel potential treatment for heart failure with preserved ejection fraction. Circ Heart Fail 2017;10(4):e003612.

45. Killu AM, Naksuk N, Desimone CV, et al. Beating heart validation of safety and efficacy of a percutaneous pericardiotomy tool. J Cardiovasc Electrophysiol 2017;28(3):357–61.

46. Killu AM, Asirvatham SJ. Percutaneous pericardial access for electrophysiological studies in patients with prior cardiac surgery: approach and understanding the risks. Expert Rev Cardiovasc Ther 2019;17(2):143–50.

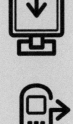

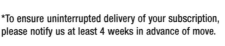

Printed and bound by CPI Group (UK) Ltd, Croydon, CR0 4YY

03/10/2024

01040306-0018